Dying, Death, and Bereavement

A Challenge for Living
2nd Edition

Inge Baer Corless, RN, PhD, FAAN, a graduate of the Bellevue Schools of Nursing in New York City, attended Hunter College and graduated from Boston University with a bachelor's degree in nursing, the University of Rhode Island with a master's degree in sociology, and from Brown University with a PhD in sociology. As a Robert Wood Johnson Clinical Scholar, Dr. Corless did postdoctoral study at the University of California, San Francisco. She has held academic positions at Russell Sage College, the University of Michigan, the University of North Carolina, Chapel Hill, as well as her current position at the MGH Institute of Health Professions at the Massachusetts General Hospital. Dr. Corless served as program director of St. Peter's Hospice in Albany, NY, and as a short-term consultant for the World Health Organization at the Western Pacific regional office. A Fellow of the American Academy of Nursing, Dr. Corless has written on hospice, end-of-life care, and HIV disease. Dr. Corless co-edited, with Dr. Mary Pittman, *AIDS: Principles, Practices, and Politics,* and, with Dr. Barbara Germino and Dr. Pittman, *Dying, Death, and Bereavement: Theoretical Perspectives and Other Ways of Knowing,* and the first edition of this book. Dr. Corless co-edited, with Zelda Foster, *The Hospice Heritage.* She coauthored, with James T. Corless, to produce their two daughters, Theresa Iola and Patricia Irene.

Barbara B. Germino, PhD, RN, FAAN, has had an eclectic career in nursing that has included patient care in three major medical centers, a community hospital, a 25-bed hospital on Kodiak Island, Alaska, and in home care; teaching in four university schools of nursing; and research on individual and family responses to life-threatening illness, including interventions to enhance their ability to manage problems and uncertainties, facilitating quality of life. Early work with chronically ill patients, and critical experiences, especially those with people who were dying with cancer, stimulated interests in life-threatening illness and dying. The opportunity to do her doctoral work with Jeanne Quint Benoliel, whose work had inspired her over many years, was a crucial experience. With colleagues in nursing and social work, she developed and teaches an interdisciplinary graduate course in death, dying, and bereavement across the life-span. She is currently Professor at the School of Nursing, University of North Carolina at Chapel Hill, and holds the Carol Ann Beerstecher-Blackwell Chair of Thanatology. She is actively involved with the Carolinas Center for End of Life Care, working on a 3-year project to enhance end-of-life care awareness, knowledge, and delivery across the Carolinas.

Mary Pittman, DrPH, is President of HRET (Hospital Research and Education Trust) and a member of the executive staff of the American Hospital Association. Prior to assuming the leadership of HRET in 1993, she was President and CEO of the California Association of Public Hospitals. Her areas of interest are community health and access to vulnerable populations. She has provided education and training on a range of issues, e.g., program evaluation, substance abuse program development, and community health program implementation. She has over 20 years experience in community-based program planning and design and has developed numerous public policy and legislative proposals to expand access and quality of health care to underserved populations. Mary has served as principal investigator on a number of research and demonstration grants. She is co-chair and founder of the Coalition for Healthier Cities and Communities. Mary has co-authored two books, *AIDS: Principles, Practices and Politics,* and *Death, Dying, and Bereavement.* She received master's degrees from the University of California–Berkeley in Public Health and City and Regional Planning, and her doctorate from UC–Berkeley in Public Health Administration. Mary serves on the boards of a number of organizations, as well as on many national advisory committees.

Dying, Death, and Bereavement

A Challenge for Living
2nd Edition

Inge Corless, RN, PhD, FAAN
Barbara B. Germino, RN, PhD, FAAN
Mary A. Pittman, DrPh
Editors

 Springer Publishing Company

Copyright © 2003 by Springer Publishing Company, Inc.

Springer Publishing Company, Inc.
536 Broadway
New York, NY 10012-3955

Acquisitions Editor: Ruth Chasek
Production Editor: Janice Stangel
Cover design by Joanne E. Honigman

03 04 05 06 07 / 5 4 3 2 1

Library of Congress Cataloging-in-Publication Data

Dying, death, and bereavement : a challenge for living / edited by Inge Corless,
    Barbara B. Germino, Mary A. Pittman. — 2nd ed.
        p. cm.
    Rev. ed. of: A challenge for living. c1995. Published by Jones & Bartlett
Publishers
    "Companion volume to Dying, death, and bereavement : theoretical
perspectives . . . "—Introd.
    Includes bibliographical references and index.
    ISBN 0-8261-2655-3
    1. Thanatology. 2. Death. 3. Bereavement. 4. Terminal care. I. Corless, Inge B.
II. Germino, Barbara B. III. Pittman, Mary. IV. Challenge for living. V. Dying,
death, and bereavement.
HQ1073.C464 2003
306.9—dc21   2003042537

Printed in the United States of America by Maple-Vail Book Manufacturing Group.

Contents

Foreword

Dame Cicely Saunders

Trained as a nurse during World War II and being invalided out, Dame Cicely Saunders obtained a war degree at Oxford and became a medical social worker. Concern for the pain control of dying patients, and the distress of their families, moved her to study medicine, and in 1958 she began work among the patients of St. Joseph's Hospice. The experience there was one of the roots of St. Christopher's Hospice, which she founded, together with a small group, and which opened in 1967. From the start, it was planned as a teaching center and a focus of research in the control of pain and other distress in 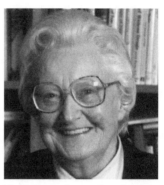 *terminal illness. This work has been recognized worldwide and was the catalyst for the hospice movement.*

Dame Cicely has received a number of honorary degrees, including Honorary Doctorate of Science from Yale in 1969, Lambeth Doctorate of Medicine from the Archbishop of Canterbury in 1977, Doctorate from the Open University in 1978, and Honorary Doctorate of Law, Columbia University, New York, in 1979. She has been a member of the Attendance Allowance Board since it started; and from 1973 to 1978 was a member of the Medical Research Council. Dame Cicely was awarded the Templeton Prize for Progress in Religion in 1981. Other honorary degrees have followed, including honorary doctorates in law and civil law from Oxford and Cambridge Universities in 1986.

Dame Cicely is an honorary fellow of the Royal College of Physicians, the Royal College of Surgeons, and the Royal College of Nurses. She was awarded the British Medical Association's Gold Medal for Distinguished Merit in July 1987, and was made a Freeman of the London Borough of Bromley in October 1987, In 1988, she was made an honorary fellow of the Royal College of Psychiatrists. In 1989, Dame Cicely was awarded the Order of Merit by Her Majesty the Queen.

Over 40 years ago, I had the opportunity and privilege of accompanying an isolated man who talked through his thoughts and feelings with me during the last 2 months of his life. A Jew from Warsaw, he had lost his family and believed that he had made no impact on the world during his short life of 40 years. The first ideas of hospice developed during our conversations, and for me they are summed up in two of his phrases. The first referred to the fact that he would leave me a small legacy—a founding gift for a then nameless place. He said, "I'll be a window in your home." The second was a response to my offer to read him something from the Old Testament, as he was quietly returning to the faith of his fathers. His response was, "No, thank you. I only want what is in your mind and in your heart." At the time, it was a specific challenge to which I tried to respond, but later I came to see it as a demand on us all for everything we could bring, of thought, experience, and skill, to the care of people facing death, to be offered together with personal concern. Setting these two demands, together with the idea of a window, challenged the beginnings of hospice to be open to many adventures and developments, focused always on close attention to individual people, their needs, and their potentials.

The story since February 1948, when David Tasma died "at peace" in the freedom of the spirit, as he told me, has been one of surprising growth. This book brings together much of the experience of many workers during these years, all facing the demands on mind and heart in a spirit of openness. The original vision seems to have the capacity to keep its recognizably addressing the same concerns in our diverse cultures and settings. Those of us who work in the field of death, dying, and bereavement have tried to listen to those people who are facing their individual journey through this part of life. From them we all continue to learn and find inspiration, whether we are concerned with researching and developing ever-improving symptom control, more understanding of psychosocial and existential tensions and possibilities, or better ways of sharing in what surely has to be the work and support of an interdisciplinary team.

Seven years as an RN volunteer in one of the early Protestant homes (St. Luke's Hospital, originally Home for the Dying Poor, opened in 1893), followed by another 7 years as a physician in St. Joseph's Hospice (opened 1905), gave me opportunities to meet and listen to innumerable patients, to observe the regular giving of oral opiates at St. Luke's, and to introduce this method of giving analgesics to St. Joseph's Hospice. It enabled me to monitor our improving clinical practice and development with a retrieval system involving 1,100 patients, and to lay the medical foundations of St. Christopher's, opened in 1967 as the first home care and teaching hospice. A Christian as well as a medical foundation, its aim was "to express the love of God to all who come, in every possible way, in skilled nursing and medical care, in the use of every scientific means of relieving suffering and distress, in understanding personal sympathy, with respect for the dignity of each person as a human being, precious to God and man" (Aim & Basis, 1965). Emphasis was laid on the fact that all those working in the hospice would give their own contribution in their own way, in a spirit of freedom, while patients would seek their own way to peace, without any pressure. Emphasized, too, was that it would be group work, open to further development.

It was not long before such a religious foundation was challenged by those wishing to enter this field without any such commitment. Certain of our own calling, but concerned to open doors as well as windows, we refused to be dogmatic, concerned only that anyone in this field must expect his or her own philosophy to be challenged and to be faced with the difficult questions that may arise from people who are calling on their own resources in crisis. That the spiritual element of the "total pain" complex included far more than any form of personal religion became obvious, as its physical, emotional, and social elements were also addressed with developing experience.

From the beginning, hospice learning and attitudes have formed bridges. First, the bridges between people as staff and volunteers have enabled these people to listen to their patients and families. The way forward must surely come in the same fashion. Patients are the true founders of the hospice movement and the field of related studies and development. Our moves into the future will be safeguarded if we go on listening, aware that the words of one individual or family may open up a whole new scene.

Building a bridge to researchers, and, in due course, to enter this field ourselves has also been important. Early meetings with such pioneers as Beecher, Eddy, and Houde were followed by productive contact with Melzack and Wall. In an editorial in the influential journal *Pain,* Wall (1986) wrote, "The immediate origins of pain and suffering need immediate attention while the long-term search for basic care proceeds. The old methods of care and caring had to be rediscovered and the best of modern medicine had to be turned to the task of new study and therapy specifically directed at pain" (p. 1). The challenge to continue to look at all aspects of suffering still faces us, and we have to back up our demonstrations of effective relief with research studies that are widely published. Our teaching must be objectively based, and we should be offering our patients continually improving understanding and therapy, all focused on their own personal possibilities of growth through loss.

Workers in the field addressed in this comprehensive book also have a responsibility to build bridges into the community, both professional and general. That so many dying people all over the world are ineptly treated faces us with an almost overwhelming challenge, as does the isolation enforced on them and their bereaved families by the disregard of the public. Hospice is about living until the end, still as part of the community. And perhaps developed countries have much to learn from projects in developing countries around the world.

As we learned to demonstrate something of what could be done by what has come to be termed *palliative medicine,* we could begin to build effective bridges with the acute services. We have had to discover when and how to draw in other specialties and learn from them, as well as to educate from our standpoint. In no way are we to take the high moral ground, but we need to meet effectively as we come from our different professional backgrounds and across the disciplines.

We will often have appropriate treatment to offer between the two extremes of all life-prolonging intervention possible and the threat of legalized, active shortening of life, with all its social dangers. We have to earn the attention and respect that will draw us in for the right patients at the right time. The hospital support or palliative care team can have a central role in this area, and is charting an important way forward.

Our whole field has not only been about need, but, above all, about achievement. We are concerned that a person should live this part of life, whether in dying or in bereavement, to the maximum potential, not only in physical ease or activity, but also in family relationships and in addressing the most important inner values. A time of crisis can be a time of growth, often at surprising speed, of resolving long-standing problems and of reconciliation, both with oneself and with those around. Hospice workers find that the freedom from distress they aim to give, by their treatment and hospitality, opens up new space for personal development. Bridges are built among the conflicted families who are more and more often referred to us, in recognition of what we try to offer.

Good communication can facilitate unexpected sharing and response and develop the growth through loss we so often see. Here, I believe we reach the central and most positive area of our concerns. We have all been inspired by those we have seen bringing unexpected gains out of loss, whether it be of health, life, or bereavement. It may come out of distress that is painful to share as we try to maintain the bridge between us. The rewards come from the resolutions that happen surprisingly frequently— but not always. At times, we can only stay beside unresolved problems or, at best, trust that what we have offered is the best we can, hoping it is good enough. A lifetime's difficulties may remain unchanged, and it would be unrealistic to expect anything else.

It is the individual's inner values that matter when there is only a limited time left, or when the most important person has died. The spiritual dimension encompasses searches for meaning in many varied ways. We have never been concerned that the people we serve should see things our way; rather, they should discover or reinforce their own way, asking for help if they wish, with freedom from any pressure or obligation. We have found that not only is our own search for meaning continually stimulated by the often desperate situations we face, but also that this constant challenge helps develop a climate of shared discovery and hope.

References

Wall, P. D. (1986). 25 Volumes of Pain [Editorial]. *Pain, 25,* 1–4.

Introduction

Inge Corless

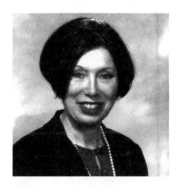

Dying, Death, and Bereavement: A Challenge for Living: has been developed at a time when individuals, by dint of geographical and circumstantial placement, are confronted by many problems not of their own making. Whether it be malnutrition created by the sequestering of food stuffs by rival war lords, the ethnic cleansing of former neighbors by individuals called to arms under the religio/political banners of leaders with xenophobic motives, violence and terror brought by anticipated and unanticipated attack, or death by disaffection and neglect of the homeless in the inner city or the rural poor, modification of the external environment has a direct effect on the well-being of every individual.

When the source of the disability is chronic, long-standing disease, the manipulation of the external environment is less significant than the readjustment of the internal environment—whether by surgery, drugs, radiotherapy, or some other means. When such mechanisms are ineffective the individual and concerned others are confronted with a challenge for living—dying, death, and bereavement.

It is the more constrained, less problematic world condition, sans the chaos of military and political machinations, that primarily, is the context for the consideration of dying, death, and bereavement in this volume. All of the complexity of dying as a result of a chronic disease is magnified by poverty, homelessness, starvation, and fratricidal battle.

Perhaps it is only when the right to live is vouchsafed that the right to die can become an issue. Were the right to die taken for granted, there would be a need to rally for the right to live.

The sanctity of life under-girds a number of practices. The call for assisted suicide while recognizing the right of the individual to self-determination contributes to the erosion of the responsibility of the citizen and the state not to engage in life-depriving activities. Furthermore, the shift from determination by self to determination by others is subtle. Given that most individuals do not wish to burden family members, partners, or friends with the care required as a result of prolonged illness, assisted suicide may seem obligatory (even noble!) to the dying person. These questions have been given renewed attention as a consequence of the efforts of Dr. Jack Kevorkian and others to assist suicides of individuals with various diseases, some in the early stages, others chronic rather than characterized by immediate decline.

The concern of persons who contemplate death by their own hands is one of doing an ineffective job of it and thereby not dying. Presence of a responsible individual assures completion but makes the survivor vulnerable to prosecution if complicity involved assistance. These issues are not easily resolved, nor should they be. Both Churchill and Corless and Nicholas touch on these issues. Related to these questions of control of the end of life is the concern that individuals neither be kept alive interminably in a persistent vegetative state nor resuscitated when there is no hope of recovery. Various mechanisms for advance directives have been instituted so that the individual's wishes may be heeded, thus relieving the family and health-care providers of concerns and litigation that either too much or too little was done. These directives, which Lund Person addresses in her chapter on regulatory issues, are a response to technological capability of life extension in situations without the capacity for meaningful interaction.

The impact of politics and economics as well as history on these issues is significant. These influences are present in some of the other subjects addressed in this book. The ever-present politics of care is explicitly addressed by Preston, Tang and McCorkle in their chapter on symptom management. The constraints imposed by shrinking resources aggravates some of the tensions between different professions. Issues resulting from reduced resources and different care-giving stances are discussed by Foster and Davidson.

Issues and approaches in working with the terminally ill and subsequently with the bereaved constitute the major focus of this book. Whether the topic is communication, life review, helping children, or the role of physiotherapy, the authors share their visions of how and what is helpful to those who are dying and those who are or will become bereaved.

Prognosticating is always a hazardous activity. The future of thanatology and of palliative care are elaborated by Churchill and Doyle, a respected philosopher and a medical educator. If in fact their future becomes our present, we are likely not to remember their foresight. If, however, events unfold in ways considerably different from what was foretold, then these chapters are most likely to seem out of step even though a number of the other chapters examine current and future issues. Thus Churchill and Doyle deserve special appreciation for their willingness to help us prepare for the future, along with Lund Person, who examines regulatory issues, and Wass and Corr, who discuss death education for children and for adults.

Indeed death education for children and for adults may enable us to meet the challenges of death and bereavement and our own dying with equanimity and grace, with hollering and bellowing, and with gratitude for the gift of life. All of this presumes a life fully lived and not foreshortened by acts of personal violence, war, or the scourge of disease. That is not to say that individuals who have not lived long have not lived life fully. Rather that the challenge for the dying person and the bereaved is greater than under more sanguine circumstances. Whatever the circumstances, dying, death, and bereavement constitute a challenge both to and for living. *Dying, Death, and Bereavement: A Challenge for Living* has the immodest aim of equipping individuals to confront these challenges effectively. Fortunately, we do so together with other concerned individuals in the context of an increasing interest in meeting these challenges.

Each for his own memorial
Earned praise that will never die
And with it
The greatest of all sepulchers
Not that in which
His Mortal Bones are laid
But a home
In the Minds of Men

Netherlands American Cemetery
Margraten, The Netherlands

As this is being written, Americans, the British, and Iraquis, as well as others, are dying in the many wars around the globe. We look forward to the day when the concern of the day is once more focused not on creating new cemeteries for the remains of fallen soldiers and civilians caught in war, but on death due to old age. May the challenge for living be one of living a productive life so that the dying, death and bereavement is for a life well and fully lived.

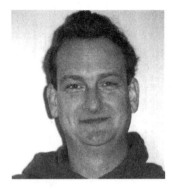

Richard T. Sabo
Born August 4, 1964
Younger brother of Donna
Elder brother of Christopher
Born and raised in northwestern New Jersey
Graduated high school in 1982
Served in the United States Navy 1982–1984
Currently living in Bangor, Maine
What else can I tell you?
I'm a self-professed gear head; I enjoy riding motor
Cycles, snowmobiles, and any other gas-powered con-
veyances. Spent 8 years
Working in healthcare as a certified sterile-processing
and distribution
Technician.
Have spent most of my adult life doing construction (labor/heavy
Equipment operator/mechanic).
My brother committed suicide on December 9, 2001.
I love and miss him!!!

Pain

Richard T. Sabo

Today I died of a broken heart
My world
My life
Ripped apart

Forever now your soul is freed
Forevermore mine will bleed

Never again to feel your touch
The need I have is oh so much

You are the one who is my brother
In this life there will be no other

A river of pain runs through my soul
Today I died of a broken heart

Acknowledgments

We acknowledge all of those who contributed to this book directly and indirectly. We are grateful for the ongoing support of our families—Inge's daughters Theresa and Patricia and "son" Rick; Barbara's husband Vic, daughter Laurie, son Michael, and granddaughter Talia; Mary's husband David and sons Mark and Scott and daughter Kate. We are also grateful to Ruth Chasek, our editor, for her unstinting support, as well as Matt Fenton, Skip Wright, Janice Stangel, and Joanne Honigman and the unnamed others who resuscitated a project that faced interminable challenges including the loss of diskettes enroute to the printer while the first author (I. B. Corless) was on sabbatical in South Africa. While dying, death and bereavement are truely challenges for living, bringing this book to life entailed its own set of challenges. As with living, there is an end—in this case publication. Thank you to all who made it happen.

Part One

The Challenge of Understanding Death

Artists

Deb Holtorf

Deborah Lees Holtorf became interested in health care when she served in the Peace Corps in West Africa in the mid 1960's. She graduated from Massachusetts General Hospital School of Nursing in 1970, and received her Master of Public Health degree from the University of Pittsburgh in 1979. After spending a number of years working in community and school health, Deborah returned to MGH Institute of Health Professions, graduating with her Master of Science in Nursing and becoming certified as a pediatric nurse practitioner. She currently works in the pediatric and adolescent unit of the Joslin Diabetes Center in Boston, MA.

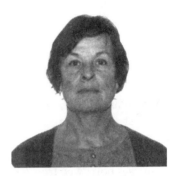

I wrote "Artists" while taking a course taught by Dr. Corless. My father-in-law died the same week a required journal entry was due. When I sat down to write the entry, "Artists" emerged instead. Thankfully, Dr. Corless accepted the substitution for the usual journal entry.

The nurses called Dorothy to tell her that you were doing poorly. Dorothy needs to get dressed and eat some breakfast. She is 83 years old and sensible. She will probably even bring a sandwich for the long haul. I will go ahead, leaving Dorothy with her capable sons. In the hospital parking lot, summoning strength to leave her car, sits your daughter, Mary. I speak to the front seat window: "Let's go."

The doctor is quiet and kind, addressing Mary: "Maybe Ed had a little stroke or a seizure, because he is no longer responding to us. We aren't having any luck keeping the fluid out of his lungs. We could take him downstairs to the ICU for more aggressive treatment, but I don't think that will add to his quality of life. Will your mother be here soon?"

You lie still in white sheets, your breathing rapid and ragged. Overnight your arms and hands have swollen with the fluid that your heart no longer has the energy to keep pumping. The doctor says you respond only to pain, but he is not sure why. I speak into your ear. "Ed, it's Deb. I'm here with Mary. Dorothy and the boys are coming. You are very sick." You pause in your labored breathing. A grunt, a nod—we know you are with us.

The little room fills with your children. Mary, your youngest, is a blower of glass. Gently curved vases and riotously spotted ornaments grace our lives. Bob, the middle child, takes the wood of trees and smoothes it into tables and cabinets. Gerry, the oldest, my husband, is a painter of woodland scenes with autumn-colored grouse camouflaged by leaves. He is a writer of stories in which gnomes and men fish from deep dark country streams side-by-side.

Dorothy, your wife of 55 years, photographer of our world, is perched beside you, on the arm of a recliner. If she sits in the chair, her arthritic knees will betray her when it is time to get up again. Her eyes contact mine. "Well, Deb, what do you think?"

Who am I to stand in the wings and coach your family in playing out this last act? My hands too often break glass. I am the lusty alto in a choir of angels, the fledgling ice skater of small leaps and big bruises. My best thoughts are inclined to be trailing just behind my spoken words. My mantra is borrowed from a Buddhist nun, Pema Chodron. "Refrain, refrain," I chant to myself, to restrain the energy that so often rules.

The other day, you reminded me of the many hours we have spent in emergency rooms together during the past couple of years. You know I am your advocate. You know I will not lie to you, even if my translation of the truth of the moment is blunt and clumsy. But you are still there. This act is for you to direct, not me. You are the fixer of things. Your creations have always been symbolic of a more profound role. Your big hands are now too swollen to hold the gadgets you have crafted to glue our daily lives together. You have been a wonderful husband and father, Ed. Don't leave yet, we still need you. A small voice in me giggles when I think of the legacy you left your oldest. "No, Gerry, I don't think that old pot looks good as a lampshade, even if you do paint it green." You have been a wonderful husband and father, Ed. Don't leave yet, we still need you.

I speak in your ear again, not to intrude, but to break through your concentration on breathing and being. It is important that you hear me now. "Ed, your heart is very weak, and your body is filling up with fluid. We can move you down to the ICU and try to get rid of the fluid, but we don't know if we can keep it off. There probably is not a lot the doctors can do to make you feel better for very long. Do you want to try?"

The final act has its hero. You are emphatic. "No!" you grunt, shaking your head side to side. You have spoken eloquently to everyone in the room, including the gentle doctor who stands in the doorway. Thank you, Ed.

I now have clear words for Dorothy. "Ed is dying. I think you need to sit with him, touch him, and tell him how much you love him." My assumption arises from so many years of knowing the two of you.

The rest of us huddle with the doctor, while Dorothy holds your hand and tells you what she needs to. There will be morphine if you are in pain or very anxious. Later in the day you will ask for it, but right now you indicate that you are comfortable. Would you like your IVs removed? You nod your approval. We leave little heparin locks to use if you need the morphine. I don't think they will bother you.

The trappings of acute illness are carried out of the room. IV poles, monitors, and nebulizers are replaced by chairs and ice chips. Your nurse checks in frequently. You and she communicate well. She wants you to be comfortable and safe, and you seem to understand that.

Your family is not sure what to do now that the scenery has been changed. Modern medicine has departed, leaving your family to a communion as old as life itself. Now what?

I look at the faces of your wife and children. You have eased their suffering by making your wishes so very clear. The remaining time will be devoted to your dying. Will it be hours or a day or two? We cannot accompany you into death, but we want to be with you as long as possible. Can I help, or should I refrain? Too late, the words are already flowing. To my own ear, their loudness shatters the air.

"I will miss having Ed next door. When we first moved in beside your folks, thinking I was all alone, I would vent my frustration at the various obstacles in my path with a stream of words that no woman of Ed's generation was supposed have heard. His laughter would ring back at me from across the field. Moments later, I would be laughing too."

Your children's faces are surprised at first, then animate. "Do you remember the time . . . ?" "I'll never forget the. . . . " "Dad was there when. . . . " "Ed was always. . . . "

We know you are there. We know you are listening. We tell our stories, and we speak to you directly. Dorothy cradles your hand. As it turns out, you have only a few hours left to live. Soon you will let us know that you are uncomfortable and would like medication. I leave you with your wife and children. Your breathing becomes relaxed and peaceful as you slip away from your family. Conversation quiets and focuses more on those who will continue to live for a time. You have kept your family with you as long as possible. It is time to say good-bye.

One

Communicating About Death and Dying

Albert Lee Strickland and Lynne Ann DeSpelder

Albert Lee Strickland is a professional writer whose multidisciplinary interests in thanatology are reflected in his coauthorship of The Last Dance: Encountering Death and Dying, *a college text now in its sixth edition. He is a former editor of* The Forum Newsletter, *published by the Association for Death Education and Counseling, and is a member of the International Work Group on Death, Dying, and Bereavement and of the Authors Guild. His publications on death and dying include* The Path Ahead: Readings in Death and Dying, *an anthology co-edited with Lynne DeSpelder.*

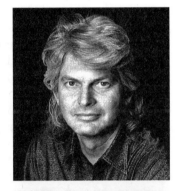

Lynne Ann DeSpelder is an educator, author, and counselor. A professor at Cabrillo College, she developed and taught one of the first interdisciplinary courses on death and dying in California. Certified by the Association for Death Education and Counseling as a death educator and as a grief counselor, she was instrumental in developing that organization's Education for Certification program. Her first nationally published popular writing on death appeared in the November 1977 issue of New Age *magazine. She is coauthor of* The Last Dance: Encountering Death and Dying *(6th ed.), as well as*

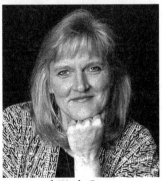

numerous other publications, and is a member of the International Work Group on Death, Dying, and Bereavement.

Waiting to speak with a patient who has completed a series of diagnostic tests, a physician ponders how to break the news of a potentially fatal condition. A parent wonders how to tell a young child about the unexpected death of a beloved relative. Reviewing videotaped coverage of an airliner crash, the editor of a television news program contemplates which segments should be broadcast on the evening news. On the job, the death of an associate's spouse causes co-workers to question how to express their condolences. Before entering the room of a patient nearing death, a nurse hesitates for a moment to consider how to frame the words that express sensitivity to the family's situation. Encounters with dying, death, and bereavement present special challenges to us as communicators.

The Communication Process

Our understanding of the world is generated through communicating, which is an ongoing process that involves the exchange of messages and meanings between individuals (Penman, 2000). Communication is not merely a series of incidents pasted together like photographs in a scrapbook; rather, it is like a motion picture in which meaning is derived from the unfolding of an interrelated series of images (Adler & Rodman, 1991).

Communication is a two-way, interactive, and transactional process (Williams, 1989). To say that it is interactive means that messages can be readily, or even simultaneously, exchanged between parties to the communication. To say that it is transactional refers to the evolutionary nature of the process by which the present message influences subsequent exchanges. Communication is a process of give-and-take, an ongoing activity between persons who function alternately as the source and the receiver of meanings or messages. In broad terms, it is a process that includes a source, a message, and a receiver (Littlejohn, 1999).

Communicating effectively requires attention to nurturing and maintaining the communication process (Luckmann, 1999). Especially important are developing the requisite trust, achieving clarity about motives, and establishing an appropriate context for successful communication. A person's attitudes, beliefs, values, needs, preferences, goals, capabilities, experiences, and communication styles all influence how he or she will send or receive a particular message (Kaplan, 1989; White & Robillard, 1989). As a result, people of different cultures sometimes experience difficulties in communicating clearly with one another. The key to overcoming these difficulties is to accept the other person's fundamental humanness and to continue efforts to communicate. Understanding the styles of communicating used by others makes it possible to create shared experiences and meanings (Smith, Hernandez, & Allen, 1971).

The ability to alternate between different styles of communicating is termed *code switching* or *style switching*. This involves identifying what is appropriate in different situations and modifying one's speech, as well as nonverbal and other communication behaviors, to achieve a good fit within the interactional context (Robinson, 1998). Having an awareness of each other's "codes" is vital for achieving clear communication. Effective communicators have positive self-concept, assertiveness, open-mindedness, empathy, and the ability to use a variety of communication strategies appropriately.

Consider the case of a young widow who was referred for counseling by her physician because she was reportedly "not doing too well." When the young woman entered the counselor's office for her initial session, she sat down rigidly on the couch, bracing herself, with legs extended and her arms crossed. The counselor opened the session by saying, "I understand you've experienced a big change in your life recently." Through clenched teeth, the young woman said, "Yeah, my old man ate it on Highway 17." Matching the young woman's language and communication style, the counselor said, "It sounds like that really pissed you off." Exploding out of her rigid position, the young woman let go with a volcanic torrent of expletives: "Yes, I'm damned angry; he was drunk and ran off the road, leaving me alone with four kids under the age of five and no insurance or any kind of security." Then, breaking down into tears, she sobbed, "God, I must be going crazy; how can I be furious at someone who's dead?"

Matching the young woman's language and communication style allowed the counselor to quickly establish a rapport that promoted effective communication. It readily became evident that this young widow was very much in touch with her feelings about the circumstances of her husband's death, even though her feelings were conflicted and confused. By paying close attention to the communication process, the counselor facilitated the expression of these feelings—a crucial step on the path to resolving grief.

Nonverbal Communication

It has been said that one cannot *not* communicate (Bavelas, 1984; Watzlawick, 1984). The truth of this statement is evident when we consider the broad range of nonverbal as well as verbal modes of communicating. Indeed, nonverbal communication is an inseparable part of the total communication process (Knapp & Hall, 1997; Phillippot, Feldman, & Coats, 1999). Although we usually think of nonverbal communication as applying only to the sphere of interpersonal interactions, it actually functions in a broader context. For example, in the international arena, nonverbal communication is used by hostile states without diplomatic relations as a means of signaling intentions and desires (Berridge, 1994). Relaxing restrictions on trade may signal a desire to improve relations; the movement of military forces may send a threatening message.

Nonverbal communication is typically divided into three components: paralanguage (features of speech beyond the basic language symbols, including tone of voice and rate of speech), kinesics (gestures, eye gaze, facial expression, touch, body posture, and movement), and iconics (objects that convey meaningful information, such as clothes and jewelry). Labels such as MD and RN, as well as titles such as doctor, nurse, and patient, are examples of symbolic identifiers that influence the process of communication. Space and time (proxemics) can be added to this list of nonverbal cues. Consider, for example, the time it takes a caregiver to respond to a patient's request for help, or the physical distance established when a physician stands behind a desk while conversing with a seated patient.

When a nonverbal message contradicts the verbal message, it creates a sense of inconsistent or incongruous communication. Because nonverbal cues tend to operate at an unconscious level, they are commonly assumed to be more trustworthy than words. Nonverbal messages are difficult to censor or falsify. Therefore, the nonverbal component of a communication may determine the ultimate impact of a message.

Verbal Communication

In considering the relationship between verbal and nonverbal communication, being aware of the distinction between low-context and high-context cultures is helpful (Hall, 1976; Robinson, 1998). Low-context communication cultures rely heavily on the verbal part of a message, which is often elaborate, highly specific, and detailed. People tend to communicate in a direct fashion, paying little attention to the nonverbal and contextual aspects of a communication. In low-context cultures, a high value is placed on individualism, independence, autonomy, and self-reliance.

In contrast, high-context communication cultures rely heavily on non-verbals and the circumstances or context of a message, which involves letting the point of the message evolve indirectly, rather than stating it explicitly. By "stalking" the issues, rather than directly stating them, the speaker demonstrates skill and arouses the hearer's interest (Asante, 1998).

People in high-context cultures attend to nuances of behavior (or "vibes") and to social context, as well as the "group identification" or understanding shared by those who are communicating. High-context cultures value collectivism, cooperation, harmony, and loyalty to the group.

It is easy to imagine how these differences in communication styles might lead to misperception and misunderstanding when people with contrasting styles interact. People from high-context cultures often view those from low-context cultures as excessively talkative, whereas people from low-context cultures often view those from high-context cultures as nondisclosing, mysterious, and even sneaky (Robinson, 1998). Caregivers, in particular, need to appreciate that communication styles differ, especially as they relate to cultural distinctions, and resist evaluating a person's way of communicating on the basis of ethnocentric judgments that interfere with effective communication.

Turning to the language people use when talking about dying or death, we find that euphemisms, metaphors, and slang comprise a large part of "death talk" (DeSpelder & Strickland, 2002, pp. 13–14). Substitutions of vague words or phrases for ones considered harsh or blunt are often used to keep death at arm's length by masking its reality. Loved ones "pass away," and the deceased is "laid to rest." However, the use of euphemisms and metaphors does not necessarily imply an impulse to deny death or avoid talking about it. Sometimes they express subtler, deeper meanings. Terms like "passing," for example, convey an understanding of death as a spiritual transition within some religious and ethnic traditions. Nevertheless, plain talk about death is subverted when euphemisms devalue and depersonalize death. Instances of this occur, for example, when soldiers killed in battle are described as "being wasted" or when civilian deaths are termed "collateral damage." Listening carefully to how language is used provides information about the speaker's attitudes, beliefs, and emotional state. Becoming aware of the metaphors, euphemisms, and other linguistic devices that people use when talking about dying and death allows for greater appreciation of the wide range of attitudes toward death and promotes flexibility in communication.

The horrific events of September 11, 2001, provide an instructive case study. Despite heroic efforts to find survivors alive and trapped in the rubble of the World Trade Center and the Pentagon, the lack of success was revealed in the linguistic shift from *rescue* to *recovery*. In daily conversations, people struggled to find the right word or phrase to adequately describe the events. Some called them "the terrorist attacks"; others spoke of "the events of September 11," "the bombing," "the tragedy," or simply "it." Every word or phrase carries its own framework of associations, and different words or phrases may be appropriate for different groups of people. For example, whereas the word *tragedy* might be appropriate for the workplace, where people are focused on recovery, the word *attack* resonates more with police officers, firefighters, and military personnel, who viewed the experience as a direct assault. For some people, "September 11" or "9–11" became a shorthand way of referring to the sequence of events involving the World Trade Center, the Pentagon, and the airliner crash in Pennsylvania. One man said: "I've called it an attack, a tragedy, and a bombing. . . . But, in the end, the name which resonates the most for me is simply the date, September 11, because it was all of those things and more" (quoted in Angwin, 2001, p. A8). This groping for the right word or phrase is part of the natural evolution of language as people try to make sense of an event or situation for which they have no adequate conceptual framework; indeed, this search can be important to the process of coping with traumatic events.

Humor is another aspect of communication that can function as a way of coping with death (DeSpelder & Strickland, 2002; Hall & Rappe, 1995). Death-related humor comes in many different forms, from ironic epitaphs to so-called black or gallows humor, which may reflect a thumbing of one's nose at death, as if attempting to minimize its power and gain a sense of mastery over it. For caregivers, humor offers relief from stressful duties that involve frequent contact with dying and death. For example, emergency workers, and others who deal with life-or-death situations, tend to form communities within which insider or "backstage" humor is used as a strategy to cope with the emotional labor of their jobs (Shuler, 2001). At one teaching hospital, doctors avoided the word "death" when a patient died, because of concern that other patients might be alarmed if the news were to be communicated openly (DeSpelder & Strickland, 2002). One day, as a medical team was examining a patient, an intern came to the door with information about another patient's death. Knowing that the word "death" was taboo and finding no ready substitute, the intern stood in the doorway and announced, "Guess who's not going to shop at Wal-Mart anymore." Soon, this phrase became the standard way for staff members to convey the news that a patient had died.

Communication About Death in the Mass Media

Newspapers, magazines, books, television, and movies are the secondhand sources from which many people learn about death. The daily news usually includes an assortment of accidents, murders, suicides, and disasters (Nimmo & Combs, 1985). Although the brief reports of death-related events on television or in newspapers seldom do justice to the actual range and depth of the human response to loss, sometimes media coverage of catastrophic events does provide a focal point for the grief of a community or nation. In the wake of the assassination of President John F. Kennedy or the explosion of the space shuttle *Challenger*, as well as, more recently, the terrorist attacks of September 11, 2001, television became a kind of "national hearth" around which viewers were symbolically gathered to contemplate the meaning of these tragedies. It is important to note, however, that coverage of death-related events by the media is sometimes accompanied by unwarranted intrusions on the bereaved. The journalistic impulse to "capture the experience" for viewers or readers may result in a second trauma for survivors, restimulating or possibly amplifying the pain brought about by the event itself. The line between public event and private loss is not always easily drawn.

Perhaps unavoidably, the media tend to present an incomplete picture of the human response to death and its meaning. Entertainment programs, for example, rarely deal with how people actually cope with a loved one's death or confront their own dying. Generally, such programs present a depersonalized image of death, an image that is usually characterized by violence (Gerbner, 1980; Tate, 1989). Consider the western or the detective drama, which glazes over the reality of death and leaves the impression that death need not be mourned. Or recall the Saturday morning cartoon as Daffy Duck is pressed to a thin sheet by a steamroller, only to pop up again a moment later good as new—reversible death! When told of his grandfather's death, one modern 7-year-old asked, "Who did it to him?" The image of death found in the media usually communicates the notion that death comes from outside, often violently. Death is portrayed as an accidental rather than a natural process.

Communicating with Children About Death

The attitudes toward death found in the media and in society generally play a major role in the socialization of children relative to dying and death (DeSpelder & Strickland, 2002). Parents and other adults sometimes communicate specific instruction about attitudes: "This is how we behave in relation to death." One woman recalled her mother's message that she should not look at the dead animals on the highway—"Put your head down, children shouldn't see that"—a clear communication about this mother's attitude about what constitutes appropriate behavior toward death. At other times, the message is less specific: "Let's not talk about it . . . ," or the message is communicated subliminally, as with the notion of replaceability. A child's pet dies, and the parent says, "It's okay, dear, we'll get another one." Such messages may have unintended consequences, as when a woman, recently bereaved by her husband's death, was approached by her young child, who said, "Don't worry, Mommy, we'll get you another one."

In communicating with children about death, honesty is foremost. Second, don't put off introducing the topic. When the experience of a close death precedes discussion, the explanation is charged with all the emotions generated by the crisis, making the attainment of clear communication more difficult. Third, set the level of explanation to the child's powers of understanding. By using as a guide the child's interest and ability to comprehend, an explanation appropriate to the child's circumstances can be provided.

Children tend to be very literal-minded. Metaphorical explanations can be used to present a child-sized picture that aids understanding, but, unless fact is separated from fantasy, a child may grasp the literal details rather than the underlying message the analogy was intended to convey. A child, told that her goldfish "went to heaven," may make an elaborate picture of the pearly gates and different sections of heaven—"Here is goldfish heaven, this is cat heaven, and over here is people heaven"—an organized concept that makes sense to a young child, but one that may cause confusion. If you tell a 4-year-old that a person who has died is "up there," and you also remark that Santa Claus lands on the roof, the child may decide that Santa Claus and the deceased person are great buddies. Children are apt to point out any inconsistencies in what we tell them. When discussing death with children, it is important to verify what they think you have told them. Ask the child to tell you what he or she learned or heard you saying about death. Indeed, the essence of these guidelines for discussing death with children has broad application in other contexts involving communication about death, dying, and bereavement.

Communication in the Context of Bereavement

When a death occurs, the first to learn about it, beyond the attending medical team or emergency personnel, are usually members of the deceased's immediate family. Those with the closest relationships to the deceased are notified first, followed by those with less intimate relationships. Ideally, this process of notification—a gradually widening circle of relatives, friends, and acquaintances—continues until everyone affected by the death is notified (Sudnow, 1967).

Death notices and obituaries published in newspapers are an important means of death notification for the wider community. People expect death announcements to appear in a timely fashion. When this does not occur, the results can be emotionally upsetting to those who knew the deceased. The person who learns about a death only after the final disposition of the body may regret not having been a participant in the communal ceremonies marking the death. Human beings experience a need to respond appropriately to the death of significant others. Because the mutual support offered by a community of bereaved persons is not likely to be as readily available to individuals after the initial mourning period, the belatedly notified person may feel isolated and alone in coping with his or her grief.

Death notification initiates expressions of mourning that communicate the fact that a person has been bereaved. Black armbands or distinctive mourning garb, as well as other signs and symbols, have been employed by various societies to distinguish the recently bereaved. Although many of these traditional signs of mourning are vanishing from modern societies, most people still believe that the bereaved deserve special consideration. A woman who became involved in an automobile accident just a few days after the death of her child reported that she wished she could have had a banner proclaiming her status as a "mother whose child has just died." Having no outward sign or symbol of her bereavement, she was subjected, as any of us would be, to the strain of waiting around and filling in seemingly endless forms. The social support elicited by nonverbal or symbolic signs of mourning can be helpful to survivors as they begin to cope with loss.

As people learn about the death of someone who has been significant to them, they tend to gather together for comfort and support in their mutual bereavement. The act of coming together is itself a symbolic communication that offers solace and attests to the reality that the bereaved are members of a caring community (Young, 1978). Gathering together for mutual support is integral to the events surrounding the funeral. This pattern of social interaction has important psychological implications for the bereaved. By corroborating the fact of a loved one's death and expressing the reality that the community has experienced a change of status, because of the death of one of its members, such social interaction facilitates the expression of grief.

The experience of loss is conditioned by a person's model of the world, that is, by his or her perception of reality and understanding about how the world works. An individual's personality and values, social roles and expectations, and relationship to the deceased all warrant consideration in determining how to communicate support in bereavement (Jackson, 1957). Giving the bereaved permission to experience and express complex and possibly conflicting thoughts and feelings is especially important. A person's response to loss encompasses myriad personal, family, and social factors.

During the early period of bereavement, a survivor's perceptions may be disorganized and events may seem unreal. This sense of disorganization or unreality is likely to be reflected in communication patterns. The bereaved may wish to talk incessantly about the deceased or may seemingly talk about everything but the confrontation with loss and circumstances surrounding the death. The response to loss is multifaceted and can be highly variable. Besides sadness, longing, loneliness, and sorrow, the bereaved may express strong feelings of guilt or anger (Bugen, 1977; Lindemann, 1944; Osterweis, Solomon, & Green, 1984). Movement toward healing in the wake of loss is facilitated by communication that takes into account the changing moods and circumstances of the bereaved. Being aware of the variety of responses associated with grief enhances our ability to cope with losses in our own lives, as well as to care for others who are bereaved. When loss is situated within a context of growth, so that what is lost can be integrated into one's ongoing life story, grief becomes a unifying rather than alienating human experience (Schneider, 1984).

Communication in the Context of Terminal Care

Physicians and other health professionals occupy a place of honor in society. Aesculapius, the first physician, according to Greek legend, was elevated to the pantheon of gods. Because of an intimate connection with the elemental human experiences of birth, life, and death, medicine and its practitioners enjoy symbolic importance (Hingson, Scotch, Sorenson, & Swazey, 1981). The lab coat of the attending physician, and the distinguishing uniforms of the nursing staff, are symbols that nonverbally communicate a sense of authority and power. Caregivers and patients may unwittingly conspire to perpetuate a pattern of paternalism in health care, whereby the caregiver assumes a parent-like authority over decisions affecting patients (Raffler-Engel, 1989; West, 1984).

One truism in medicine is that hope and a positive attitude play key roles in a patient's ability to cope with illness (Bessinger, 1988). Indeed, physicians may withhold certain facts about serious illness, out of concern that a full, open disclosure could lessen the patient's hopes of recovery. However, it is important to distinguish between framing a communication so that it corresponds to the patient's ability or willingness to learn the truth and glossing over or neglecting a full disclosure of the facts, out of a medical paternalism that subverts the patient's prerogatives.

When a medical condition involves a life-threatening diagnosis, the nature of the conversations between physician and patient has a significant bearing on the patient's decisions about treatment, as well as his or her ability to cope. From initially breaking bad news about a likely fatal diagnosis, until the last moments of life, patient–caregiver communications involve two interrelated tasks: one in which medical information is provided to the patient, and the other in which supportive dialogue centers on the patient's emotions and responses to the situation (Buckman, 2000). Physicians are obligated to provide information about the disease or threatening condition, offering details to the extent the patient wishes, so that the patient understands what to expect and the options that may be considered as treatment proceeds (Rosenbaum, 1978). Important to this process is establishing an atmosphere of openness and trust, to help mobilize the patient's will to live, which is a key element in any therapeutic effort (Gray & Doan, 1990a, 1990b; LeShan, 1969).

Most people say they would want to be informed if diagnosed with a life-threatening illness, and physicians generally acknowledge a responsibility to inform patients about the facts of a life-threatening condition. However, the question of when and how to tell can be difficult to answer (President's Commission for the Study of Ethical Problems in Medicine and Biomedical and Behavioral Research, 1982a, 1982b). Presenting bad news in a way that avoids harming the patient's interests requires physicians to consider such factors as the patient's personality, emotional constitution, and capacity to function under stress. A survey conducted in the early 1960s showed a strong tendency on the part of physicians to withhold information about a potentially fatal diagnosis involving cancer (Oken, 1961). Descriptions of the disease were often couched in euphemisms, to temper the impact of the diagnosis, or adjectives were used to suggest that the cancer was benign. Accordingly, patients were told they had a "lesion" or "mass," or they were given a more precise description, such as "growth," "tumor," or "hyperplastic tissue." The tumor might be described as "suspicious" or "degenerated." In short, physicians explained the medical situation in very general terms intended to elicit the patient's cooperation in the proposed course of treatment.

Today, patients diagnosed with a potentially terminal condition are likely to learn the truth about their illness, and to learn sooner, than was the case in the past (Novack et al., 1979). Nevertheless, some details about an illness may not be disclosed unless the patient or a family member takes the initiative by asking specific questions. Furthermore, physicians are generally reticent when it comes to speculating about prognosis or outcome—matters that tend to be much less certain (Novack et al., 1989).

The trend toward greater disclosure is related to the importance now placed on obtaining a patient's informed consent to a plan of treatment. Informed consent is based on three principles (President's Commission, 1982a, 1982c): First, the patient must be competent to give his or her consent; second, consent must be given freely; third, consent must be based on an adequate understanding of the proposed treatment and its potential side effects. The values underlying informed consent include serving the well-being of patients and respecting their right of self-determination. Realizing these values requires that attention be given to the processes of communication between patient and practitioner.

Although coercive treatment is rare, caregivers may unwittingly exert undue influence on patients by means of subtle or overt manipulation. Routine medical care is often provided without explicit consent. When a patient enters a medical institution, his or her cooperation with caregivers is expected. The tacit communication may be that the patient has no choice about following the treatment plan. Thus, the nature of the communication process between patient and provider may determine the presence or absence of informed consent.

Patients vary about the degree of disclosure with which they feel comfortable. Some patients prefer to "let the doctor decide"; others seek to gain sophisticated medical knowledge by searching the literature regarding a treatment plan. Ultimately, informed consent does not mean inundating patients with a flood of facts; rather, it means treating patients as whole persons and respecting their unique preferences. The capacity to maintain healthy self-concept; to set goals and strive to meet them; to exercise choice, out of awareness of one's power to meet challenges; to engage in interactions with one's environment—all of these reflect a "coping capacity" that can sustain the will to live, even in the face of death (Weisman, 1984).

In an institutional medical setting, where patients are supposed to get well, the dying person may be treated as a deviant. Death may be seen as less a natural event than a medical failure. In this cultural context, biological death may be preceded by social death (Blauner, 1966; Cassell, 1974;

Sudnow, 1967). A pattern of avoidance, resulting from premature social death, is seen in the example of nurses taking longer to answer the bedside calls of terminally ill patients than to answer the calls of less severely ill patients (Bowers, Jackson, Knight, & LeShan, 1964). Avoidance is also evident in the evasive responses of some caregivers when patients attempt to initiate discussions about dying or death. These responses include reassurance ("You're doing fine"), denial ("You've got nothing to worry about"), changing the subject ("Let's talk about something more cheerful"), and fatalism ("We all have to die sometime"). Such responses present a marked contrast to the more helpful response of caregivers who display a willingness to discuss issues that concern patients who find themselves facing death ("What is happening to make you feel that way?").

Contact that bridges the usual professional distance reduces the alienation that patients may experience in an institutional setting. Establishing continuity of care between at least one caregiver and the patient is an important step toward eliciting the trust and confidence that forms a foundation for effective communication (Donovan & Pierce, 1976; Quint, 1967).

A century ago, physicians and nurses did perhaps as much to console as to cure the patient. Indeed, consolation and palliative measures were sometimes all the practitioner could offer the patient. A caregiver who steps into the room, sits by the patient's bedside, and demonstrates a willingness to listen, is likely to be more successful in providing solace and aid than the one who breezes in, remains standing, and quips, "How're we today? Did we sleep well?"

Skillful communication is a key to caring for the whole person. Caring is not always synonymous with doing. Nor is effective communication synonymous with having "something to say." The death of the body is a physical phenomenon, but the passing of a person is essentially nonphysical (social, emotional, psychological, spiritual); yet, these phenomena tend to become confused. Effective communication goes beyond caring for the person as a physical entity. It encompasses nonverbal as well as verbal communication. Actions, as well as words, are important. These insights about the communication process have application in all our relationships, whether or not the immediate context involves dying or death.

Communicating Social Support

We cannot communicate without giving of ourselves, nor can we communicate without benefitting from the gifts of others (Shepherd, 2001). The idea that communities are welded together by communication goes back at least to Aristotle's *Politics* (Depew & Peters). Thinking about the relationship between community and communication naturally leads to a consideration of social support, which refers to a process intended to help distressed individuals through the anxiety and uncertainty of difficult or painful life events (Albrecht & Adelman, 1987a). Figuring out the best way to support another person is not always easy or obvious. Nevertheless, in helping others make sense of themselves, their actions, and their situations during a crisis, the phrase "beginning to have an ear" is a helpful image (Albrecht & Adelman, 1987b, p. 255). Taking as a hint the fact that humans are endowed with two ears and only one mouth, listening is usually more important than talking.

When it is time to talk, saying what you mean is important. Being evasive, dishonest, or deceptive puts clear communication at risk. Effective communication does not require that the people who are communicating always agree with each other, but it does require a willingness to drop the protective guard that screens one's self and feelings from others.

Because communication is a two-way process, it takes a willingness to give as well as take from the interaction. This involves being open to each other's needs, as well as a readiness to not only hear the other person's spoken words, but also to "tune in" on unspoken levels of meaning that may be communicated by nonverbal and other behavioral "languages." When uncertainty exists about what the other person means, asking for clarification is better than to guess and guess wrong.

Although social support is usually conceived of as occurring at the level of interpersonal relationships, its aims and methods can be extended to encompass the larger community. Cynicism and radical individualism not only thwarts the giving and receiving of social support when people are in crisis, but it also undermines public dialogue about critical social and political issues that affect the common welfare. These unfruitful forces can be counteracted by a commitment to the common good and to a "dialogic civility" that respects multiple perspectives, with the goal of "keeping the conversation going" (Wood, 1999, p. xiii).

Modern technologies are expanding our options for communicating social support. Conventional face-to-face encounters are being augmented by the option of "reaching out and touching someone" via the Internet and electronic mail. Memorial pages and virtual cemeteries on the World Wide Web make it possible for individuals remote from one another to share their stories and acknowledge their losses. Soon after the collapse of the World Trade Center, many of the individuals who escaped wrote personal accounts of their experiences and e-mailed them to friends and family members as a way of coping with grief and helping others (Davis, 2001). These personal essays were swiftly shared with millions of people, by virtue of lightning-fast e-mail chains that forged a global community. In some instances, persons unknown to the writers gained helpful information about loved ones through the e-mailed accounts.

In this time of horror, electronic mail was also used by groups of friends who set up e-mail circles to make sure people were accounted for, as well as to give and receive reassurance (Peterson, 2001). Children, too, made their voices heard in e-mails and on Internet Web sites. "Talking things through" on the Internet became a way for children, as well as adults, to begin coping with an unsettling tragedy. Reflecting on the various ways that individuals and communities communicated social support in the minutes, hours, and days following the terrorist attacks, one writer noted that it gave "proof that a great, vast net of humanity exists, a net of friendship and abiding concern" (Varadarajan, 2001, p. W13).

Discussion Questions

1. How does matching language and communication styles promote effectiveness in interactions involving dying, death, and bereavement?
2. Which components of the communication process do you believe are most significant in interactions involving dying, death, and bereavement?

References

Adler, R. B., & Rodman, G. (1991). *Understanding human communication* (4th ed.). Fort Worth, TX: Harcourt Brace Jovanovich.

Albrecht, T. L., & Adelman, M. B. (1987a). Rethinking the relationship between communication and social support. In T. L. Albrecht & M. B. Adelman (Eds.), *Communicating social support* (pp. 13–16). Newbury Park, CA: Sage.

Albrecht, T. L., & Adelman, M. B. (1987b). Intervention strategies for building support. In T. L. Albrecht & M. B. Adelman (Eds.), *Communicating social support* (pp. 255–269). Newbury Park, CA: Sage.

Angwin, J. (2001, October 8). After the cataclysm, Americans grope for the words to describe "it." *Wall Street Journal*, p. A8.

Asante, M. K. (1998). *The Afrocentric idea* (Rev. ed.). Philadelphia: Temple University Press.

Bavelas, J. B. (1984, April). *Reviewing pragmatics sixteen years later.* Paper presented at the meeting of the International Communication Association, San Francisco, CA.

Berridge, G. R. (1994). *Talking to the enemy: How states without "diplomatic relations" communicate.* New York: St. Martin's Press.

Bessinger, C. D. (1988). Doctoring: The philosophic milieu. *Southern Medical Journal, 81,* 1558–1562.

Blauner, R. (1966). Death and social structure. *Psychiatry, 29,* 378–394.

Bowers, M. K., Jackson, E. N., Knight, J. A., & LeShan, L. (1964). *Counseling the dying.* New York: Thomas Nelson.

Buckman, R. (2000). Communication in palliative care. In D. Dickenson, M. Johnson, & J. S. Katz (Eds.), *Death, dying, and bereavement* (2nd ed.) (pp. 146–173). London: Open University/Sage.

Bugen, L. A. (1977). Human grief: A model for prediction and intervention. *American Journal of Orthopsychiatry, 47,* 196–206.

Cassell, E. J. (1974). Dying in a technological society. In P. Steinfels & R. M. Veatch (Eds.), *Death inside out: The Hastings Center report* (pp. 43–48). New York: Harper & Row.

Davis, A. (2001, September 18). Personal essays on tower terror circle the globe. *Wall Street Journal,* pp. B1, B6.

Depew, D., & Peters, J. D. (2001). Community and communication: The conceptual background. In G. J. Shepherd & E. W. Rothenbuhler (Eds.), *Communication and community* (pp. 3–21). Mahwah, NJ: Lawrence Erlbaum.

DeSpelder, L. A., & Strickland, A. L. (2002). *The last dance: Encountering death and dying* (6th ed.). Boston: McGraw-Hill.

Donovan, M. I., & Pierce, S. G. (1976). *Cancer care nursing.* New York: Appleton-Century-Crofts.

Gerbner, G. (1980). Death in prime time: Notes on the symbolic functions of dying in the mass media. *Annals of the American Academy of Political and Social Science, 447,* 64–70.

Gray, R. E., & Doan, B. D. (1990a). Empowerment and persons with cancer: Politics in cancer medicine. *Journal of Palliative Care, 6*(2), 33–45.

Gray, R. E., & Doan, B. D. (1990b). Heroic self-healing and cancer: Clinical issues for the health professions. *Journal of Palliative Care, 6*(1), 32–41.

Hall, E. T. (1976). *Beyond culture.* New York: Anchor-Doubleday.

Hall, M. N., & Rappe, P. T. (1995). Humor and critical incident stress. In L. A. DeSpelder & A. L. Strickland (Eds.), *The path ahead: Readings in death and dying* (pp. 289–294). Mountain View, CA: Mayfield.

Hingson, R., Scotch, N. A., Sorenson, J., & Swazey, J. P. (1981). *In sickness and in health: Social dimensions of medical care.* St. Louis: Mosby.

Jackson, E. N. (1957). *Understanding grief: Its roots, dynamics, and treatment.* Nashville: Abingdon Press.

Kaplan, T. (1989). An intercultural communication gap: North American Indians vs. the mainstream medical profession. In W. von Raffler-Engel (Ed.), *Doctor–patient interactions* (pp. 45–59). Philadelphia: John Benjamins.

Knapp, M. L., & Hall, J. A. (1997). *Nonverbal communication in human interaction* (4th ed.). Fort Worth, TX: Harcourt Brace.

LeShan, L. (1969). Mobilizing the life force. *Annals of the New York Academy of Science, 164*, 847–861.

Lindemann, E. (1944). Symptomatology and management of acute grief. *American Journal of Psychiatry, 101*, 141–148.

Littlejohn, S. W. (1999). *Theories of human communication* (6th ed.). Belmont, CA: Wadsworth.

Luckmann, J. (1999). *Transcultural communication in nursing*. Albany, NY: Delmar.

Nimmo, D., & Combs, J. E. (1985). *Nightly horrors: Crisis coverage by television network news*. Knoxville: University of Tennessee Press.

Novack, D. H., Detering, B. J., Arnold, R., Forrow, L., Ladinsky, M., & Pezzullo, J. C. (1989). Physicians' attitudes toward using deception to resolve difficult ethical problems. *Journal of the American Medical Association, 261*, 2980–2985.

Novack, D. H., Plumer, R., Smith, R. L., Ochitill, H., Morrow, G. R., & Bennett, J. M. (1979). Changes in physicians' attitudes toward telling the cancer patient. *Journal of the American Medical Association, 241*, 897–900.

Oken, D. (1961). What to tell cancer patients: A study of medical attitudes. *Journal of the American Medical Association, 175*, 1120–1128.

Osterweis, M., Solomon, F., & Green, M. (Eds.). (1984). *Bereavement: Reactions, consequences, and care*. Washington, DC: National Academy Press.

Penman, R. (2000). *Reconstructing communication: Looking to a future*. Mahwah, NJ: Lawrence Erlbaum.

Peterson, A. (2001, September 13). Old friends reach out to New Yorkers. *Wall Street Journal*, p. B5.

Phillippot, P., Feldman, R. S., & Coats, E. J. (Eds.). (1999). *The social context of nonverbal behavior*. Cambridge, England: Cambridge University Press.

President's Commission for the Study of Ethical Problems in Medicine and Biomedical and Behavioral Research. (1982a). *Making health care decisions: The ethical and legal implications of informed consent in the patient–practitioner relationship: Vol. 1. Report*. Washington, DC: Government Printing Office.

President's Commission for the Study of Ethical Problems in Medicine and Biomedical and Behavioral Research. (1982b). *Making health care decisions: The ethical and legal implications of informed consent in the patient–practitioner relationship: Vol. 2. Empirical studies of informed consent*. Washington, DC: Government Printing Office.

President's Commission for the Study of Ethical Problems in Medicine and Biomedical and Behavioral Research. (1982c). *Making health care decisions: The ethical and legal implications of informed consent in the patient–practitioner relationship: Vol. 3. Studies on the foundations of informed consent*. Washington, DC: Government Printing Office.

Quint, J. (1967). *The nurse and the dying patient*. New York: Macmillan.

Raffler-Engel, W. Von (1989). Doctor–patient relationships in the 1980s. In W. von Raffler-Engel (Ed.), *Doctor–patient interaction*. Philadelphia: John Benjamins.

Robinson, L. (1998). *"Race," communication, and the caring professions*. Philadelphia: Open University Press.

Rosenbaum, E. (1978). Oncology/hematology and psychosocial support of the cancer patient. In C. A. Garfield (Ed.), *Psychosocial care of the dying patient* (pp. 169–184). New York: McGraw-Hill.

Schneider, J. (1984). *Stress, loss, and grief: Understanding their origins and growth potential*. Baltimore: University Park Press.

Shepherd, G. J. (2001). Community as the interpersonal accomplishment of communication. In G. J. Shepherd & E. W. Rothenbuhler (Eds.), *Communication and community* (pp. 25–35). Mahwah, NJ: Lawrence Erlbaum.

Shuler, S. (2001). Talking community at 911: The centrality of communication in coping with emotional labor. In G. J. Shepherd & E. W. Rothenbuhler (Eds.), *Communication and community* (pp. 53–77). Mahwah, NJ: Lawrence Erlbaum.

Smith, A. L., Hernandez, D., & Allen, A. (1971). *How to talk with people of other races, ethnic groups, and cultures*. Los Angeles: Trans-Ethnic Foundation.

Sudnow, D. (1967). *The social organization of dying*. Englewood Cliffs, NJ: Prentice-Hall.

Tate, F. B. (1989). Impoverishment of death symbolism: The negative consequences. *Death Studies, 13,* 305–317.

Varadarajan, T. (2001, September 14). De gustibus. *Wall Street Journal*, p. W13.

Watzlawick, P. (1984). *Self-reference and world views*. Paper presented at the meeting of the International Communication Association, San Francisco, CA.

Weisman, A. (1984). *The coping capacity: On the nature of being mortal*. New York: Human Sciences.

West, C. (1984). *Routine complications: Troubles with talk between doctors and patients*. Bloomington: Indiana University Press.

White, G. M., & Robillard, A. B. (1989). Doctor talk and Hawaiian 'talk story': The conversational organization of a clinical encounter. In W. von Raffler-Engel (Ed.), *Doctor–patient interaction* (pp. 197–211). Philadelphia: John Benjamins.

Williams, F. (1989). *The new communications* (2nd ed.). Belmont, CA: Wadsworth.

Wood, J. T. (1999). Foreword. In R. C. Arnett & P. Arneson (Eds.), *Dialogic civility in a cynical age: Community, hope and interpersonal relationships* (pp. xi–xv). Albany: State University of New York.

Young, J. Z. (1978). *Programs of the brain*. New York: Oxford University Press.

Two

Death Education for Children

Hannelore Wass

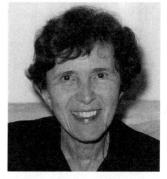

Dr. Hannelore Wass is professor emeritus of educational psychology at the University of Florida. She is the founding editor of Death Studies, *one of the two leading journals in the field, which she edited for 14 years, and which has been instrumental in defining the field of death, dying, and bereavement and its application in education, counseling, and care. She has published more than 70 research papers and chapters and 11 books.*

Much of her research has focused on the development of children's understanding of death, and on destructive themes in the media, and their socializing impact on perceptions, attitudes, and behaviors. Findings prompted her to propose ways in which homes and schools may provide effective antidotes to the cultural violence and the distorted views of death they engender, thereby helping children develop more realistic perceptions and to help them cope with death-related experiences and concerns.

Dr. Wass served for 15 years as the consulting editor of the pioneering Series on Death Education, Aging, and Health Care, in which 40 books on death were published under her editorship. Dr. Wass developed and taught two graduate courses on death at the University of Florida and has lectured and consulted widely in the United States and abroad. She served several terms on the board of directors of the International Work Group on Death, Dying, and Bereavement and the Association for Death Education and Counseling. She received two awards for outstanding contributions to the field.

Education has been a major component of the field, dating back to its beginnings. The death awareness movement challenged individuals to acknowledge their personal mortality, suggesting that it is essential for a meaningful life. Such consciousness-raising itself can be seen as an educational effort. There are, essentially, two reasons for providing death education. Just as education is an integral part of any field of study, so death education is critical for preparing professionals to advance the field and accomplish its purposes. Death education is also important for providing the general public with basic knowledge, wisdom, and skills helpful for coping and transcending death-related problems. It can address individuals at different educational levels and ages, can be formal or informal, and can be provided by various agencies, such as family and educational institutions.

Education in general is, of course, a major vehicle for communicating information and for facilitating understandings. Knowledge is important for developing and changing attitudes and values. Education also directly influences attitudes and values. It is intended to help define, strengthen, or modify them. Education also seeks to address the range of feelings experienced in learning processes and helps to manage them.

The aims of death education in the broadest sense are identical to those of the death movement and the field that evolved from it, as well as the agencies and organizations concerned with application in practice and policy making. These aims are to promote quality of life and living for ourselves and others, and to help create and maintain the conditions that bring them about. The aims are of special significance today, and to achieve them is urgent.

Rapid advances in science and technology have led to more and more specialization and fragmentation in matters of people's welfare, such as health care, child care, social services, and education, depersonalizing important aspects of these functions. Medical, biomedical, and technological advances have raised new questions and created uncertainties and controversies over such fundamental aspects of existence as when life begins and ends, what constitutes medical treatment, what are individuals' rights, compared to the obligations of the state, in determining the manner of their dying or the timing of it, and whether health care for the elderly should be rationed or withheld to meet rising health care costs. Spectacular advances in genomics raise even more fundamental questions about human "nature," and call for a redefinition of humanness and human purposes. They may also raise unrealistic hopes for eternal youth (Wass, 2001).

Meanwhile, there is much suffering, hardship, and untimely death experienced by many people in many parts of the world and in our own society. Genocide, starvation, the spread of AIDS, substance abuse, and destructive behavior against self and others, are among the deeply troubling aspects of our time. The question is not only of the quality of life, but of life itself.

There is need for informed, thoughtful people who are emotionally healthy, who care for themselves, and who are caring of others, to help work out solutions to these problems. Education is a major vehicle for producing such people. Children represent society's potential. Today's children are tomorrow's adults working in factories and offices, hospitals and research labs, are tomorrow's judges and juries, parents, and policy makers. They are the link to future generations. Survival and betterment are inevitably bound up with them. Any education about death, dying, and bereavement needs to begin with children.

Culture as Death Educator

Whether we know it or not, agree or disagree, children are recipients of death education from our actions as well as inaction. Children grow up in society, learn from it, absorb its wisdom, myths, and practices, its ambivalence, and its anxieties. Bandura, the pioneer in social learning theory (e.g., 1986), formulated and researched the well-established principle of observational learning called *modeling*. Models can be physical, involving real people and objects, or symbolic, involving verbal, audio, or visual representations. Modeling is recognized as one of the most powerful means of transmitting values, attitudes, and patterns of thought and behavior. Children adopt many values and beliefs from significant adults in their world, such as parents, teachers, public figures, sports heroes, and famous entertainers, through modeling. In similar manner, they learn from their physical and symbolic environments. Thus, inevitably, children learn fundamental lessons and develop basic attitudes about death, when they visit a cemetery, take part in a memorial service, or observe adults discussing the subject among themselves. Children learn from myriads of nonverbal behaviors that accompany speech, such as the tone of voice, an expression on the face, the tightening of a face muscle, a gesture, or an abrupt silence when adults become aware of the child's presence. Children learn by watching the evening news, a television war movie, a crime series, when playing with their toys and video games, and by observing dead animals in their backyard or experiencing the death of a pet.

This kind of education is informal and unplanned, but powerful nonetheless. It is an ongoing process, and part of the child's "enculturation" or socialization. It takes place at various times, in a variety of circumstances, and with varying degrees of emotional intensity. This learning prepares children for their functioning and interaction as adults.

Whether a personal encounter with death is the loss of a family member or peer through violence or illness, or the more remote experience of daily deaths on the evening news, children experience deaths as much as adults do, although not necessarily with the same meanings. If these experiences are troubling to adults, they are also troubling to children. How children are helped to understand and make sense of such experiences, and how they are comforted in the face of them, are important questions for a society to answer.

Because today's average life expectancy is higher than in previous eras, because in the social structure of our society young adults form their own nuclear families, and because most people die away from home, many children do not experience the death of a family member, such as a grandparent, during their formative years. Often, grandparents or other relatives live and die in distant geographic regions. Ironically, in the same society, at a time of personal remoteness from death, children nonetheless are continuously bombarded with death in their daily lives.

Death in the Entertainment Media

Perhaps the most powerful "death education" is delivered by the telecommunications media (Wass, 1995a). Symbolic violence is a significant issue, because the media have become a pervasive feature of American family life and thus a force in the child's socialization and cultural upbringing. A recent survey (Woodard & Gridina, 2000) indicates that nearly all families with children have a television set and a VCR, the majority have a computer and video game equipment. More than one half of the children have a television set in their bedrooms. Children spend an average of $4^{1}/_{2}$ hours a day in front of some sort of video screen. Analyses of violent programming content (e.g., Gerbner et al., 1980; Wilson et al., 1998) show that the amount of television violence has been consistently high and rising over the years. Across the television landscape (excluding news), nearly two thirds of the programs contain violence—an average of seven violent incidents per hour. One third of violent programming contains nine or more violent interactions. Concerning contexts, most violent incidents involve acts of physical aggression that threaten to kill or do kill. Perpetrators are portrayed as heroes more often than villains. Most violent acts are committed for personal gain or out of anger, have no consequences (portray little or no observable pain and suffering by the victims), and in nearly three fourths of the violent scenes, there is no punishment of the perpetrators (e.g., remorse, condemnation).

From 40 years of studies on the effects of violent media on children, with findings consistent across time, methods, child populations, and funding sources (e.g., federal agencies, media industries, independent research), clearly there is a causal link between heavy viewing of televised violence and subsequent aggressive behavior, and that frequent viewing of television violence leads to the belief that such violence is an accurate portrayal of reality, resulting in the fear of becoming a victim of violence. And prolonged viewing of filmed and televised violence appears to lead to emotional desensitization toward real-world violence, and to lessening of empathy and willingness to help those who are victimized (Wass, 2003).

Even though the electronic games industry has voluntarily rated its products, such ratings are commonly disregarded by distributors and retailers. Children make up 60% of the video game audience. Parents are often unaware of the extent of violence in many games. Health officials and child advocates familiar with video games are alarmed by their extreme violence. Interactive media may have an even greater impact on children than the more passive media forms. The graphics in video games are approaching motion picture quality, and evermore powerful platforms are being developed to process these images, thus making them more realistic and exciting (Federal Trade Commission, 2000).

The recording industry also labels music releases containing explicit lyrics, violence and/or sex (Wass, 1995a). However, with a few notable exceptions, as with the electronic games industry, distributors and retailers largely ignore them. Rap/hip hop and rock are popular music genres among older children. Many of the best-selling CDs have explicit content labels. Even though a few large retailers refuse to sell such records, children with Internet connection have no difficulty accessing and downloading lyrics from Web sites.

Real Violence

For a number of children in our society, the question is not what kind of cultural "death education" they receive, unintended or intended, but rather how to keep alive. Violence is now the primary cause of death in young people, following accidents. Youth violence is no longer viewed only as an issue of the criminal justice system, but is now designated as a high-priority public health issue. No community, whether affluent or poor, urban, suburban, or rural, is immune from its devastating effects. In the decade 1983–1993, arrest rates for violent crimes by children between ages 10 and 17 years increased by about 70%. Both the rates and actual numbers of homicide arrests nearly tripled (Cook & Laub, 1998). This epidemic of violent, often lethal behavior has alarmed families, psychologists, lawmakers, and children. Even though youth violence has decreased from 1993 to 1999, arrests for aggravated assault have declined only slightly, and another key indicator of violence, youths' confidential reports about their violent behavior, reveals no change in the proportion of young people who have committed physically injurious and potentially lethal acts (Snyder & Sickmund, 1999). Arrest records give only a partial picture of youth violence. For every youth arrested in any given year in the late 1990s, at least 10 were engaged in some form of violent behavior that could have seriously injured or killed another person, according to these reports (Snyder & Sickmund, 1999).

Following the Columbine High School tragedy in Colorado, the administration and Congress asked the surgeon general to develop a report on youth violence in our country. The resulting report, *Youth Violence: A Report of the Surgeon General* (2000), reviews a large body of research on where, when, and how much youth violence occurs, what causes it, and which of today's many preventive strategies are effective. The most important conclusion of this report is that youth violence is a preventable problem. A second conclusion, however, is that, after years of effort and expenditures of public and private resources, the search for real solutions remains an enormous challenge.

Many young people live with the trauma of having been a witness to deadly violence. Even larger numbers are victims of violence because they live in fear for their lives. Across the country, thousands of children and adolescents carry guns and other weapons. Metal detectors, security guards, and locked buildings in schools are daily reminders of potential threats to students' lives, and so, although giving a certain sense of security, are also keeping fears high, even though school shootings are far less frequent than one would expect, based on the publicity they receive. The new contexts of youth violence make the concern that death education may arouse fears and anxieties seem somewhat naïve, and require new thinking and new approaches to educational efforts.

Parents as Death Educators

As the primary social institution, the family informally teaches children the basic facts and values about themselves, the world, and about life and death. Parents have a fundamental role in helping their children to understand, evaluate, and manage their death experiences, through mediation, reassurance, and emotional support. But even today parents often are uncomfortable discussing death with their children, and tend to avoid it when possible. There is still a tendency among parents and the general public to believe that children are uninterested, unaware, and unaffected by death, and that, therefore, the topic is best left for later years.

Answering Questions

We have known for some time, however, that children, even at young ages, are curious, thoughtful, and concerned about death. They observe and gather data, interpret and misinterpret them, assimilate or accommodate them, and store what they have learned. They are as interested in death as they are in almost everything. They ask fundamental questions, to which philosophers and theologians have sought answers through the ages, such as "Why did the hamster die?" or "Where was I before I was born?" They also ask questions related to the processes of death and decomposition that tend to disturb adults. "How long does it take for a body to rot to the bones?" "Why do people die with their eyes open?" "What is rigor mortis?" The nature of the questions reflects the child's level of cognitive development. Study suggests that the child's understanding of death (as of other concepts) advances from immature to more mature, from ego-centered to ego-decentered, and from concrete to abstract, in discernible patterns. We know, for instance, that the preschool child's understanding of death is guided by reasoning processes that are qualitatively different from those of the adult, or even older child. The child's immature reasoning leads to understanding death as a state of immobility or sleep, a condition that can be reversed (Wass, 1984a, 1995b). It is important for parents to know this and to avoid reinforcing such thinking by their own explanations. Knowing the young child's thinking pattern is particularly important when a parent or sibling dies and parents and others are trying to help the child comprehend what has happened and reassure the child that his or her own life, care, and well-being are not threatened (Wass, 1984b).

Giving Comfort and Reassurance

Children also develop and learn different kinds of fears and concerns, depending on their developmental stage, life circumstances, and experience. Children fear the dark, monsters, vampires, werewolves, and the devil. They fear being dropped, abandoned, and buried alive. They fear losing parents, grandparents, and their own lives, through accidents, individual violence, war, or disease. Children also appear to develop mechanisms and behavior patterns of their own for managing some of their death-related fears, such as magic practices and superstitions, humor, and denial (Wass & Cason, 1984; Wass, 1998). But parents can do much to put their child's fears in perspective and to reassure and comfort the child. The first priority is for parents to provide a physically safe environment. In addition, the child needs a social environment that is psychologically "safe" and supportive. In an atmosphere of love, trust, and openness, in which joyful and distressing events and all kinds of thoughts and feelings are shared, children are more likely to express fears they may have about death, to share disturbing thoughts, and to ask questions about the subject. By keeping open lines of communication, parents can encourage such expression and serve as sounding boards, comforters, and guides.

Parents can find many "teachable moments," occasions that can serve to teach children important lessons about life and death. Keeping a pet, especially one with a short life expectancy, helps the child to learn firsthand about the life cycle and gives the child an opportunity to tend, love, and grieve for another creature, all with the caring guidance of parents.

When a family member or relative is ill and dies, it is up to the family whether or not children are allowed to visit this ill or dying loved one, or have the choice to attend the funeral or memorial service, and it is the parents' choice to include the child in the family's grieving. Hopefully, it is parents, along with other family members and friends, who are available and able to provide comfort and reassurance to the child.

Parents can be important resource persons, guiding their children toward vicarious experiences with death, through literature (Wass, 1984c). There are many excellent books on the market written by sensitive writers for children of all ages, which deal with the death of a pet, grandparent, friend, sibling, or parent [see Chapter 13 for some suggestions]. Psychologists have long noted the striking power such experiences can have for changing children's attitudes, as well as informing, comforting, and entertaining the child.

Mediating and Moderating Violence in the Media

Most scientists conclude that children learn aggressive attitudes and behavior from violent content, but they also agree that parents can be a powerful force in moderating, mediating, and perhaps preventing such influence. To do this, it is helpful for parents to be informed about the major risk factors associated with media violence, to be aware of their children's developmental levels and the programs, video games, and music lyrics their children favor. In addition, parents need to be informed about existing parental guidelines, ratings, and advisories. The Federal Communications Commission publishes the *TV Parental Guidelines*, V-chip information, and other assistance, on its Web site. The National Institute on Media and the Family (2002a), an independent nonprofit organization, has developed "KidScore," a rating system that applies to video games, TV programs, and films, which it offers on its web site. The National Institute on Media and the Family (2002b) also annually prepares an extensive "video and computer game report card", which parents may find useful. The V-chip, manufactured with all new television sets sold since January 1, 2000, gives parents new control over the television content that enters their homes, by letting them block programs. Information on activating and programming the V-chip is available through the V-Chip Education Web site (<http://www.vchipeducation.org/pages/using.html>).

Mediation and intervention are perhaps the most effective approaches to the problem. Parents may watch television with their children, and ask specific questions about their understanding and why they like a particular show or character. This will provide an opportunity to counteract violent messages in drama programs by pointing to their fictional nature. Watching the news with children enables parents to assist by providing perspective and comfort. Parents may discuss the potential negative effects of media violence with their children, communicate their own values, and encourage their children to watch programs that demonstrate helping, caring, and cooperation.

Parents can be role models for helping the child to develop healthy habits and constructive recreational activities and play, and to engage in family-oriented activities with their children. They can help their children to manage anger and frustration, learn constructive ways to settle interpersonal conflicts, and develop empathy and cooperative attitudes toward others. All this is best accomplished in an atmosphere of acceptance and support. As more parents become informed about their children's intellectual capacities, interests, fears, and needs with respect to death, as they become more comfortable with the subject and more aware of the important function they can serve, they will be more likely to interact in helpful ways with their children.

Death Education in the Schools

The pioneers in the death movement recognized the need for education about death, dying, and bereavement for all levels and age groups, and proposed systematic approaches to helping children learn about death. Leviton (1969) and Knott (1979), among others, offered guidelines for specific goals, curriculum design, methods of instruction, and resources. By then, studies of children's concepts and attitudes toward death, including those of dying and bereaved children, had established that even at young ages children are curious, have some understanding of death, and are able to grieve. These insights gave further impetus to educational efforts. Death education was approached from the perspective of preventive health education, as preparation for living, and as personal experience gained through literature. Leading educators suggested ways to incorporate discussions of death into various subject areas at secondary and primary levels or to design independent units of instruction (e.g., Ulin, 1977; Crase & Crase, 1984; Stevenson & Stevenson, 1996).

Judging from the considerable number of publications in the 1970s and early 1980s, death education seems to have been successful in health education at the high school level. But, by the mid 1980s, progress seemed to have slowed, and programs declined (Pine, 1986). A national survey of U.S. public schools supported this assessment (Wass, Miller, & Thornton, 1990a). It was found that 20% of high schools, 15% of middle schools, and less than 10% of elementary schools incorporated the study of death into their curricula. Those who did, tended to include it in health science or family life. Goals were to better prepare for life, to appreciate life and health, and to be less afraid of death. Teachers reported they had received inadequate preparation and would welcome continuing education workshops on the subject. However, there have also been encouraging developments indicating that schools are responding to children's needs.

Crisis Intervention

We know today that children's responses to the loss of a loved one are not unlike those of adults, except for those specifically related to their cognitive–developmental level. The kinds of things that help adults with their grief also help children. Because bereaved children are in school for most of the day, it helps when teachers, counselors and other staff, and classmates are supportive, understanding, and caring. When a child's parent or sibling has died, parents, who normally nurture the child, are often so devastated by the loss that they are unable to provide any kind of comfort or care for the bereaved sibling. It is therefore especially important that the school assist the child during the crisis period.

Sometimes a classmate or other member of the school community dies. The dramatic increase in the rates of suicide, homicide, and other risk-taking behavior, make it more likely that children lose a schoolmate through death sometime during their school years. The school can help children to grieve these deaths also. A schoolmate's death, especially when it is sudden and violent, affects surviving children deeply. Often this is the first personal encounter with a human death. The death of a peer can destroy the sense of invincibility with which children tend to shield themselves, and make them aware of their own vulnerability, a discovery that may be extremely threatening. Children may react with a host of feelings, from rage to agitation, from denial to despair, and a range of behaviors, from aggression to withdrawal. In such situations, crisis intervention is essential for helping children to manage their reactions. Help is now available in many school systems, thanks to the efforts of educators (e.g., Stevenson, 1994) and psychologists (e.g., Leenaars & Wenckstern, 1991), who helped design programs and protocols for intervention in schools. Highly publicized recent tragedies involving students have shown that communities mobilize all their resources to provide support and counseling for students in such circumstances.

Grief support and suicide/homicide intervention are special programs designed to go into operation when a crisis occurs. They are not part of the regular curriculum. Nonetheless, they are planned responses by the schools to death events that affect students. All schools should have policies and plans to deal with crises. But, in addition to programs in crisis intervention, schools can provide systematic education that is *preventive* and future-oriented, as well as *intervent*ive.

AIDS and Other Health-Related Education as Prevention

One of the notable efforts toward classroom-based prevention is AIDS education. The U.S. Department of Health and Human Services, in collaboration with the Centers for Disease Control (CDC), the National Center for Chronic Disease Control and Health Promotion, and other health agencies and professional organizations, in 1987, established the Coordinated School Health Program. By the year 2000, 20 states had been funded under the program (CDC, 2001a). This program was originally established to address the risk of adolescents contracting the human immunodeficiency virus (HIV), that causes AIDS, from risky sexual behavior or drug use, or both. In a national survey of public schools (Wass, Miller, & Thornton, 1990b), 46% of the schools reported providing such education, at least at the high school level, and nearly all the parents in those schools supported such education. An earlier study showed that three fourths of the states either required or encouraged sex/AIDS education, and nearly 9 of 10 large school districts in the United States supported it (Kenney, Guardado, & Brown, 1989). Various health officials, commissions, and committees at federal and state levels, and professional associations, have continued to urge schools to provide instruction about AIDS as part of a comprehensive health education program for all grade levels.

In 1992, CDC's Coordinated School Health Program was expanded to include health promotion through other healthy habits, physical activity, drug education, and constructive behavior. The National Center for Chronic Disease Prevention and Health Promotion conducts biannual youth risk behavior surveys assessing the progress of these efforts in terms of (self-reported) behavioral outcomes. An examination of the trends in youth risk behaviors 1991–1999 (CDC, 2001b), shows that some behaviors have improved (e.g., fewer physical fights, carrying a weapon to school, and suicidal thoughts, and increased use of condoms), but many have remained unchanged or worsened (e.g., frequent cigarette use, drug use, episodic heavy drinking, use of birth control pills).

These developments indicate that agencies and organizations can mobilize and collaborate effectively to introduce health-promoting programs in the schools, but that, at the same time, efforts must be intensified to achieve greater benefit for children and society.

Education to Prevent Violence

Proponents of death education for children insist that there is an urgent need for schools to address the life and people problems of today, and to help students to learn skills to solve them. Such education can be incorporated into various subject matters and made suitable for different developmental levels. Learning ways to manage anger and frustration, developing attitudes of tolerance and respect, empathy and compassion, and developing skills needed to communicate effectively, are all essential tools for helping young people to become sensitive, responsive, and responsible adults.This kind of education contains basic ingredients of long-term primary prevention of destructive behavior. It can serve as an antidote to the distorted perceptions children form from the entertainment media, while at the same time contributing to a high quality of life.

Additionally, teaching media literacy, such as video production (stunt men, fake wrestling, animation), the relationship between advertisement and programming, competition for audiences, target marketing, methods of persuasion, cost of advertising, among other topics, may help to countermand negative influences of violent media content (Wass, 1995b). Together, such educational efforts may help to reduce the fears and anxieties children already have.

Death Education as Preparation

Although most schools have established protocols for crisis intervention and have introduced AIDS education and other preventive education in health education curricula, teaching about death, dying, and bereavement in a systematic manner has remained a controversial issue. Some parents say it infringes on their and the church's domain. Some critics point to inadequate teacher preparation. There has been a concern that such study would induce fears and anxieties in students. These concerns, combined with increasing pressures to teach complex technological and other basic skills, make it less likely that the subject of death will be viewed as a needed part of the school's curriculum. Yet such education may now be more important than ever.

Schools are probably the most effective vehicle for public education about death in the long term. The public is offered information about death in various forums, through books, the press, the electronic media, and by word of mouth. But such education is not systematic or comprehensive. It can become so through the processes and mechanisms of the public schools. Children in their own right can benefit. They are entitled to learn about the facts of life and death, funerals, the sorrow of grieving, and skills for coping and overcoming grief, just as they are about other facts, skills, and practices in our culture. Schools are logical places for such education. They are the only social institution that can reach the more than 50 million children of school age in this country, and whose function is to educate. The schools's role is to teach the young about all aspects of life, to prepare them for a future of personal well-being and responsible social behavior.

The goals of death education are essentially those articulated by Leviton and others in the 1960s and 1970s. Those goals are to inform and help children gain insights and understanding; to help them develop constructive views and values by learning to weigh issues, based on observation, reason, and compassion; and to assist them in learning coping skills, and caring attitudes and behavior toward self, others, and life. These goals reflect society's needs, as well as those of the individual child. In systematic death education, the study of death, dying, and grieving is integrated into the various subject areas of the school curriculum, such as social studies, psychology, health sciences, family life, biology, earth sciences, literature, and art.

A natural topic for the life sciences, for example, is to study not only the life cycle of plants and small animals, but that of humans as well, from conception, birth, growth, and maturity, to old age and death. Here, or in the study of the earth sciences, students can learn how industrialization and unchecked population growth are causing the slow but steady deterioration of the earth, such as the destruction of rain forests, pollution of air, land, and water, and the depletion of the ozone layer. They can also learn about available means and measures to halt this process.

Psychology or family planning are natural subject areas for discussing how people respond to the crisis of dying and death; what feelings, thoughts, and behaviors such experiences evoke; and how one can cope and transcend them, and support others in this process.

In art class, the teacher might encourage students to choose painting projects, such as grief. In art appreciation, the teacher can point to some of the famous art works created through the centuries that treat death. After all, many artists have chosen this fundamental experience as a theme for their work, and millions of people have been enriched by seeing such creations.

One of my former students teaches literature in a high school. Once, when her students were studying Shakespeare's *Romeo and Juliet*, she challenged them by saying: "Suppose Romeo were Rick and Juliet were Stacy, and they were both eleventh graders living in Jacksonville. Would they feel the same way or differently? What could they do? How could they get help? Do *you* ever have suicidal thoughts and impulses?" The discussion that followed was an eye opener for the teacher. She was surprised about how deeply her students felt, and how interested they were in the discussion.

At the elementary level, teachers can fit death-related topics into their teaching even more easily. Because they have more time with the students, they have a wider range of possibilities and options. In the study of the community, for example, younger students often are taken on field trips to city hall, the fire station, supermarket, and the museum. They could also visit the cemetery and the funeral home in this context. The possibilities are numerous. Thoughtful teachers who are comfortable with the subject, and have basic knowledge about it, find ways to incorporate it naturally into their teaching.

There are several advantages of such integrated education. For one thing, the topic is naturally imbedded in its larger context, rather than separated from it, and is thus less likely to be distorted. Additionally, the long-term approach is developmental, that is, children learn about death-related matters in ways appropriate to their developmental levels, learn about the subject from different perspectives, and in small doses at a time. Because such teaching is foresighted and *proactive*, rather than *reactive*, it is likely to be more low-keyed and less stressful and emotionally taxing.

Health professionals, and others in the helping fields, can assist in different ways, through their work, organizations, and at the community level, to help families to deal with death-related concerns at home, to make death education more acceptable in the schools, to participate in efforts to persuade the entertainment industries to lower levels of violence, and to engage in long-term efforts to prevent actual violence. When family, schools, and other agencies and organizations all work together to help the young develop knowledge and skills for coping and transcending, and to instill in them motivations and values of caring and compassion, there may be a future of full humanity.

Discussion Questions

1. How may prior knowledge about death, dying, and bereavement help children to cope more effectively when they encounter a death in their own lives?
2. Does death education in the schools, as discussed in this chapter, interfere with parents' rights and religious beliefs about life after death?
3. How might parents be helped to become more informed about possible negative influences of violent media and peer pressure to engage in risky behavior?
4. How might the entertainment industries be persuaded to reduce the levels of violence in their products?

References

Bandura, A. (1986). *Social foundations of thought and action—A social cognitive theory* (pp. 47–80). Englewood Cliffs, NJ: Prentice-Hall.

Centers for Disease Control. (2001a). *Adolescent school health programs: An investment in our nation's future.* Retrieved Dec. 15, 2002, from http://www.cdc.gov/nccdphp/bb_healthyyouth/index.htm

Centers for Disease Control. (2001b). Trends in Youth Risk Behaviors 1991–1999. http://www.cdc.gov/mmwr/preview/mmrhtml/ss4905a1.htm (Accessed December 15, 2002.)

Cook, P. J., & Laub, J. H. (1998). The unprecedented epidemic in youth violence. In M. Tonry & M. H. Moore (Eds.), *Youth violence. Crime and justice: A review of research* (Vol. 24, pp. 27–64). Chicago: University of Chicago Press.

Crase, D. R., & Crase, D. (1984). Death education in the schools. In H. Wass & C. A. Corr (Eds.), *Childhood and death* (pp. 345–363). New York: Hemisphere.

Federal Communications Commission. (2001). V-chip: Viewing television responsibly. <http://www.fcc.gov/vchip> (Accessed December 13, 2002.)

Federal Trade Commission. (2000). *Marketing violent entertainment to children.* Washington, DC. http://www.ftc.gov/opa/2000/09/youthviol.htm (Retrieved March 2, 2001).

Gerbner, G., Gross, L., Morgan, M., & Signorielli, N. (1980). The "mainstreaming" of American violence—Profile Nr. 11. *Journal of Communication, 30,* 10–29.

Kenney, A. M., Guardado, S., & Brown, L. (1989, March/April). Sex education and AIDS education in the schools: What states and large school districts are doing. *Family Planning Perspectives, 21,* 56–64.

Knott, J. E. (1979). Death education for all. In H. Wass (Ed.), *Dying: Facing the facts* (pp. 385–403). Washington, DC: Hemisphere.

Leenaars, A. A., & Wenckstern, S. (1991). *Suicide prevention in schools.* Washington, DC: Hemisphere.

Leviton, D. (1969). The need for education on death and suicide. *Journal of School Health, 39,* 270–274.

Leviton, D. (1977). The scope of death education. *Death Education, 1,* 41–56.

National Institute on Media and the Family. (2002a). <http://www.mediafamily/org/kidscore/index.shtml>. (Accessed December 13, 2002.)

National Institute on Media and the Family. (2002b). <http://www.mediafamily/org/research/report_vgrc20001-2.shtml>. (Accessed December 13, 2002.)

Pine, V. R. (1986). The age of maturity for death education: A socio-historical portrait of the era 1976–1985. *Death Studies, 10,* 209–231.

Snyder, H. N., & Sickmund, M. (1999). *Juvenile offenders and victims: 1999 National Report (NCJ 178257).* Washington, DC: U.S. Department of Justice, Office of Justice Programs, Office of Juvenile Justice and Delinquency Prevention.

Surgeon General. (2001). Youth Violence: A report of the U.S. Surgeon General. Retrieved from http://www.surgeongeneral.gov/library/youthviolence/youvioreport.html (Accessed December 14, 2002.)

Stevenson, R. G. (Ed.). (1994). *What will we do? Preparing a school community to cope with crises.* Amityville, NY: Baywood.

Stevenson, R. G., & Stevenson E. P. (Eds.). (1996). *Teaching students about death.* Philadelphia: Charles Press.

Ulin, R. O. (1977). *Death and dying education.* Washington, DC: National Education Association.

Wass, H. (1984a). Concepts of death: A developmental perspective. In H. Wass & C. A. Corr (Eds.), *Childhood and death* (pp. 3–24). New York: Hemisphere and McGraw-Hill.

Wass, H. (1984b). Parents, teachers, and health professionals as helpers. In H. Wass & C. A. Corr (Eds.), *Helping children cope with death* (2nd ed., pp. 75–130). New York: Hemisphere McGraw-Hill.

Wass, H. (1984c). Books for children. In H. Wass & C. A. Corr (Eds.), *Helping children cope with death: Guidelines and resources* (2nd ed., pp. 151–207). Washington, DC: Hemisphere.

Wass, H. (1995a). Appetite for destruction: Children and violent death in popular culture. In D. W. Adams & E. J. Deveau (Eds.), *Beyond the Innocence of childhood: Factors influencing children and adolescents* (pp. 95–108.) Amityville, NY: Baywood.

Wass, H. (1995b). Death in the lives of children and adolescents. In H. Wass & R. A. Neimeyer (Eds.), *Dying: Facing the facts* (3rd ed., pp. 269–301). Washington, DC: Taylor & Francis.

Wass, H. (1998). Healthy children and fears about death. *Illness, Crisis, & Loss, 6,* 114–126.

Wass, H. (2001). Past, present, and future of dying. *Illness, Crisis & Loss, 9,* 90–110.

Wass, H. (2003). Children and media violence. In R. Kastenbaum (Ed.), *Macmillan encyclopedia of death and dying* (Vol. 1). New York: Macmillan Reference.

Wass, H., & Cason, L. (1984). Fears and anxieties about death. In H. Wass & C. A. Corr (Eds.), *Childhood and death* (pp. 25–45). New York: Hemisphere and McGraw-Hill.

Wass, H., Miller, M. D., & Thornton, G. (1990a). Death education and grief/suicide intervention in the public schools. *Death Studies, 14*(3), 253–268.

Wass, H., Miller, M. D., & Thornton, G. (1990b). AIDS education in the U.S. public schools. *AIDS Education and Prevention, 2*(3), 213–219.

Wilson, B. J., et al. (1998). Violence in television programming overall: University of California, Santa Barbara study. In *National Television Violence Study* (2nd ed.). Center For Communication and Social Policy. Thousand Oaks, CA: Sage Publications.

Woodard, E. H. & Gridina, N. (2000). Media in the home: The fifth annual survey of parents and children. Philadelphia, PA: The Annenberg Public Policy Center of the University of Pennsylvania.

Three

Death Education for Adults

Charles A. Corr

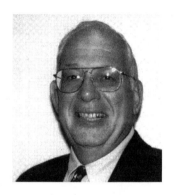

Charles A. Corr is professor emeritus, Southern Illinois University, Edwardsville, and a volunteer with the Executive Committee of the National Donor Family Council, National Kidney Foundation (1992–present).

Dr. Corr has been a member of the boards of directors of the Association for Death Education and Counseling (1980–1983), the Illinois State Hospice Organization (1981–1984), and the International Work Group on Death, Dying, and Bereavement (1987–1993; chairperson, 1989–1993).

In addition to more than 60 articles and chapters, Dr. Corr's publications include numerous books, including: Hospice Care: Principles and Practice *(Springer, 1983);* Helping Children Cope with Death: Guidelines and Resources *(2nd ed., Hemisphere, 1984);* Handbook of Childhood Death and Bereavement *(Springer, 1996); and* Death and Dying, Life and Living *(4th ed., Wadsworth, 2003).*

In the late 1950s and early 1960s, death was commonly said to be a taboo topic (Feifel, 1963). Gorer (1965) went so far as to say that death had changed places with sex, and that death was the "new pornography." This did not mean that issues related to dying, death, and bereavement had gone completely without discussion. To mention just one example, Plato's (1961) famous portraits of the trial, imprisonment, and death of Socrates in the *Apology*, *Crito*, and *Phaedo* are classics of Western literature, and they include Socrates' observation that the whole of philosophy or human wisdom can rightly be construed as a preparation for death (*Phaedo*, 67e).

But at the middle of the twentieth century, research and writing on dying, death, and bereavement were limited, and there were few educational opportunities in this field. In this context, Feifel's book, *The Meaning of Death* (1959), is a landmark that helped to encourage behavioral scientists, clinicians, and humanists to direct attention to these topics, study and do research, write articles and books, found journals and organizations, and engage in education of all sorts (Pine, 1977). That had led to educational programs for preschool and church-school groups, children and adolescents in elementary and secondary schools, college and preprofessional students, postgraduate and professional audiences, and hospice volunteers, members of support groups, and the general public (Wass, Corr, Pacholski, & Sanders, 1980; Wass, Corr, Pacholski, & Forfar, 1985).

Early historical developments in the field of death education have been reviewed by Pine (1977, 1986) in two concise, informed, and effective articles. Our task in this chapter is to understand the phenomenon of death education, that is, education specifically concerned with death-related issues, with special relationship to adult audiences. In order to do this, we need to think first about societal relationships with, and attitudes toward, death. Much of this applies to all of society's citizens—children, adolescents, adults, and the elderly—but our specific concern in this chapter is death education for adults.

Societal Death Systems

Every society has its own death system (Kastenbaum, 1972). That is, every society develops ways in which, as an organized entity, it deals with the implications of dying, death, and bereavement. In technical terms, a death system is the "sociophysical network by which we mediate and express our relationship to mortality" (p. 310). In other words, in response to the implications of death, every society seeks to organize itself in various ways, on behalf of both the collective entity and its individual members. It does this by erecting a functional structure that it puts between death and its implications, on the one hand, and itself and its members, on the other hand—a structure that interprets death to the society and its members.

One society's death system might be formally or explicitly organized in some or all of its aspects. By contrast, another death system might be informally expressed in the ways in which the society conducts its everyday affairs. In practice, most death systems are likely to combine formal and informal elements.

Until recently, not much attention had been paid to the overall structure and patterns of societal death systems. But when individuals are asked to reflect on their own society's death system, they usually can easily identify its components and recognize ways in which they function. This suggests that most of us are familiar with the workings of our own society's death system, although we may not have thought of it in those terms.

Elements of a death system include:

1. People—individuals defined by their more-or-less permanent or stable roles in the death system, such as funeral directors, lawyers, florists, and life insurance agents, in our society;
2. Places—specific locations that have assumed a death-related character, such as cemeteries, funeral homes, health care institutions, and the "hallowed ground" of a battlefield or disaster;
3. Times—occasions that a society associates with death, such as Memorial Day, Good Friday, or the anniversary of the death of a loved one;
4. Objects—things whose character is somehow linked to death, such as death certificates, hearses, obituaries and death notices in the newspaper, weapons, tombstones, a gallows, or an electric chair; and
5. Symbols—things that have come to signify death, such as black armband, a skull and crossbones, certain solemn organ music, and certain words or phrases.

Functions of a death system are:

1. to give warnings and predictions, as in the case of civil defense sirens or hurricane warning systems;
2. to prevent death, as in the case of emergency medical care and other rapid response systems;
3. to care for the dying, as in the case of modern hospice programs;
4. to dispose of the dead, as in the case of funeral directors, cemeteries, and crematories;
5. to work toward social consolidation after death, as in the case of funeral ritual or self-help groups for the bereaved;
6. to help make sense of death, as in the case of certain religious or philosophical systems; and
7. to bring about socially sanctioned killing, as in the case of some aspects of police protection, training for war, and capital punishment.

The important point about the notion of a death system is that such a system will be found in some form in every society. No society is without a system for coping with the fundamental realities that death presents to human existence. Much can therefore be learned about any society by considering the nature of its death system and the ways in which it functions.

A Death-Denying Society?

Some have argued that the death system in American society functions largely to deny the presence of death, to exile or exclude death as a social or public reality (e.g., Kübler-Ross, 1969). Many things can be said in support of that view. For example, through a process of institutionalization, professionalization, and specialization, we have tended in our society to move death away from the mainstream of living. And we are often unwilling to speak openly or directly about death, preferring to employ oblique, evasive, or euphemistic language, instead. Surely, it is true that the death system in our society functions in many important ways to keep death at a distance from the mainstream of life and to gloss over many of its harsh aspects.

That may be either good or bad (or perhaps a bit of both), but it is too simple to say that ours is solely a death-denying society (Corr & Corr, 2003; Corr, Nabe, & Corr, 2000). It is that, in many respects, but it is also more than that. Death is. It cannot be defined or avoided everywhere and at all times. Life, death, and societies are more complex than they are made to appear in the catchphrase of a "death-denying society." For that matter, it has long been recognized that denial and acceptance are themselves complicated phenomena that can coexist in individuals and in societies, by functioning on several different levels at the same time (Dumont & Foss, 1972; Weisman, 1972).

We need not think only of a contrast between acceptance and denial when we seek to characterize the death system in our society or in any other society. Instead, we will do better to think of the many ways—often different, sometimes contrasting or contradictory—in which a given society relates to the many-sided issues associated with dying, death, and bereavement. If so, we will ask ourselves questions of the following sort: What is the nature of our death system? How does it function? How well does it serve our needs?

Societal Groups, Their Members, and Protection

One judgment about death systems in the modern, developed societies of North America and Western Europe is the following: "We have created systems which protect us in the aggregate from facing up to the very things that as individuals we most need to know" (Evans, 1971, p. 83). There are two important elements in this judgment: the interests of the group or aggregate against those of the individual, and the theme of "protection."

Groups do tend to serve their own interests. They will argue that this is done precisely in order that they can serve the interests of the largest number of their members. Or they will say that serving the interests of their members is best achieved through serving the interests of the group. This is a noble ideal. It is often true. But not always. Conflicts do arise, as when society exercises powers of eminent domain to take the private property of individuals for public (group) purposes, or when society sends its youth abroad to fight and die in wars on behalf of communal rather than individual interests. So we need to inquire whether our death system maintains an appropriate balance between the interests of the society and of the individual.

How will we judge the value of the desire to "protect" people from the realities of dying, death, and bereavement? The issue here is the danger of misguided protection, of "doing all the wrong things for all the right reasons." Many years ago, the French essayist La Rochefoucauld (1665/ 1868) wrote that "one can no more look steadily at death than at the sun" (I, p. 41). This is certainly true. To gaze directly and without filters at the sun is to run the risk of loss of one's vision, just as immersion in death without some redeeming perspective can numb and overwhelm vitality in living. But we do live our lives in the warmth and light of the sun, and we inspect it, often obliquely or through some sort of screen. Similarly, it is the privilege and obligation of human beings to be able to conduct their lives with an awareness of their own mortality. We cannot expect to cope effectively with loss, grief, and death when they break into our lives, if we have not prepared ourselves to do so. Too much protection, or protection of the wrong sort, may not be conducive to maximizing quality in living.

Society and Education

All of the mediating and expressive functions of a societal death system involve education. To give warnings and predictions about death, or to try to prevent death, is to alert people to the dangers of death and to advise them how to behave to avoid or minimize those dangers. To care for the dying and to support the bereaved is to draw attention to the needs of vulnerable people and to emphasize both how and why others should help such people. To dispose of the dead is to acknowledge that the corpse is no longer a living person, but still remains an object for special treatment. To help make sense of death and to sanction certain sorts of killings is to affirm an intellectual and value framework within which both life and death find their appropriate places.

Death systems are not neutral. They reflect attitudes and express positions through which messages are conveyed. Through its death system, a society says: This is how we are coping with death; this is how we will cope with death; this is how we ought to cope with death. Individuals are free to accept and internalize these messages, or to resist and reject them. But it is foolish and probably a doomed cause to ignore or try to remain ignorant of them. The death system in our society is the milieu in which we live. Its messages are powerful and omnipresent.

Education for Adults: Four Levels

In the field of dying, death, and bereavement, education for adults is conducted at four distinguishable levels: cognitive, affective, behavioral, and valuational. Death education is a cognitive or intellectual enterprise, in the sense that it provides information about death-related experiences and aids in understanding those experiences. Information of this sort takes many forms. For example, it is important to know that towards the end of the 1980s lung cancer surpassed breast cancer as the leading cancer cause of death for women in our society. This tragic fact is clearly related to patterns of smoking cigarettes, and is, in part, an ironic outcome of cigarette advertising that tells women, "You've come a long way, baby." Similarly, during the early 1980s, it was the recognition of an unusually high incidence among young males in New York City of a relatively rare form of skin cancer, Kaposi's sarcoma, which had hitherto been confined largely to elderly males of Mediterranean descent, that helped to identify a new cause of death—acquired immune deficiency syndrome (AIDS).

The cognitive dimensions of death education parallel similar dimensions in all academic or classroom education, although these are not the only ways such dimensions can be addressed. In addition to facts, this dimension of education includes new ways of organizing or interpreting the data of our experience. In the field of thanatology, for example, Elisabeth Kübler-Ross (1969) and Maria Nagy (1948) are both well known for stage-based theories they advanced to explicate coping with dying (in the case of Kübler-Ross) and cognitive development in children (in the case of Nagy). Each of these theories has helped to draw attention to and illuminate an important field of study, although each also has its limits and has been challenged, either in itself or in the ways in which it has been applied (Corr, 1992, 1993, 1995, 1997).

The affective dimensions of death education have to do with feelings and emotions about dying, death, and bereavement. For example, a wide range of feelings is involved in experiences of loss and bereavement. Research and education in this area helps to sensitize the nonbereaved to the depth, intensity, duration, and complexities of grief following a death. Much of this has yet to be communicated to the public at large, which may still wrongly think that a few days or weeks may be more than adequate to "forget" or "get over" the death of an important person in one's life (Osterweis, Solomon, & Green, 1984). In fact, mourning is far more like a process of coping with stress and striving to achieve an ongoing adaptation, or learning to live with one's loss, than it is like ending a process or resolving a problem. For this reason, researchers have suggested that it is important for at least some bereaved persons to sustain "continuing bonds" with the deceased, maintain the "empty space" in their lives, and not "finish grieving" (Klass, Silverman, & Nickman, 1996; McClowry, Davies, May, Kulencamp, & Martinson, 1987).

In its affective dimensions, death education seeks to appreciate the feelings of those who have been affected by death, as well as the feelings of those who have not been so affected. For example, we have learned that it is always wrong for someone who has not been bereaved to say to a bereaved person, "I know how you feel." Not only is this impossible, but bereaved persons have told us how arrogant it appears to them and how it seems to diminish the uniqueness and poignancy of their loss. Similarly, instead of dismissing grief associated with miscarriage or stillbirth, on the false assumption that no bonding had yet occurred, we have learned to appreciate the many forms of bonding during pregnancy and the legitimacy of parental grief in cases of perinatal death (Lamb, 1988). This has led to widespread recognition in professional pediatric circles of the value of permitting parents to see and hold the dead infant, take pictures or retain other mementoes, and obtain follow-up postmortem information—all as ways of completing the bonding process and laying the foundation for healthy mourning (e.g., Johnson, Johnson, Cunningham, & Weinfeld, 1985). In light of realistic education, what might have seemed ghoulish or repugnant to the uninformed can now be seen as part of a healthy process.

The third important dimension of death education has to do with behavioral considerations. Why do people act as they do in death-related situations? How should or could people act in such situations? Behavior is the outward expression of what we feel and believe. In our society, much behavior, both public and private, seeks to avoid contact with dying, death, and bereavement. Often, that is because people do not know what to say or what to do in such situations. They pull back from contact with the dying or the bereaved, leaving the latter alone and without support or companionship at a time when sharing and solace are most needed (Klass, 1988). Similarly, many people hesitate to mention the name of a deceased person, leaving survivors to experience a kind of double loss of both the presence and the memory of that person.

In contrast to all of this, the hospice movement in recent years has taught us how much can be done to help people cope with dying (Connor, 1998; Corr & Corr, 1983; Lattanzi-Licht, Mahoney, & Miller, 1998), much as research on funeral ritual (e.g., Fulton, 1995) and studies of self-help groups (Hughes, 1995) have shown the way to assist people in coping with bereavement. Education arising from these sources affirms the great value to be found in the presence of a caring person, and it directs us not so much to speak as to practice active listening. Sometimes it gives us confidence to be comfortable when we are only sitting quietly alongside a dying or bereaved person with our discomfort. For many, it has led to the development of skills in interacting. None of this eliminates the sadness of death, but it can help to recreate the caring communities that all vulnerable people need, but that seem too frequently to have atrophied in many modern societies.

The fourth or valuational dimension of death education lies in its role in helping us to identify, articulate, and affirm the basic values that govern our lives. The only life we know in this world is inextricably bound up with death. We would not have this life if death were not one of its essential parts, and we struggle in our imaginations to conceive what any sort of life without death might be like. Life and death, living and dying, happiness and sadness, attachments and loss—neither pole in these and many other similar dyads stands alone in our experience. For this reason, the perspective of death is an essential one (but not the only one) in helping us to achieve an adequate understanding of life.

Many of the things already mentioned point toward what we value: sensitivity, vulnerability, resilience, temporality, finitude, and community. But perhaps our values come to the fore most sharply when we are asked what shall we tell our children about death, and how shall we respond to the moral problems of our time. Shall we hide death from children and beguile them with tales of an unending journey without shadows or tears? Can we sustain such a charade for long? And will it enable our children to cope with life on their own when we are gone (dead?) or unavailable? Or shall we introduce children to the realities of death in ways that are appropriate to their developmental level and capacities, and with the support of mature values that enable us to live a meaningful life and cope in constructive ways with death (Corr & Corr, 1996; Wass & Corr, 1984a, 1984b)?

Death-related values are often prominent in many of the moral problems of our time: nuclear warfare, epidemic, famine and malnutrition, dislocation of populations, capital punishment, and all of the quandaries posed by modern medicine and its complex technologies. For example, is life the ultimate value? I think not. Others might disagree. Certainly, human life is a value and, for the most part, an important one. This is part of what is meant by saying that life is sacred. But that is not the same as the assertion that human life is absolute. I might sacrifice my life for the sake of the lives of others, or perhaps for some transcendent value. And, although I might act to sustain life when the life itself retained the potential to engage in human relationships and when its sustenance required no more than my presence and ordinary modes of care, would I do so when there was no longer the potential for any human relationship and when its sustenance depended on extraordinary interventions of medical technology?

Is there a "right to die"? In 1997, the U.S. Supreme Court ruled that no such right could be found in or grounded in the U.S. Constitution, although it indicated that individual states had the constitutional right to make laws that provide for physician-assisted suicide. The voters of Oregon approved such a law, entitled a "Death with Dignity Act," in 1994, and reaffirmed it on a 1997 ballot (Haley & Lee, 1998). Education about assisted suicide should explore its meaning, implications, and the values that might lead individuals and groups to favor or oppose such behavior.

Education for Adults: Goals

Our fundamental goals in death education for adults are of three general types. The first has to do with individuals themselves; the second concerns individuals in their personal transactions with society; and the third concerns individuals in their public roles as citizens within the society. First, education about dying, death, and bereavement is intended to enrich the personal lives of those to whom it is directed. It helps them understand themselves and appreciate both their strengths and their limitations as finite human beings. Most of us wish to control every aspect of our lives. This is not a goal we can expect to achieve. Instead, we can only realistically hope to influence those aspects of our lives that fall within the scope of our autonomy. That may not seem like enough: We want more. But, although accidents (most involving motor vehicles) are the fifth leading cause of death in our society, and even though we cannot prevent all accidental deaths, it is nevertheless important to fasten our seatbelts and drive defensively whenever we are on the road. So we can exert some positive influence on accidental deaths.

Orville Kelly (1975) once founded a self-help group called "Make Today Count" (MTC) for those who have a life-threatening illness. Its members are living under the threat of death. (Is that not true in some sense for all of us, although perhaps moreso for many MTC members?) In response to this realization, members of MTC chapters find meaning and fulfillment in each day they are alive. Against this, think how many people are merely "killing time." Death education encourages every individual to make each day of his or her life as satisfying as it can be. This is not a hedonism of the moment, which gives no thought to the consequences of one's actions. That would lead to a hedonism that is blind to the future, in just the way that so much living for the future is blind to the passing present. When we make today count, we do not exclude memories from the past or hopes for the future, but we emphasize that the past is gone, the future may not come, and the present is all that we really have right now to treasure and enjoy.

The second goal of death education is to inform and guide individuals in their personal transactions with society. For our purposes, this goal can be illustrated by considering transactions with two major components of our societal death system: health care services and the funeral industry. From birth to death, we are all consumers of health care, but statistics show that we draw upon such services most during the last 6 months of our lives. Care of those who have far-advanced illnesses, who are chronically ill and unable to take care of themselves, or who are terminally ill, is big business in modern societies.

In recent years, the death awareness movement has drawn attention to the fact that even those who are within days or hours of death are alive. Dying patients, we have come to realize, are living human beings. As such, dying persons and their family members need to be informed about services that are available to them and options they might select. Should one continue to seek a cure to forestall death, or is it appropriate to place greater emphasis on the management of distressing symptoms? Who should provide services and where should they be provided, for example, at home or in an institution? Education acquaints us with alternatives and enables us to select for ourselves those that most satisfy the needs and preferences of the individuals involved.

Similarly, education speaks to the importance of funeral ritual as a means to help the bereaved achieve at least three important tasks: (1) to dispose of the body in appropriate ways, (2) to contribute to realization of the implications of the death, and (3) to assist in reintegration and meaningful ongoing living (Corr, Nabe, & Corr, 1994). But different societies, groups, and individuals address these tasks in different ways. In our own society, common postdeath practices include embalming and viewing the body, burying the corpse underground or entombing it in an aboveground mausoleum, cremating and disposing of the remains in various ways (burial, entombment, inurnment, or scattering of ashes), donating the body to scientific research and/or education, and conducting a memorial service in the absence of a body. Each of these options has served the needs of some people at some time; any one of them may be unsatisfactory to a particular person or group. Education in this area is intended to inform people about alternatives and to help them choose which might best serve their needs.

A funeral is frequently said to represent the third largest expenditure (after the purchase of a house and an automobile) that most individuals will make in their lives. And health care towards the end of life is also a major expense, although federal funding and private insurance may amortize its burden over many years of premiums and income from a group of beneficiaries. If death education only resulted in an informed consumer in these two areas, it would have done much to improve the ways in which individuals relate to their societies.

The third goal of death education is to prepare individuals for their public roles as citizens within a society. Once upon a time, when questions were raised about the legal meaning of death, society turned to common law, the common body of knowledge and wisdom about any subject. Common law was often represented by a legal dictionary, such as *Black's Law Dictionary* (Black, 1979), which defined death as "the cessation of life" (p. 360). Such a definition is true enough, but it seems to lack specificity and is not very explicit in its guidance. Recognizing that, the dictionary went on to offer a further explication of the concept of death as "permanent cessation of all vital functions and signs" (ibid.). The vital functions in question were usually identified as involving the respiratory and circulatory systems, and the signs were typically expressed in terms of bodily fluids, that is, air (or, more specifically, oxygen) and blood.

Some difficulties arose with the introduction of mechanical devices like the respirator, which forced air into and out of the lungs, and which could often in this way stimulate the action of the heart. Was this "flow of vital bodily fluids" (and thus, life), or was it merely ventilation and mimicry of such vitality? When these questions arose in civil or criminal litigation, judges and juries were forced to make decisions that led to case law. In the absence of legal rule or precedent, such decisions were not always consistent.

The natural progression of things leads to the enactment of legislation on such difficult points, in order to guide the courts. Such legislation may take into account the views of various experts, but in the end it is the work of a political process on the part of those who represent the people. Clearly, when the populace and its representatives are informed and articulate, one might have a better basis on which to hope for sound public policy. The task of education is to contribute to policy making on issues like definition of death, natural death or living wills, durable power of attorney in health care matters, assisted suicide and euthanasia, organ and tissue donation, organ and tissue transplantation, capital punishment, and a variety of other matters. No one can expect a democratic system to function effectively when its educational underpinnings on matters such as these are inadequate.

Adult Audiences for Death Education

Kalish (1989) described four types of concern in individuals who express interest in death education:

> (1) personal concern because of some previous experience that has not been resolved; (2) personal concern because of some ongoing experience, such as the critical illness or very recent death of a close family member; (3) involvement with a relevant form of work, such as nursing, medicine, social work, the ministry, or volunteer service through a hospice organization; or (4) a wish to understand better what death means or how to cope more effectively with one's own death or the death or grief of others. (p. 75)

People with each of these types of concern can readily be identified in classes, workshops, or presentations on dying, death, and bereavement. Those who are dealing with a current death-related experience, or with the aftermath of an unresolved death-related experience, deserve special sensitivity. They may be very tender in their feelings and vulnerable to added pain. Many have chosen to come to an educational forum in order to use the information and other resources it provides in coping with their own experiences. But it is important to keep in mind the distinctions between education, support, counseling, and therapy, and to be alert to individuals who need intervention beyond education or simple support.

Two examples come to mind in this connection. The first was a young man who enrolled in our college course called "Children and Death." In introducing himself, he explained that he had been planning to marry a divorced woman who had three young sons. Unfortunately, she was killed in a motor vehicle accident before the marriage could take place. Her three boys were then returned to the custody of their natural father. Our student explained that he felt a tie to these boys and had enrolled in this course to learn how he might help them. As the course developed, however, it became clear that his own needs were also a very prominent part of his motivation. A second example was a young woman who enrolled in our college course called "Death and Dying." After the first class, she talked to the two instructors and told them that her sister's fiancé had been killed in an auto accident just 1 week earlier. We asked her to consider whether she might wish to withdraw from our class at this time. Had she selected that option, we promised to arrange for her enrollment in another term. In the end, she chose to stay in the course, but did not find that an easy decision with which to live. She managed to get through the term only because she was very determined and because she sought the help of several private conferences with the instructors, during which she was free to cry and express her grief in other ways.

Individuals who enroll in death-related educational offerings for vocational reasons usually express their desire to improve their competencies to help those whom they serve, as patients or clients. For example, it was nurses who first flocked to seminars in this field offered by Dr. Elisabeth Kübler-Ross (1969), because they knew that they needed assistance and that they would likely be the ones who would find themselves alone in the middle of the night with a dying person or calling up family members to report a death. Some who linked death education to their work speak only of what the education will mean for their clients. Others realize that it also applies to them, both as professionals in coping with their work-related responsibilities and as persons in their own right. With Kübler-Ross, death education seeks to show its relevance in all of these ways: to the client who is coping with dying or bereavement, to the helper in his or her work-related role, and to the helper as a person in his or her own right. As Shneidman (1978) noted, death-related interactions are the only ones of which it can never be said that the problem being faced by the client are not also problems to be faced by the helper.

A fourth group of people turns to death education for a different sort of reason. They do not have the immediate pressure of a past or present death-related experience, nor are they primarily associated with work-related concerns. Rather, their motivation involves curiosity about the subject, which may be combined with a desire to prepare themselves for personal experiences that might arise in the future. Sometimes people like this will say, "No one important to me in my life has yet died. But my grandparents are getting pretty old." These individuals are proactive. They prefer to act ahead of time to prepare themselves (insofar as that is possible), and not just wait until events demand a reaction. Individuals of this sort have benefited from the longer average life expectancies of recent generations, but they are sufficiently alert to realize that their advantage cannot be endless, and that no human life is completely "death free."

Conclusion

During the seventeenth century, Francis Bacon (1620/1960) described three kinds of philosophers. His description is relevant here, because he meant, by *philosopher*, a person who seeks wisdom, a combination of knowledge and practical relevance. For his model, Bacon proposed that philosophers were like ants, spiders, or bees. We can think of these images as suggesting three views of death education for adults.

Ants are empiricists who gather lots of raw materials, but often without much selectiveness and without modifying what they have gathered for constructive exploitation. The caricature of this is the idiot savant, who retains and can recall huge masses of information about some limited or arcane subject, for example, baseball batting averages. A more contemporary example is the Internet, which is full of information, but often is unclear about its soundness and/or meanings. Gathering information in death education is important, but the information must be reliable and the learner must do more than simply amass data. At best, the empiricist ant acts only to acquire information, then to produce it or repeat it back when required. But that is the end of the process. In this model, education might be described in terms of writing on a blank tablet or filling up an empty vessel. If this is so, then learners are essentially passive. As a result, their education is primarily determined by the nature of the external forces that act upon them and does not go much beyond repeating what others have told them.

According to Bacon, spiders represent philosophers of a different sort, who spin theories of marvelous ingenuity and formal perfection out of their own innards. Here, one simply offers opinions without any foundation in the external world. This reflects a popular view of philosophy as the mere dreaming up of plausible theories, but it also describes a large group of people in our society who base their attitudes on their feelings, rather than on information or evidence. Such people may act to put forward or state their views, but they are essentially uneducated, because, even when their theories are cleverly constructed, they lack effective links to the realities of life. And often they are unable to reflect critically on the strengths and weaknesses of the views they hold.

By contrast with ants and spiders, Bacon reminds us that bees both gather materials and transform them in satisfying and productive ways. Without the pollen gathered by worker bees that venture out of the hive into the countryside, there would be no honey. But, without the contribution of the bees' internal organs, even the nectar of the sweetest flower would never be transformed into honey. Humans who proceed in the manner of bees both gather data obtained through their encounters with the world, and reflect upon it in ways that convert it from a brute given to an intelligent aspect of a larger mosaic of knowledge and appreciation. Fostering this sort of process ought to be our real goal in education about dying, death, and bereavement.

In all of its many forms, death education for adults is intended to provide the materials, to suggest insights, and to guide the reflective self-understandings that help us to cope in more effective ways, as individuals, as consumers, and as citizens, with our own death, with the deaths of those close to us, and with all of the other implications of death throughout our lives. To the degree that this process is successful, our lives, our societies, and our death systems will be energized and enriched.

Discussion Questions

1. After reading this account of societal death systems, how would you characterize the effectiveness of the American death system in relationship to any specific death-related topic in which you are particularly interested?

2. This chapter's discussion indicated that there are four levels of death education for adults: cognitive, affective, behavioral, and valuational. How might these four educational levels apply to a specific death-related topic in which you are particularly interested?

3.   The discussion in this chapter identified three general types of goals in death education for adults. Have you had any prior experience with death education? If so, how did it serve any or all of these three general goals? If not, what types of goals do you think death education might serve in your own life?

4.   Following Kalish, this chapter described four types of concerns that might lead individuals to express an interest in death education. Why did you become interested in death education and how do you think it might help you?

References

Bacon, F. (1620/1960). *The new organon and related writings* (F. H. Anderson, Ed.). New York: Bobbs-Merrill.

Black, H. C. (1979). *Black's law dictionary* (5th ed.). St. Paul, MN: West.

Connor, S. R. (1998). *Hospice: Practice, pitfalls, and promise*. Bristol, PA: Taylor & Francis.

Corr, C. A. (1992). A task-based approach to coping with dying. *Omega, 24*, 81–94.

Corr, C. A. (1993). Coping with dying: Lessons that we should and should not learn from the work of Elisabeth Kübler-Ross. *Death Studies, 17*, 69–83.

Corr, C. A. (1995). Children's understandings of death: Striving to understand death. In K. J. Doka (Ed.), *Children mourning, mourning children* (pp. 3–16). Washington, DC: Hospice Foundation of America.

Corr, C. A. (1997). Children and questions about death. In S. Strack (Ed.), *Death and the quest for meaning: Essays in honor of Herman Feifel* (pp. 217–238). Northvale, NJ: Jason Aronson.

Corr, C. A., & Corr, D. M. (Eds.). (1983). *Hospice care: Principles and practice*. New York: Springer.

Corr, C. A., & Corr, D. M. (1996). *Handbook of childhood death and bereavement*. New York: Springer.

Corr, C. A., & Corr, D. M. (2003). Death and bereavement around the world: Death and bereavement in the americas. In J. D. Morgan & P. Laungani (Eds.), *Cross cultural issues in the care of the dying and the grieving* (pp. 37–55, vol. 2). Amityville, NY: Baywood.

Corr, C. A., Nabe, C. M., & Corr, D. M. (1994). A task-based approach for understanding and evaluating funeral practices. *Thanatos, 19*(2), 10–15.

Corr, C. A., Nabe, C. M., & Corr, D. M. (2003). *Death and dying, life and living* (4th ed.). Belmont, CA: Wadsworth.

Dumont, R., & Foss, D. (1972). *The American view of death: Acceptance or denial?* Cambridge, MA: Schenkman.

Evans, J. (1971). *Living with a man who is dying*. New York: Taplinger.

Feifel, H. (Ed.). (1959). *The meaning of death*. New York: McGraw-Hill.

Feifel, H. (1963). Death. In N. L. Farberow (Ed.), *Taboo topics* (pp. 8–21). New York: Atherton.

Fulton, R. (1995). The contemporary funeral: Functional or dysfunctional? In H. Wass & R. A. Neimeyer (Eds.), *Dying: Facing the facts* (3rd ed., pp. 185–209). Washington, DC: Taylor & Francis.

Gorer, G. (1965). The pornography of death. In G. Gorer, *Death, grief, and mourning* (pp. 192–199). Garden City, NY: Doubleday. (Originally in *Encounter*, Oct. 1955, 5(4), 49–52).

Haley, K., & Lee, M. (Eds.). (1998). *The Oregon Death with Dignity Act: A guidebook for health care providers*. Portland, OR: The Center for Ethics in Health Care, Oregon Health Sciences University.

Hughes, M. (1995). *Bereavement and support: Healing in a group environment*. Washington, DC: Taylor & Francis.

Johnson, J., Johnson, S. M., Cunningham, J. H., & Weinfeld, I. J. (1985). *A most important picture: A very tender manual for taking pictures of stillborn babies and infants who die*. Omaha, NE: Centering.

Kalish, R. A. (1989). Death education. In R. Kastenbaum & B. Kastenbaum (Eds.), *Encyclopedia of death* (pp. 75–79). Phoenix, AZ: Oryx.

Kastenbaum, R. (1972). On the future of death: Some images and options. *Omega, 3*, 306–318.

Kelly, O. (1975). *Make today count*. New York: Delacorte.

Klass, D. (1988). *Parental grief: Solace and resolution*. New York: Springer.

Klass, D., Silverman, P. R., & Nickman, S. L. (Eds.). (1996). *Continuing bonds: New understandings of grief*. Washington, DC: Taylor & Francis.

Kübler-Ross, E. (1969). *On death and dying*. New York: Macmillan.

Lamb, Sr. J. M. (Ed.). (1988). *Bittersweet . . . hellogoodbye: A resource in planning farewell rituals when a baby dies*. Belleville, IL: SHARE National Office.

La Rochefoucauld (1665/1868–1881). Réflexions ou sentences et maxims morales. In his *Oeuvres* (3 vols.) (D. Gilbert & J. Gourdault, Eds.). Paris: Hachette.

Lattanzi-Licht, M. E., Mahoney, J. J., & Miller, G. W. (1998). *The hospice choice: In pursuit of a peaceful death*. New York: Simon & Schuster.

McClowry, S., Davies, E. B., May, K. A., Kulenkamp, E. J., & Martinson, I. M. (1987). The empty space phenomenon: The process of grief in the bereaved family. *Death Studies, 11*, 361–374.

Nagy, M. (1948). The child's theories concerning death. *The Journal of Genetic Psychology, 73*, 3–27.

Osterweis, M., Solomon, F., & Green, M. (Eds.). (1984). *Bereavement: Reactions, consequences, and care*. Washington, DC: National Academy Press.

Pine, V. A. (1977). A socio-historical portrait of death education. *Death Education, 1*, 57–84.

Pine, V. R. (1986). The age of maturity for death education: A sociohistorical portrait of the era 1976–1985. *Death Studies, 10*, 209–231.

Plato. (1961). *The collected dialogues of Plato including the letters* (E. Hamilton & H. Cairns, Eds.). New York: Bollingen.

Shneidman, E. S. (1978). Some aspects of psychotherapy with dying persons. In C. A. Garfield (Ed.), *Psychosocial care of the dying patient* (pp. 201–218). New York: McGraw-Hill.

Wass, H., & Corr, C. A. (1984a). *Childhood and death.* Washington, DC: Hemisphere.

Wass, H., & Corr, C. A. (1984b). *Helping children cope with death: Guidelines and resources* (2nd ed.). Washington, DC: Hemisphere.

Wass, H., Corr, C. A., Pacholski, R. A., & Sanders, C. M. (1980). *Death education: An annotated resource guide.* Washington, DC: Hemisphere.

Wass, H., Corr, C. A., Pacholski, R. A., & Forfar, C. S. (1985). *Death education II: An annotated resource guide.* Washington, DC: Hemisphere.

Weisman, A. (1972). *On dying and denying: A psychiatric study of terminality.* New York: Behavioral Publications.

Four

Respecting the Spiritual Beliefs of the Dying and the Bereaved*

Thomas Attig

Thomas Attig is the author of The Heart of Grief: Death and the Search for Lasting Love *(Oxford University Press, 2000),* How We Grieve: Relearning the World *(Oxford University Press, 1996), and numerous articles and reviews on grief and loss, care of the dying, suicide intervention, death education, expert witnessing in wrongful death cases, the ethics of interactions with the dying, and the nature of applied philosophy. He spent the greater part of his career (1972–1995) as professor of philosophy at Bowling Green State University, where he served as department chair for 11 years* 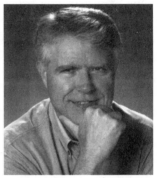 *and established the first PhD in applied philosophy in the world in 1987. A past president of the Association for Death Education and Counseling, he served as vice-chair of the board of directors of the International Work Group on Death, Dying, and Bereavement. He holds degrees in philosophy from Northwestern University (BA) and Washington University in St. Louis (MA and PhD). He currently resides in the San Francisco area and devotes his time to writing, speaking, and consulting.*

When persons are dying, grieving, or responding to others facing death, their spiritual beliefs are commonly challenged. Perhaps then, more than at any other time, they are prompted to wonder about the meanings of their lives, of the lives of those they love and care for, and of living in general. Confrontation with death casts life and its meaning in stark relief.

---

*An earlier and far less detailed treatment of this theme was published previously as "Respect for the Dying and the Bereaved as Believers" in the *Newsletter* of the Forum for Death Education and Counseling, 1983.

Persons' beliefs play an extremely important role in their spiritual lives. I have in mind beliefs about life and death, immortality, suffering, meaning and purpose, God, and the like. It is possible to ask what respect for the beliefs and for persons as believers requires, while the issue of the validity of the beliefs is held in suspension. This question of respect is my concern here, with emphasis upon respecting the dying and the bereaved. What does respect for the spiritual beliefs of persons require, when they are struggling to make sense of, and to find a way of sustaining meaning and purpose in, living in the shadow of death?

Beliefs as Worthy of Respect

First, consider why beliefs about death and dying, life and its meaning, God and immortality, are worthy of respect. By definition, beliefs that we call spiritual are those which have bearing upon persons' perceptions of the very meaning of their lives. Beliefs of such importance, understandably, are held as precious by their possessors. Minimally, respecting believers requires acknowledging the centrality of the beliefs in the persons' own self-definition and identity. Not only do persons often have firm convictions about spiritual matters, but they often think of these beliefs as defining their deepest selves. To profess "I am a Christian," "I am a Jew," or "I am Hindu" is often to speak volumes concerning perception of place and purpose in the universe, heritage, place in the community, personal integrity, orientation or posture in the face of challenge, fond hopes and aspirations, personal destiny, and so on. All of these matters are intimately related to persons' most cherished values, that is, what they care about, most fundamentally. To the extent that persons are what they care about and these beliefs importantly define what they care about, personal identity is intimately connected with personal spiritual belief.

Moreover, many derive self-esteem, both in the sense of self-confidence and in the sense of self-worth, from the understandings of themselves, their experiences, and their place in the world, which the beliefs provide. Their beliefs can be a principal source of the confidence required (a) to affirm the meaning of their lives and of living a human life in general, (b) to carry on day to day, (c) to maintain hope for the future, (d) to sustain faith in the face of adversity, and (e) to meet life's greatest challenges without despairing. When life is most difficult and the temptation to conclude that it is of little worth is the greatest, spiritual beliefs can support people in believing that individual human lives cannot be reduced to insignificance, that they can and do make a difference worth making, that the world is better for their existing, or that they have worth, even if those around them may not fully acknowledge it. Derivatively, such spiritual beliefs can and often do define fundamental life-styles, courses of purposeful action, and patterns of social interaction for individuals, within communities and throughout entire cultures.

This much, then, can be said for the value of spiritual beliefs in general. They have the power to profoundly influence and shape individual and collective life.

Beliefs as Bases for Coping

More specifically, in considering respectful response to the dying and the bereaved, spiritual concepts and beliefs constitute the principal means of their intellectual coping with reality. It is too easy to forget and underestimate the importance of the capacities of the mind and spirit to orient persons within reality and to support their discerning meanings in living within it. This may be especially so in a culture which is at least impatient with things intellectual, if not decidedly anti-intellectual. How persons think and believe decisively colors their experiences of themselves, others, and the world they share.

If people also cope emotionally, behaviorally, and socially, these other dimensions of coping are often decisively influenced by the manner of coping through believing. That is, what persons believe has great impact upon what they feel, their evaluation of their feelings, and their choices about their appropriate expression, their choices of action and reaction, and their interactions with others. There is even a developing speculative literature which suggests that there are profoundly important and too-little-understood mutual influences of beliefs and humans' organic or physical reactions to stress and crises, such as those presented by dying and bereavement (e.g., see the works of Bernie Siegel, Karl Symington, Norman Cousins, and James Lynch).

To be sure, the dimension of coping through spiritual belief, that is, struggling to understand reality and to discern meanings within it, is inappropriately isolated from emotional, behavioral, and social coping. People cope as whole persons, in all dimensions of their lives at once. An important purpose is served in focusing upon the dimension of coping through spiritual belief, to clarify and to deepen understanding of its significance, but it would be untrue to human reality to suppose that such coping is anything but intimately linked with each of the other dimensions.

One principal function of coping through belief is to help persons, through concepts and beliefs, to orient themselves to reality. Persons experience reality and their lives within it as presenting profoundly challenging questions of understanding. What is the true nature of reality? How is it organized? What are its fundamental dynamics, and what makes it change as it does? What is my place and that of my fellows within physical and spiritual reality? What kinds of creatures are we, and what differences does that fundamental human nature make? How are we to understand the peculiar mix of physical and spiritual existence that we seem to enjoy? Are we free or determined? How am I and others affected by forces beyond our control, and where, if anywhere, may we possibly have some influence? Are we alone in the universe? Is there divine influence on the course of events in reality and within our own lives? Does human life end in death or does all or part of us survive? What kind of different life, if any, might follow? Many concepts and beliefs at the heart of traditional philosophies and religions serve to enable persons to orient themselves within reality by providing answers to questions such as these.

A second principal function of coping through belief is to help persons, through their concepts and beliefs, to discern the meaning(s) of reality and of their lives within it. Questions of meaning have to do less with the shape and structure of reality and human life, and more with the sense it makes that reality and life have such shape and structure. They are questions of value and purpose, of the potential for such things as satisfaction and fulfillment, the realization of value, experienced meaningfulness, or salvation. "Why" questions of a distinct sort hold a prominent place in human wondering about meaning. Here, the question is not one of the cause, so much as the reason or purpose for that in question. In this spirit, persons have, for nearly as long as language has been recorded, wondered about such matters as: Why do we live? (What is [are] the purpose[s] of human life? What is [are] the purpose[s] of this individual human life?) Why is there suffering? (What is [are] the reason[s] for suffering for this particular suffering?) Why is there death? Why this particular death, here and now?

In coping spiritually with challenges to understanding the meaning(s) of life, people are struggling with at least these four pivotal issues, in an attempt to say "Yes" to life:

1. Is small OK? That is, how is the supposed meaningfulness of human life compatible with our being so small and insignificant on a cosmic scale, that is, with our being so tiny in a vast universe and our lives lasting so little time in universal history?

2. Is change OK? That is, how is the supposed meaningfulness of human life compatible with there seemingly being nothing permanent and lasting either in reality or in our lives?
3. Is suffering OK? That is, how is the supposed meaningfulness of human life compatible with the prevalence of suffering, because all beginnings have endings, all attachments are fleeting, and all commitments are impermanent?
4. Is uncertainty OK? That is, how is faith in the meaningfulness of living to be sustained when our grip on answers to questions such as these seems tenuous at best (if and when we have answers that are at all satisfying), that is, when our attempts to discern answers to these most pressing questions seem so clouded with uncertainty?

Such questions of meaning take on added poignancy and urgency as persons encounter death and bereavement. Again, many concepts and beliefs at the heart of traditional philosophies and religions serve to enable persons to discern the meaning(s) of reality and their lives within it, by providing answers to questions such as these.

Shneidman, in the last chapter of *Voices of Death* (1980, pp. 183–193) (and many others, in other contexts), affirms that the firmness of conviction, and not the content of conviction itself, is the most significant factor when beliefs help persons to cope either with dying or with bereavement. The key factor is that the dying or bereaved be sustained by some means or other in the conviction that the life in question (be it their own or that of one for whom they care) has meaning. Caregivers dare not underestimate the power of spiritual concepts and beliefs in addressing fundamental questions of the nature of reality and its meaning, because they serve this end. The human need here is palpable.

Respect Generally Conceived

Surely, part of respecting the spiritual beliefs of the dying and the bereaved involves cultivating a deep appreciation of the importance of the coping through spiritual belief in their lives, which has just been sketched. That is, respect for the spiritual beliefs of the dying and the bereaved requires understanding of how, in part, their thriving as the individuals they are derives from their being able to find their lives to be meaningful.

But there is more to the notion of respect than simply understanding how it is that persons thrive or flourish through belief, when they do.

Caregivers must also develop understanding of the ways in which thriving through belief can be inhibited, hindered, or undermined. In other words, such spiritual thriving is vulnerable, and caregivers must be acutely aware of that vulnerability.

Spiritual thriving can be adversely affected simply by the introduction of crisis events, such as dying and bereavement, into otherwise relatively untroubled living. With physical debilitation and enervation, disruption of daily routine, interruption of normal patterns of interaction with others, and the like, come stresses that test persons' capacities to maintain satisfying life-styles, to remain engaged in meaningful activities and projects, to uphold fulfilling relationships, and to sustain faith and confidence that life is meaningful and worth living.

Moreover, the foregoing sections suggest that one of the major tasks confronting the dying and the bereaved is that of coming to terms with, or making sense of, both the event of death itself and living in the shadow of the event, that is, of thinking it through. If this is so, then the dying and bereaved are vulnerable to underappreciation of the significance of that task and to compromise of their motivation to address it.

But, surely, respecting persons (as spiritual believers or otherwise) is not simply a matter of understanding or appreciating something about them, even something as important as how they can thrive and how that thriving can be undermined. Rather, respect involves acting in the light of such understanding, that is, translating such understanding into respectful response and behavior. The actions or omissions of caregivers themselves can affect significantly the spiritual thriving, through belief of those for whom they care. Minimally, respect requires that caregivers not interfere in the spiritual thriving of others, and that they not exacerbate their vulnerability. A higher order of respect involves caregivers in finding ways to actively support, sustain, or facilitate spiritual thriving, and to effectively and sensitively minimize that vulnerability.

The dying and the bereaved can experience considerable disorientation and confusion, and caregivers can cultivate abilities to support and promote their coming to understand the dimensions of spiritual belief of their experiences and coping needs. They can learn means of helping them to sustain the motivation to meet the challenges to their beliefs. They can develop skills for supporting them in choosing alternative means of meeting these challenges and in acting on those choices. Finally, they can cultivate sensitivity and abilities to respond flexibly to the spiritual individuality of those in their care.

Specific Dimensions of Respect

The spiritual thriving of the dying and the bereaved may be hindered by intolerance or even proselytizing by caregivers. When beliefs matter as much as spiritual beliefs do, and in particular beliefs about life, death, and suffering and their meaning, possibly dogmatism and defensiveness will take root and flourish. Where they do flourish, tolerance for, much less appreciation of the sustaining power of, alternative beliefs is not likely. If deathbed conversions are rare, especially where there is already firm conviction in place, and if firmness of conviction is crucial for spiritual thriving in such circumstances, then tolerance of alternative beliefs is essential, if that thriving is not to be thwarted.

Caregivers, too, are struggling to come to terms with, and to make sense of, the deaths and suffering in the lives of those for whom they care. They are also affected by those deaths, albeit not, in most cases, as powerfully as immediate family and close friends. As with anyone who is confronting death, dying, and suffering, caregivers can find it disturbing to discover that they, too, are intellectually and spiritually challenged in the midst of circumstances, when supposedly, they have been prepared to function in a fully professional manner. They, too, rely upon concepts and beliefs to orient and sustain them. It can be especially challenging for them to resist the tendencies toward dogmatism and defensiveness in themselves, which derive from their own intellectual and spiritual needs and vulnerability. Recognizing that they may be tempted by such tendencies may well be a key to their avoiding the further temptations of intolerance or proselytizing, when they find that their views differ from those of the persons in their care.

There is an unfortunate tendency concerning beliefs about life, death, and suffering and their meanings. The tendency is to confuse believing with knowing. While not underestimating the importance of beliefs in the lives of individual believers, one must be ever aware of the difference between conviction (however firm) and knowledge. Caregiver pretension to knowing here is especially dangerous. Humility is crucial as a firm base for the tolerance that is required.

In attending to the needs of the dying and the bereaved as spiritual believers, respect would come easier if all involved could remember that, in coming to terms with death, we are interpreting mysteries and not simply solving problems. When confronting ultimate human limitation, it is salutary to remember the words of John Stuart Mill:

Human existence is girt round with mystery: the narrow region of our existence is a small island in the midst of a boundless sea. To add to the mystery, the domain of our earthly existence is not only an island in infinite space, but also in infinite time. The past and the future are alike shrouded from us: we neither know the origin of anything which is, nor its final destination. (Mill, 1874/1969)

The distinction between mysteries and problems is most useful here. Problems are, by definition, the kinds of challenges that cry for and often yield to definitive solution. When confronted with problems, persons seek solutions that will transform the reality, which is problematic, typically through decisive action. Mysteries, by contrast, do not yield. Rather, mysteries pervade the reality with which we must come to terms. The mysterious dimensions of reality transcend both our conceptual grasp and our control. Yet, they command our attention and compel us to respond. However, our responses are not comprised of reality-transforming actions. Rather, the mysteries remain as factors defining the human condition, and, instead, we transform ourselves as we come to terms and attempt to make sense of them. In response, we transform elements of our perspective, understanding, and life pattern.

Definitive answers to the most important questions of life, death, and their meanings are beyond our grasp. Questions of the meanings of life, death, and suffering are questions about centrally important mysteries of life. Objective certainty is simply unattainable here. Acceptable answers to these mysteries are elusive and our hold upon them tentative, at best. Yet many, if not most, are moved to continue the quest for answers that orient them within reality and sustain coping with such mysteries. Caregiver appreciation of this aspect of the human condition, that is, that we are together challenged by life's fundamental mysteries, can serve to promote the humility and tolerance required, if the alternative perspectives and beliefs of those in their care are to be respected.

In the dimension of spiritual belief, as in the other dimensions of their experiences, the dying and bereaved are vulnerable to influences that encourage passivity and helplessness. Davidson has identified a pattern in caregiving that tends to have just such an effect, which he terms "the surrogate suffering syndrome" (1980). This syndrome is a pervasive pattern in caregiving among professionals and nonprofessionals alike. It encompasses all attempts to shield persons subject to care from painful or otherwise difficult experiences. The idea is to bear the burden for the cared-for person, whether that person is a friend, relative, or someone for whom one has professional responsibility. It is an attempt to run interference on pain. It is a well-intentioned strategy for caregiving. Tragically, as with many other well-intentioned modes of interaction, the intention is seldom realized. Indeed, there is room to doubt whether it could ever be realized. Can one person cry the tears of another? Can one person face the mortality of another? Can one person do the grief work for another?

Caregivers must realize that they can no more carry the burdens of coping, through belief, for those in their care than they can carry the physical, emotional, or social burden. The dying and the bereaved themselves face the challenges of coming to terms with and making sense of the challenging events in their lives. At most, helping here can take the form of supporting persons in finding or sustaining confidence in answers and beliefs that they find to be functional.

A case study well illustrates this point. In his well-known film entitled *Death of the Wished-For Child* (1980), Davidson focuses upon the experiences of a young woman whose child dies within hours after birth. She is on the receiving end of every form of surrogate-suffering-style caregiving imaginable, as caregivers attempt to spare her meeting the difficult challenges. Little noticed is the repetition of the pattern in others' responses to her exploring questions of the meaning of the event in her life. At one point, she recounts a scene in her hospital room. In the presence of her friend, a minister offers a "10-minute sermon" on why she should not be asking the "Why?" questions she is asking, since failing to find definitive answers will only be frustrating. When the minister leaves, her friend offers a counter-sermon on the importance of her continuing to question, and urges acceptance of a particular answer having to do with the supposed connection of the inadequacy of her faith and that of her husband with the death of her child. The exchanges left her angry and frustrated, with her questions yet unanswered.

Clearly, part of what is happening here is both the minister and her friend are attempting to spare her the difficulty of coping in her own way with the challenges to her spiritual beliefs by the death. Also clear is the futility of any such attempts to spiritually cope for another. Each must find his or her own path, and any helping efforts provided by others can only be helpful if they encourage and support the first-person exploration of the issues by those they hope to help.

There may be potentially inhibiting factors blocking the full and meaningful expression of spiritual values or exploration of spiritually pressing questions, in medical and social contexts. In some circumstances, access to spiritual leaders and counselors is limited or restricted, or access to spiritual community is compromised. In others, for example, in an intensive care unit, space and privacy are limited. In others, medical procedures, including the use of drugs or apparatus, undermine lucidity or inhibit full expression. In still others, exploration of spiritual territory that is perceived to be too painful or stressful is discouraged by other persons, for example, family members. In all of these cases (and others like them), the respectful caregiver can at least minimize the hindrances and perhaps take positive steps to circumvent or overcome the obstacles to spiritual functioning, for example, by providing access to spiritual guides or community members, encouraging delays or relocation of ritual events to make participation possible, making space available, promoting at least temporary lucidity, compensating for reduced expressive functioning, or encouraging exploration of difficult questions.

In some instances, full spiritual thriving is blocked by underappreciation, by the believers themselves, of the value and power of the beliefs in question. Persons often have firm convictions without fully comprehending the range of implications and applications of their belief. That is, they sometimes do not see how their beliefs speak to their current circumstances. Here, it is probably vital that the dying or bereaved be placed in the hands of one who is skilled in helping them to see the connections, so that they may derive from their beliefs the sustaining power within them. Priests, rabbis, ministers, chaplains, lay ministers, and so on should be among those most adept at doing at least this much, even without extensive training in pastoral counseling.

I am confident that, when properly interpreted, all of the major religious traditions speak powerfully to the questions of the sustainability of confidence in the meaningfulness of life in spite of profound human limitation. The path to salvation that each defines marks the way to gentle but firm affirmation of meaningful life and the ultimate acceptability of our lives being small and insignificant and pervaded with change, suffering, vulnerability, and uncertainty.

People may come to experience dying or bereavement with no previously held firm convictions on spiritual matters. If Shneidman is correct, such a lack of conviction can be one of the most disturbing factors in such persons' experiences (1980). What is a respectful response if one is concerned about the confusion and distress so often apparent or expressed? Again, imposition of the beliefs of the caregiver is just that: an imposition. Instead, encouraging and supporting exploration of spiritual issues of meaning, in an effort to help the persons to discover or develop for themselves sustaining convictions that are congruent with their values and life patterns, is more respectful.

The convictions that matter most at the times in question are convictions concerning the meaningfulness of lives lived and now ending or ended, and of lives that now must be lived following significant loss. The variety of beliefs that can be sustaining here should not be conceived too narrowly. For some, to be sure, the conviction will take root in traditional religious doctrine, be it theistic or nontheistic. For some, however, the conviction that life is meaningful may derive from less formal or creedal sources.

Victor Frankl, in *Man's Search for Meaning* (1984), has suggested that persons can derive conviction of the meaningfulness of life from (a) creative or productive activity that gives them a sense of contributing to others and the world around them, (b) experiences that they find to be meaningful in themselves, including especially the experiences of loving and being loved, as well as such things as aesthetic and other pleasures and satisfactions, the experience of communing with nature, and encounters in reverence with the divine, and (c) experiences of penetrating their own suffering with meaning other than being overwhelmed or defeated by it. All of these sources of meaning can potentially be supported to some degree in the lives of both the dying and the bereaved.

Robert Lifton has urged, in *The Broken Connection* (1983), that persons derive a sense of meaningfulness in their lives from beliefs that their lives are connected with something that is transcending. Although some sources for such conviction are traditionally religious, some are not. Sources of such conviction can, according to Lifton, derive from perceived connectedness with a life to follow (literal immortality in various forms), or through such means to symbolic immortality as living on through one's works, in the memories of others, through the ongoing life of one's people, and the like.

Again, Shneidman, in his *Voices of Death*, prompts reflection on these matters through recounting the story of a young Russian woman, Marie Bashkirtseff, who died in nineteenth-century Paris, leaving the following remark in her diary:

> This is the thought that has always terrified me: to live, to be so filled with ambition, to suffer, to weep, to struggle, and, at the end, oblivion! as if I had never existed. (p. 5)

Clearly, Frankl, in writing of making a contribution; Lifton, in writing of symbolic immortality; and this young woman, are all underscoring the potential of deriving a sense of meaningfulness in life from a belief that one's life has made a nontrivial difference, that the world is somehow a better place for one's having been here, or at least that all of the effort and struggles do not come to nothing when death comes.

Such differences as one might make and take satisfaction in need not be earthshaking. Part of accepting the human condition, and affirming life and its meaningfulness, may entail accepting the idea that few if any make differences noticed by all. Rather, we all have opportunity to make differences where we are with what resources we have. Such differences can be known and appreciated by a few or even many, and faith in having made a difference can be sustained, even if not all who have been touched by a life acknowledge such differences. Some may be content with having made a difference in the lives of family, friends, and peers, and may be convinced that that difference will continue to matter to their survivors, even after death.

Having said this much about the kinds of convictions that people might find sustaining, what kind of respectful response to the dying and bereaved might be in order? First, remember that not all will find traditional religious doctrine to be attractive, even when issues of the meaningfulness of their lives seen unaddressed. To be sure, offering to bring the dying or the bereaved into contact with representatives of various religious orders may be appropriate and effective. However, should such offers be declined, there are other options yet available, if distress about such spiritual matters persists. Life review is common among the dying and the bereaved. Reviewing lives to discern the presence of meaningful contributions, legacies given and embraced, differences made, rewarding experiences, rewarding relationships with others, overcomings of tragedy, and so on can encourage and support a sense of meaningfulness. Assurances can be given that the dying will not be lost in oblivion, that the differences they have made will be remembered and appreciated after they have gone. Helping persons to renew, deepen, and maintain connections with others, and to address unfinished business within relationships or in projects of significance to them can be very sustaining. Addressing issues of guilt and forgiveness (including self-forgiveness) may well be an important part of this process. Helping the bereaved to learn to sustain a loving relationship with those who have died can speak to this same spiritual need (see Attig, T. (2000). *The Heart of Grief: Death and the Search for Lasting Love*. New York: Oxford University Press).

Thriving through spiritual belief may also be blocked by the presence of dominating emotions, such as anger or guilt, which may in fact be deeply rooted in the beliefs of the dying or the bereaved. That is, the emotions may be so controlling in the situation that exploration of the underlying spiritual values and questions may be inhibited or stifled. For example, a person may be angry at God for what is believed to be an unfair or unjust death, or another might feel guilty based upon a belief in God as punishing for some unknown but presumably justified reason. In order to facilitate spiritual thriving in such cases, a skilled counselor must overcome the resistance that allows the emotions to dominate, and gently but firmly invite, encourage, and support exploration of the validity of the beliefs which are the basis of the emotions.

Perhaps the circumstances within which it is most difficult to define a respectful response are those in which the dying or the bereaved have firm convictions that are clearly dysfunctional. That is, quite possibly, beliefs themselves may impoverish the lives of believers, compromise or deaden their appreciation of the value and meaning of living, and ultimately undermine or inhibit their thriving as individuals and in their relation with others.

In such cases, respect requires extreme caution about judgment that the firmly held conviction is in fact dysfunctional. Such judgment is not to be confused with or supplanted by a judgment (a) that the belief "could not possibly be functional," simply because it is different from the belief of the caregiver, or (b) that the belief is serving a function that the caregiver finds undesirable, unpalatable, or the like.

Rather, the judgment that the belief is dysfunctional must be based on caregiver perception that the belief is in fact contributing to the disorientation of the person, or is clearly undermining the person's own sense of meaningfulness in the experience. For example, a person may believe that a sufficiently strong faith will reverse the inevitability of a loved one's death. Or, a person may be convinced that he or she is responsible for the death of another from cancer, simply by virtue of a moral failing, and the person may be driven toward suicide by this guilt. In these cases, unrealistic or meaning-destroying beliefs are dominant, human suffering is compounded, and such persons are headed for disaster.

Here, it is good to remember that conviction, no matter how firm, neither changes the fundamental contours of reality and the human condition nor provides believers with immunity from suffering or death. At best, it supplies means of coping with or living in the face of death and suffering. This was as much true for the founders of the great religions as it is for followers among the dying and bereaved today.

When dysfunctional beliefs are present, respect for the believer requires recognition of the dysfunctional character of the belief and the courage to intervene caringly in the name of the person's own thriving. Again, imposition of alternative beliefs is inappropriate. Yet, encouragement of exploration of alternative interpretations of the beliefs in question or of alternative beliefs that are compatible with the person's values and life patterns is appropriate and respectful. For example, the caregiver may invite a religious believer to examine how the central figures in the great religions themselves found faith to be sustaining in their own encounters with death and suffering. A most compelling and powerful instance of this in interaction with Christians, for example, could be exploration of the story of the passion of Jesus, in which he confronted the prospect of dying, asked that his friends be close by, experienced and expressed fear, sorrow, and grief, and yet found his faith to be sustaining. The literatures of the great religions are filled with comparable and compelling accounts of central figures wrestling with issues of the compatibility of human limitation and finiteness and the meaningfulness of human life. Exploration of such texts and spiritual counseling can help the dying and the bereaved to consider how the meaningfulness of lives now ending or ended, or yet to be lived by survivors, is not nullified or cancelled by death.

Yet another fruitful approach might be to respectfully and sensitively explore and address the underlying emotions at the base of the believer's seemingly desperate attempt to control or manipulate reality with faith. Clearly, part of what seems so distressing in the typical case is the feeling of helplessness and powerlessness in the face of a reality or chain of events over which one has little or no influence. This helplessness and powerlessness, as well as feelings such as fear, anxiety, despair, extreme sadness, abandonment, or guilt, may well be present. Inviting expression of such feelings can be a vital first step. Helping persons to find things to do and say, short of changing the realities of death and inevitable loss, may address the feelings and to some extent dissipate the felt need to magically manipulate the world through controlling belief.

These reflections on respect for the spiritual beliefs of the dying and the bereaved are neither exhaustive nor definitive. Rather, they provide a framework for understanding respect for spiritual belief in the most general terms and for beginning thoughts on specific ways of supporting and respecting the dying and the bereaved in their spiritual thriving and vulnerability in the shadow of death.

Note that these reflections focus upon only one central dimension of the spirituality of the dying and the bereaved. Spirituality is not simply a matter of belief about the mysteries that pervade the human condition. Yes, faith can sustain our thriving as we confront such mysteries, and we are vulnerable in our faith in ways I have described. But spirituality also encompasses such things as resilience, perseverance, courage, hope, and joy. These, too, can support our thriving as we face life's most profound mysteries and challenges. And we are vulnerable in each of them in ways

I have not described here. A comprehensive treatment of respecting and supporting the fullness of the spirituality of the dying and the bereaved would also cover these topics (see Attig, 2000, pp. 245–279).

Discussion Questions

1. What are the three defining features of respect for the spiritual beliefs of the dying and the bereaved?
2. What are some special challenges presented by those who have clearly dysfunctional spiritual beliefs and the means of responding respectfully to them?

References

Davidson, G. (Director). (1980). *Death of the wished-for child* [motion picture]. Available from The Order of the Golden Rule, Springfield, IL.

Frankl, V. E. (1984). *Man's search for meaning* (3rd. ed). New York: Simon and Schuster.

Lifton, R. J. (1983). *The broken connection: On death and the continuity of life.* New York: Basic Books.

Mill, J. S. (1969). *Three essays on religion.* New York: Greenwood Press.

Shneidman, E. (1980). *Voices of death.* New York: Harper & Row.

Part Two

The Challenge of Dying

The Struggle to End My Father's Life

Zelda Foster

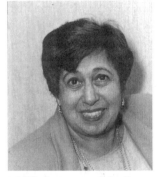

Zelda Foster, MSW, is the former director of a large social work department at the Brooklyn Veterans Affairs Medical Center. She is a cofounder and first president of the New York State Hospice Association. As a young worker in 1965, she wrote a seminal article dealing with the conspiracy of silence facing dying patients.

A graduate of Brooklyn College and the Columbia University School of Social Work, Zelda Foster has written and taught extensively on psychosocial issues. She is currently on the faculty of both the Shirley M. Ehrenkranz School of Social Work at New York University and the Smith College School of Social Work, as part of the Soros Foundation Project on Death in America grants. She is a fellow of the New York Academy of Medicine and participates in the American Red Cross disaster mental health services. She co-edited, with Inge Corless, The Hospice Heritage: Celebrating Our Future.

This could not be happening to me. All the paths taken in my adult life led me toward a different direction. It was so clear and all of it had fallen in place, up until now. I clutched my father's health care proxy in my hand as I stood in a city hospital emergency room beseeching the hospital administrator to allow the withdrawal of my father's life supports. The events of the weekend grew more unreal with each passing obstacle and dehumanization. I, a cofounder of the New York State Hospice Association, the chair of a hospital task force on the withholding and withdrawal of life-sustaining treatment, and proponent of more rational decisions regarding medical futility, stood there helpless and trapped in a bureaucratic maze of indifference.

It began on Friday night, November 5th, when my 90-year-old mother phoned for us to drive right over. My father wasn't right. I dressed quickly. As we drove on rain-slicked streets further hampered by a car accident ahead, creating delays, I felt dread. My father was 93. I knew that one day a phone call would signal his death. As my husband and I raced into the house, we found my mother sobbing, bent over him. My first thought was what a good death this was. He hadn't really been ill, only somewhat symptomatic for 2 weeks. What an easy death in his bed alongside his beloved wife of 67 years. I felt his face. He was so warm, so alive. The words crept out, words I'll always regret: "Call an ambulance." They came and they did what they were trained to do. They resuscitated him for more than 1 hour after he stopped breathing, then took him to the closest city hospital. As the four men and one woman worked over him, as the two policemen stood by, I wondered how I was going to stop what had been placed in motion.

My sister and her husband arrived. My daughter came to stay with my mother. We raced to the emergency room, and waited interminably in a room, demanding over and over that we be permitted to see my father and to speak to a physician. Finally, my sister and I were allowed in, but not the sons-in-law who had each loved my father for more than 30 years. My sister and I saw my father attached to machines and were told by the nurse that there was minimal brain function. We told her we had a health care proxy. We asked to see a physician. The physician who had examined him was no longer there. When the staff heard that we wanted to sign a do not resuscitate (DNR) order, a physician was called. This would mean that if my father's heart stopped beating again, resuscitation would not take place. The physician came after another delay, barely spoke to us, and gave us the paper to sign. We were pushed out of the emergency room after only several moments with our father, with no opportunities for us or our husbands to begin saying our goodbyes to him. How could we, his daughters, be unable to protect and safeguard him as his mind and spirit left his vacant, devoid-of-personhood body. What disrespect to force that body to breathe!

We had become our parents' caregivers, almost imperceptibly at first, then incrementally and more apparent to them than to us. These proud, immigrant parents who had devoted their lives and hopes to us became less able with time. They struggled to remain independent, and in fact, as grandparents and great grandparents, they succeeded in maintaining a caring, giving role. How he would have despised this indignity, this mindless invasion.

The emergency room administrator on duty officiously told us that treatment could not be withdrawn once started. I wanted to scream out, "Haven't you heard of the New York State Health Care Proxy Law or the Federal Self-Determination Act?" I knew there would be no way of convincing him that there was no distinction between withholding and withdrawing treatment, or that my father's health care proxy allowed us to decide on his behalf. We left at 3 a.m., deciding to return Saturday morning to see the daytime administrator. We were certain that if reason did not prevail, at least the law would. How could a New York City hospital in 1993 not obey the law? Could our father's and our rights to protect his wishes be abrogated?

We learned that yes—yes, yes, yes—they could be abrogated. Obstacle after obstacle was placed in our way. The daytime emergency room administrator sent us to the day hospital administrator. She told us that, since my mother was listed as the first proxy and the daughters as the second, we needed to prove that she was unable or unwilling to serve in that role. This felt manageable. We contacted her two geriatricians, each located at major teaching hospitals in New York City. Both called the hospital and were told they needed to put their statements regarding my mother's incapacity in writing and mail it. How absurd when one imagines the number of days that would take. Instead, I went to Manhattan to pick up one letter and brought it to a now-evening administrator.

Further obstacles were presented. An attending physician was required and none were available until Monday. This led to further endeavors on Sunday morning, but we were told by the daytime administrator after her consultation with the hospital CEO that the proxy allowed the withdrawal of only nutrition and hydration, not other life-sustaining treatment. Our explanation, that New York State law requires a separate statement regarding nutrition and hydration, and that statement was only an added proviso, not a provision standing alone, fell on deaf ears. No explanation helped. We were dealing not only with ignorance, but also with an impenetrable bureaucratic wall.

My mother only understood that my father was dead. She saw him die. There was no way she could comprehend that a machine was forcing breath. She kept asking when was the funeral, expecting it immediately, in keeping with Jewish tradition.

By Sunday afternoon, we felt desperate and began enlisting legal help. We contacted several of my daughter's law professors. I prepared a letter outlining each obstacle we had encountered. On Monday morning, at the hospital where I work, colleagues armed phones and a fax machine. We faxed my letter to Brooklyn Legal Services, where an attorney was waiting to receive it.

Brooklyn, NY
11:00 p.m., Sunday, November 7, 1993

Ms. Lauren Shapiro, Esq.
Ms. Cynthia Schneider, Esq.
Brooklyn Legal Services
105 Court Street
Brooklyn, NY 11201

Dear Ms. Schneider and Ms. Shapiro:

This letter is written to provide clear evidence of a grievous abridgement of the Federal Patient Self-Determination Act, and to express anguish created by this injurious disregard of our rights.

At this time, my father, who is 93 years old, continues to be maintained, at _____ Hospital, on a respirator, despite my continued and clear demand, acting under a proxy in his behalf according to his wishes, that he be disconnected. _____ Hospital's latest refusal, in a continuing series of changing reasons for denial, is the negation of our New York State proxy, which was executed by an attorney and indicated agreement by my father to the cessation of life support as well as nutrition and hydration in the event that he was incapacitated. _____ Hospital's insistence that there is only agreement stated in the proxy to withdrawal of hydration and nutrition, not life-sustaining treatment, thwarts my father's wishes and is patently ignorant of New York State law regarding this proxy. The attached proxy refers to nutrition and hydration only as an explicit *added proviso as per state law.* _____ *Hospital's demand that I seek a court order is a total abrogation of the intent of a health care proxy, which has as its purpose the avoidance of the need for a court order and the protection of patient rights.*

This information and hospital decisions were imparted to me November 7, 1993, at about 8 a.m. by the weekend hospital administrator, a Ms. T, who presumably was advised by the hospital CEO. The above decision was the last made by _____ Hospital in what has been a series of evolving obstacles and objections raised since Friday night, November 5, 1993, when my father was taken by EMS ambulance to the emergency room at approximately 11:30 p.m.

This is the sequence of events that has transpired until now, along with the names of hospital personnel and their decisions:

1. My father experienced a cardiac arrest in his home, late Friday evening, November 5, 1993. EMS was called, and was able to resuscitate him using CPR. He was then taken by ambulance to hospital.

2. The family—me, my sister, my husband, and my sister's husband—were not allowed to see my father, and no one was available to talk to us for around an hour. After many demands, we were able to view him and talk to the nurse caring for him. When she explained that he was not conscious or responsive, we asked to speak with the doctor who had initially seen him,

to execute a DNR and have my father removed from the respirator. We had left the proxy home in haste and were willing to get it.

We were told that this initial doctor was unavailable, and we never got to speak to him. A new physician was paged. After that doctor arrived, the ER administrator, who was then present, told us officiously that one can withhold life-sustaining treatment, but not withdraw it. The doctor said that was not so, but the administrator was disbelieving. We agreed to return the next morning with my father's health care proxy.

3. We returned the next morning, Saturday, November 6, 1993, at about 8 a.m. An ER coordinator, although pleasant, had no sense of patient rights proxy procedures and process. She advised us to speak to Ms. T.

4. We contacted Ms. T. a short time later by phone from home. Ms. T. advised us that, since my mother's name (she is 90 years old) was listed first and mine second on the proxy, we had to prove that my mother was not competent to act on this proxy, and that a physician would have to state this to Ms. T. by phone.

5. With great difficulty, two physicians, Dr. F from NYU Medical Center and Dr. L from Long Island Jewish Hospital, who had treated my mother, were located early that afternoon. Both called Ms. T, stating that my mother was not able to act on the proxy. Ms. T then advised them that they would have to put this in writing and mail it. Dr. F of NYU's geriatric practice wrote a letter, which my husband drove from Brooklyn to NYU to pick up in the late afternoon, then brought to _____ Hospital about 7:00 p.m. Saturday night.

6. On arriving, we contacted Mr. A, the evening administrator, who, upon receipt of this letter, advised me, my sister, and my husband that only an attending MD could disconnect the respirator, and no attending was available. We demanded that an attending be contacted and brought in to meet our right to not have life-prolonging treatment, and to allow our father to die with dignity. He agreed to do the best he could to meet our request.

7. At about 8 a.m. on Sunday morning, November 7, 1993, I phoned Ms. T to ask if an attending was contacted. It was then that she told me that she had been advised by the hospital CEO that our proxy was not satisfactory, despite the fact that it was drawn up and executed by a lawyer and met the terms of New York State law. She advised that the CEO insisted that we seek a court order.

The Hospital has created one obstacle after another to challenge our rightful request that our father be allowed to die with dignity. It has, in doing so, caused an abridgement of our rights to carry out our father's wishes and has cost us such considerable pain and anguish that we seek immediate relief and additionally the censure of the Hospital.

Sincerely,

ZELDA FOSTER

Attachments:
Proxy
Dr. F's letter

I and a group of colleagues gathered together using several phones. We contacted Choices for Dying, where we had an attorney who was ready to receive our letter. We called the State Department of Health's local office, only to be told by their complaint division that one cannot withdraw treatment with a heath care proxy. I called the Albany office, who had corroborated that this, of course, was erroneous. A physician colleague sat with us, waiting to see what further impediments might be thrown in our path. Finally, a call came from the hospital's patient representative. The calls from our lawyers and the New York State Department of Health had pressed the right buttons. I was asked how physicians in New York City could state that my mother was unable to act as proxy as she was in a nursing home in Florida. What total negligence! No one had said that my mother was in Florida. In fact, if she were, would this have indeed made her unable to act as a proxy? Finally, he (the patient representative) decided to call my mother and ask her if she was unwilling to act as a proxy. How is a person, judged by two physicians to be unable to act as proxy, placed in a position to receive a phone call she could not possibly comprehend? We allowed him to call, knowing that my aunt would receive the call and respond by stating that he was to deal with the daughters.

A call came soon after from a physician asking if I would like to be present when the life supports were removed. My daughter, a friend, and I drove to the hospital. In the gentle care of two physicians who extended much warmth to us, my father within moments slipped into death.

I will always associate his death with these events. The days we needed to grieve were taken from us as we struggled with an indifferent and incompetent system. The nightmare of helplessness and dehumanization stays with me. Certainly, my knowledge and power did eventually result in a response, but how hard it was to effect it. I think of others less knowledgeable, not well-connected, and know that they would have no guidance and advocate. Because of this, I wrote many letters, including official complaints to appropriate state and city departments, to the Task Force on Life and the Law, and to the Health Care Financing Administration. Certain agencies seem to bear no responsibility, politely offer tokens of apology, perhaps excuses, or agree to respond at a later date. So far, there has been only recognition that the hospital's weekend procedures needed improvement. Apparently its ethics committee made recommendations. How I would have liked to be at that meeting, but, after all, I am only the person whose rights and whose grievous loss was unacknowledged. No one addressed the emergency room procedures that allowed indifference, inhumanity, and plain crude displays of incivility.

As we consider the gravity of the Federal Patient Self-Determination Act and State proxy laws with respect to patient rights, we must be more vigilant. Rights are not assured in the absence of humane, responsive environments. Procedures have value, but the essential value is in the connection between people in a helping system of care. Unembraced by respect and concern, I said my first good-byes to my father among strangers.

Perhaps this experience will serve us well in the future. If it happened to me, it could certainly happen to any of us. This tells me that the direction I have taken almost all of my adult life with regard to death with dignity has total meaning and value. As a social work leader, I have helped instill this in others. Only I know now, in the most personal way, that we must press on. The struggle and our firm determination must and will continue.

Discussion Questions

1. How would you develop, in your setting, an approach that would ensure fuller participation of patients, families, and surrogates in completing an advance directive?

2. What would you establish in your setting to enable health care staff and colleagues to provide leadership for patients, families, and surrogates in end-of-life care planning throughout the course of a serious illness or decline?

Five

Dying in the Hospital

Patrice O'Connor

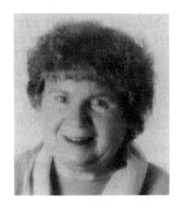

Patrice O'Connor has been an administrator in the Hospice and Palliative Care field for twenty years. She has lectured nationally and internationally and published on spiritual care, administration of hospital-based hospice/palliative care programs, patient's last hours, and dying in the hospital setting. Ms. O'Connor is currently a palliative care consultant.

> There is a season for everything, a time for every occupation under heaven.
> (Ecc. 3:1–3, *Jerusalem Bible*)

> It's not that I'm afraid to die; I just don't want to be there when it happens.
> (Allen, 1972, p. 106)

That we will all die is a fact of life. How, when, and where this event will happen is more of an uncertainty, but, clearly, the where is the most predictable. According to the Office of Technology Assessment Task Force Report of 1998, 80% of the 2 million Americans who die each year do so in hospitals (Hogan et al., 2000). The shift of place of death from home to medical setting is a result of the advances in medical care and the philosophy of doing all that is medically possible to prolong life. Denial of the event of death has been facilitated by scientific developments and a sense that death is a failure by caregivers. Death is no longer a family event, even though most people express the desire to die at home (Foley, 1996).

The question then arises, how equipped are hospitals to handle the processes of death and dying? What are the obligations of the medical personnel to patients, families, and themselves, in meeting needs of the dying in these institutions? Has education for the professional addressed these critical issues of caring for the dying patient and his or her family?

These questions, along with the shrinking health care dollar, evoke concerns in the ethical, legal, and moral arenas about such issues as do not resuscitate orders, living wills, and the "right to die." Humanistic responses have not kept pace with the rapid technological developments, creating some very difficult death-related issues. With medical technology, the body can be kept alive, but what about the quality of life? How many times can a body "die," then be restored, to be maintained by machines? Who defines life? Do the wishes of patient, family, or hospital prevail? If there is conflict in life and death decisions, what once were medical decisions become legal events, and are now settled in the courts. The meeting of all these forces has made this a challenging time in health care (Corr, 1999).

Place of Death

With the increase in proportion of deaths that occur in hospitals, there has been an increasing debate about appropriateness of the place of death. Death, in the opinion of many, should be a family affair and occur at home. It is increasingly institutionalized and hidden from public view. As people become less familiar with the process of death, they may increasingly assume that terminally ill patients receive better care in the hospital. However, this need not be the case. Most people want to die at home, but do not do so for social, rather than medical, reasons (Gilbar & Steiner, 1996).

Society is being challenged to change in order to meet the needs of a population in which the elderly are the fastest growing segment, and in which medical technology has made it more difficult for patients to die. The increase in the number of people with AIDS, the increase in the elderly population, and the Gross National Product of health care costs at 12%, raises the question of just how much can be spent on health care, let alone on care of the dying (Christakis, 2000; Emanuel & Emanuel, 1998).

Callahan has raised difficult questions concerning the medical goals in our aging society (Callahan, 1990). In particular, he examined the issue of resources being spent on the elderly, and therefore being unavailable for future generations. As an example, he compared the expenses of high-technology care for an elderly terminal patient and the limited resources allocated for prenatal care. Callahan continued his argument, offering an alternative that makes care rather than cure our societal priority (Hastings Center, 1995).

Legal Influences on Care

Increasingly, the legal system is becoming a part of the debate. Cases such as that of Nancy Cruzan have assisted in determining the rights of patients and families to influence health care delivery in certain illness situations (*Cruzan v. Director*, 1990). Still, no matter what the courts rule, and despite all the changes in medicine, the place where doctors and patients with families will struggle with the right to die and chance to live will remain rather simple and familiar—the patient's room, doctor's office, solarium, or hallway of the hospital. Family conferences are one of the most powerful tools for assisting patients' families and caregivers with understanding the concerns of all involved. As a forum for educating patients and their families, the conference can furnish reliable, accurate medical information, set realistic and reasonable expectations, clarify health care choices, and provide instructions for treatment and caregiving from the professional caregiver (American College of Physicians, 1998).

Reporting of such a conference, in the chart, would have prevented the candid tale of a mercy killing reported by a young doctor, called at 3 a.m. to see a patient he did not know, who was dying of ovarian cancer. After he assessed the situation, he proceeded to give her an injection of morphine sulfate, which depressed her respiratory center, and she died. This story might have had a different ending if a family conference had been held earlier, with staff who knew her and her family. With reporting of the conference in the chart including details of the discussion and decisions made during the conference as well as the role of palliative care, a more peaceful experience in living and dying would have occurred for the patient and the young doctor (Young, 1988; Jacobson, Francis, & Battin, 1997).

One issue that is mandated as part of hospital policy is obtaining the wishes of patients and families about resuscitation. Each patient, at the time of admission, is required to indicate his or her choice if emergency resuscitation becomes necessary. Personnel (admission clerks, medical students, nurses, resident, or attending physicians) who discuss this issue with patients vary from institution to institution, and have varied backgrounds, skills, and expertise. The response of the patient is likely to be influenced by the manner in which it is presented, and by whom. Patients have expressed the fear that, if they sign a do not resuscitate order, medical care will not be as good as if they did not sign: "Maybe the doctor will not try hard enough." The hospital personnel, who must ask the patient their wishes about resuscitation, must be sensitive to the seriousness of the process, and deal with each situation in a personalized and individual way. Examples of different situations might include a woman having a baby, a person having elective surgery, and a patient who is terminally ill. The new mother and the patient who is having elective surgery would probably want resuscitation efforts undertaken. The patient who is terminally ill may perceive that not all care will be given to him, and it may be the first time he was asked about resuscitation status since he became terminally ill. Different emotions can be expected from people in each situation (Meisel, Snyder, & Quill, 2000; Gostin, 1997; Quinn, 1997).

Another time of stress is when caregivers tell families that death has occurred. Caregivers, no matter their profession, seem to show a strong dislike for the task of delivering such news, referring to the problematic and uncertain nature of each situation. Along with telling news of the death may come the responsibility to ask for an autopsy and to request organs for transplantation. Although rare, this is also an uncomfortable part of delivering bad news, because it has to be done immediately after death. Teaching how to tell the bad news of a death is an important dimension of medical and nursing education (Buchman, 1999).

Caregivers and Dying

"A good death is one a person would choose for himself" (Weissman, 1972, p. 4). Because most people would choose to die at home, free from pain, surrounded by loved ones, this statement implies a conflict between the ideal and the reality. The role of the health care professional is that they must respect the dying person's right to choose, and honor for the person's choices, even when they differ from his or her own values and goals (Emanuel, 1995). In the event when such choices may involve illegal activities, the care provider is not required to engage in such activities. In such instances, a referral to another provider may be necessary,

The SUPPORT study was an effort to achieve a clearer understanding of the characteristics of dying in the American hospital. This $28 million dollar project enrolled over 9,000 patients suffering from life-threatening illness in five U.S. teaching hospitals over a 4-year period. The study demonstrated that physicians did not routinely query their patients about end-of-life decisions, and that they did not respond to interventions that had been designed to increase the frequency with which these discussions were held (Lynn, Teno, & Harrell, 1995). Because of the negative outcome of the study's interventions, the Hastings Center published a special supplement that analyzed areas of medical education, ethics, and cultural differences that assisted in understanding what may be some of the reasons for the negative findings (Hastings Center, 1995).

Increasingly, death takes place in a hospital, where sophisticated technological equipment and professionals focus on curing diseases and confronting emergencies. Within an organizational context, where dying carries with it the "curse" of failure, what is the role of the health care professional (Silveria & Dipiero, 2000)?

Medical literature describes how difficult it is for young medical students, interns, and residents to deal with dying patients (Billings & Block). Their experiences indicate they must respond to a wide range of situations in dealing with dying patients and families. The difficulty arises when they know the patient and feel they have been a failure if death occurs, or if they come in "cold" to pronounce a patient dead and must communicate this knowledge to the family. In addressing these situations, physicians do not want to deny their humanity, but need assistance in maintaining perspective (Cassel, 1997; Blank, 1995).

Issues of dealing with dying patients are not sufficiently addressed in medical schools and residency programs. The interest of patients and physicians alike are best served when decisions about life and death are made jointly. Medical students and residents need help in learning both attitudes and skills in this area. Medical educators have recommended that theses specific topics be included as curricula are revised (Barzansky & Veloski, 1999; American Board of Internal Medicine, 1996).

The process of dying can trigger overwhelming emotions, not only in the person and family, but also in their professional caregivers. Perhaps as a result of their education and socialization, physicians often feel helpless in the face of devastating illness, and are afraid to project hopelessness to their patients. Professional caregivers need assistance in expressing their feelings when the disease does not respond to the treatment. They need to be realistic in their expectations and communicate hope to the patient and family, while not abandoning the patient in the dying process. Patients need to be related to as human beings, not as diseased entities that have failed treatment (Cassel & Omenn, 1995).

Review of nursing textbooks indicates a lack of references regarding issues concerning the care of the dying. Some initiatives have been started to address these concerns (Ferrell & Virami, 2000; Wilson, Barnett, & Richardson, 1999; Kennedy Schwarz, 1999).

Nursing curricula through the American Association of Colleges of Nursing has started the End of Life Nursing Education Consortium (2001). The goal of this project is a peaceful death and developed recommended competencies and curricular guidelines for end of life care. There are nine modules for the project:

1. Nursing care at the end of life
2. Pain management
3. Symptom management
4. Cultural considerations in end-of-life care
5. Ethical/legal issues
6. Communication
7. Grief/loss/bereavement
8. Preparation and care for the time of death
9. Achieving quality of life at the end of life

Acute care hospitals in the United States are generally oriented toward providing aggressive treatment aimed at curing or controlling disease. The reality of dying in the hospital setting may not be addressed in reference to patient or family, let alone the professional caregiver. Stress in dealing with the dying process may be manifested in many ways, including:

1. Role ambiguity—role expectations are not clearly communicated;
2. Role conflict—expectations of various professionals are incompatible or are in conflict; and
3. Role overload—extent beyond which any person is capable of meeting multiple expectations (Vachon, 2000)

Administrators can reduce the stress by being aware of those needs during staff selection (such as identifying coping mechanisms, exploring unresolved grief, and questioning the presence of a social support system), staff training and orientation (adopting a buddy system, and offering continuing education programs), and including, as part of the hospital support systems, support groups at work, and continuing peer support using formal and informal methods.

The cumulative effect on staff, of multiple patients' deaths, may lead to emotional depletion and spiritual exhaustion. Attitudinal, behavioral, and social factors may manifest themselves in expressions of unresolved grief, the need to be perfect, projection of one's needs, overseriousness, lack of sharing, inappropriate sharing at home, norms of solemnity, lack of structured opportunities for sharing, and administrative nonresponsiveness. Workshops on death awareness can reduce anxiety about death (Grande, Todd, & Barclay, 1997).

Administrators can help staff members explore the option of leaving work without this decision being considered an admission of failure. With administrative authority, supervisors can help caregivers who develop serious maladaptive symptoms by decreasing exposure to stressors, by temporary work modification, by removing them from the job situation, and by providing professional support. One of the most important challenges facing administrators today is finding ways to motivate and adequately support frontline staff.

The advances of medical technology have raised serious and difficult questions about the delivery or withholding of life-support procedures. In the media, almost monthly, specials bring to the public such topics as "How doctors decided who shall, shall not die." The public can read in the Sunday paper that they now have the following freedoms:

1. To ask questions
2. To see records
3. To demand emergency treatment
4. To demand politeness, respect
5. To say no to X rays, laxatives, excessive examinations
6. To ignore advice
7. To demand that care continues
8. To have most illnesses kept secret
9. To refuse medication
10. To die (Hunt, 1989)

Yet, when a person is dying, the person and family, upon entering the hospital, relinquish control over the person's course of dying. The attitudes and behavior of staff determine, to a large degree, the social context in which the dying occurs. Open communication among doctor, nursing staff, relative, and patient is enhanced if all are told of the impending death. Some of the major issues surrounding the dying process may include decisions about continuing aggressive treatment, telling other significant persons of the impending death, settling unfinished business, and discussing place of death. The patient and family can be helped, if they know what options are available. Although every patient has the right to full disclosure, he or she also has the right to be treated with compassion and common sense. Although some patients may want to leave all medical decisions to their physician, the doctor's role is not one of paternalism. Patients and families may need encouragement in order to participate fully in the decision making process, and may wait for a cue from the professional caregiver in this matter (Quill, 2000; Rabow & Hardie, 2000).

Patient and Family Expectations

The dying patient and family (because of the large number of baby boomers caring for their elderly parents and looking to the future for themselves) have changed the implications of death. Society seems to be more open to exploring and trying understand the place of dying and death in the lives of individual. *Tuesday's with Morrie,* a book about the interactions between an elderly dying teacher and his former young student has been on the bestseller list for over 2 years (Albom, 1997). *On Our Own Terms,* on Public Television, reported on the intimate end of life journeys of more that a dozen individuals, their families, and their caregivers, as they struggled to infuse the end of life with compassion and caring (Moyers, 2000). In periodicals, *Time* magazine and *Modern Maturity* have featured articles concerning the issues around dying and death.

Dying persons and families represent a particularly vulnerable group, especially those dying in an acute care/cure-oriented setting. Studies of family members in the hospital have consistently reported that relatives define support in two ways: (1) honest information and clear explanation about the patient's condition and what is being done, and (2) assurance that the patient is being kept comfortable. These findings also give evidence that nonsupportive behavior includes efforts to encourage them to cry, removing them from the bedside of the patient, and reminding them that the suffering will be over soon (Bascom & Tolle, 1995). The Assumptions and Principles Underlying Standards of Terminal Care emphasizes that the patient and family have the right to expect that the hospital will respect their philosophy of life and death, assist them in maintaining their right to set goals, and treat the patient and family as the unit of care (Wald, 1979).

When relatives were asked to share concerns uppermost in their minds during hospitalization, four concerns were identified most frequently:

1. Problems created by the symptoms of the illness
2. Fear of the future
3. Waiting
4. Difficulty with obtaining information (Covinsky, 1994)

In the same study of the needs of critically ill patients, there was a need to refocus the feeling of hope, even when the relatives were acknowledging the impending death. Research on grieving spouses of chronically ill oncology patients showed that the spouse had eight needs: to be with the dying person, to be helpful to the dying person, to be assured of the comfort of the dying person, to be informed of the mate's condition, to be informed of the impending death, to express emotions, to receive comfort and support of family members, and to receive acceptance, support, and comfort from health professionals (McCormick & Conley, 1995). The review of research on families during the terminal phase found that families regarded information about their relative's condition and interventions directed at their relative's comfort as most supportive. Families regarded as least supportive interventions that encouraged families to express their own emotions. Being physically near their dying relative was very important to families whose relatives were hospitalized (Hardwig, 1995).

Friends and families have the right to expect that staff members in the hospital will be aware of, and assist with, the needs indicated in these studies. To meet these concerns, administrators may consider using the ethics committee to assist in addressing some of the difficult medical, legal, and moral issues around dying and death. Family members, as well as staff, should be encouraged to attend patient-specific meetings, because open communication is an essential part of decision making (Anershed & Ternestedt, 1998; Davis, Cherkryn Reimer, & Materns, 1994; La Puma, Schiedermayer, & Sieger, 1995).

When all understand that death is a natural part of the life cycle, death in the hospital setting will be handled in a concerned manner, with full realization that death, whether as result of a massive injury or as a consequence of terminal illness, is not a failure (O'Connor & Sendor, 1997).

Implications for Dealing with Death in the Hospital

Because most Americans are dying in an institutional health care setting, both administrators of these institutions and practitioners would be better prepared to deal with death issues if they had the opportunity to examine and understand a variety of perspectives and responsibilities in this matter. Policies and procedures might then reflect these concerns.

Death can occur in many ways in the hospital, such as sudden death on arriving at the emergency room, terminal illness on a floor for acute care, neonatal death, suicide, and death resulting from a hospital "mistake." Each of these circumstances is very different, and each response will be different, but the common thread is that they all occurred in the hospital and were responded to by hospital personnel. Support is needed in all situations for family members, and all too often forgotten for the caregivers themselves. Administrators can address some of these concerns in the following ways.

Selection of Staff

Some departments in the hospital, such as the emergency room, will deal with death more frequently than others. In screening candidates for employment, inquiries should be made about their feelings and competencies in handling situations in which persons are dying, and valuable information may be obtained about how they have previously assisted patients and families in these circumstances. This is not to rule out new or inexperienced staff, but to alert them to the realities of the employer's expectations and make them aware that administration perceives this activity as part of their job performance. During the selection process, some inquiries should be made as to recent experience with death. A person seeking employment in a cardiac unit who has just lost a family member with heart disease may need to be directed to another department during the grief and bereavement period.

Orientation of Staff

It is beneficial to address, during the process of orientation, the attitudes of all staff members on the topic of the dying patient and death. Having current employees share their experiences with new staff may be helpful, since this topic may have been handled only in an academic setting, if at all. Initial clinical experiences for new staff members, and daily exposure to dying patients, can affect staff differently. A session on death awareness may vary, from Worden and Proctor's Death Awareness Questionnaire (1982) to a video or role playing. This will depend on the needs of the department, and on the frequency of dealing with dying patients and death. The new staff members need to feel that death is not viewed as a failure of the health care system, but as a natural part of the life cycle. The skill of caring with compassion is needed in caring for all patients, but especially when the patient is dying. The caregiver learns that interaction with the dying person can continue to be fruitful by relating as one human being to another.

In-service Support for Staff

This may be done on a departmental level, but since the dying patient and death can affect many departments within the institution that have served the same patient, some thought should be given to interdisciplinary in-service sessions. These sessions could focus on having staff share their reactions and feelings about a certain patient or the circumstances of the patient's dying. For departments in which death is dealt with on a frequent basis, additional sessions may be useful. Administrators may offer these sessions, but an outside person should lead the session, because this will give the formal and informal leaders of the group the opportunity to be full participants instead of putting energy into group process and outcome.

These sessions may include, but are not limited to, covering areas such as exercises in word association, lifelines, time lines, a personal death awareness index, and "How I Want to Die," with case studies as examples, and writing one's own obituary and eulogy. It is also helpful to complete some open-ended sentences, such as:

1. My first experience with death was . . .
2. The reason I am working with this type of patient is . . .
3. A positive experience with a dying patient and family was . . .
4. A negative experience with a dying patient and family was . . .
5. I am affected by my patient's death in the following ways . . .
6. I express these feelings at work . . . at home . . .
7. I feel most comfortable working and talking with someone who is dying, when I know . . .
8. I wish there were some ways that families could be helped to . . .
9. Ways that I can help other staff working with dying patients and families are . . .
10. Ways that others can help me work with dying patients and families are . . .

The last session could be a memorial service that the staff develops with readings from different religious traditions or meaningful passages from literature. A passage used during a session for AIDS patients was "We cannot judge a biography by its length, by the number of pages in it, we must judge by the richness of the contents . . . sometimes the "unfinished are the most beautiful symphonies . . . " (Frankl, 1950).

Staff members will react differently to each session. During one series, writing the obituary and eulogy were given as a homework assignment. Twelve staff members were participating in the workshop. Only two of these completed the request and returned with the assignment. Some participants stated they had completed the forms but forgotten the papers, and one or two said it was too difficult to complete. At this point, new obituary forms were distributed. Allowing some time for completion, staff members were asked to communicate their responses if they felt comfortable. By the end of this session, all staff had shared their obituaries.

Having all questions and statements in handouts has proven helpful, allowing time for each participant to write his or her response before sharing verbal responses. This gives time for introspection. The leader should fully participate in all exercises, to reenforce the idea that we all have feelings and reactions and need to explore them for ourselves, and to benefit patients and families, and support other team members. These sessions can help team members confront the facts about themselves and ways to support one another in dealing with the dying process and how it affects patients, families, and themselves. One insight that became apparent in these sessions is how, beyond education and clinical experience, past experiences and religious traditions can affect behavior. These shared experiences assist staff in understanding one another's frames of reference when dealing with the dying process.

After the memorial service, a group of night nurses, working with persons with AIDS, expressed their concern for a number of patients who were alone and had no one to plan a formal memorial service. The night nurses decided to have a tape with some music ("Amazing Grace," "You'll Never Walk Alone") and a few Psalms (Psalm 23, "The Lord is my Shepherd . . . ") ready, so they could have a remembrance at the bedside. By having the service on a tape, it could be played even if only one person could be present, and it gave them a feeling of closure for the patient and for themselves. This in no way imposes a religious element to the death, but declares that the patient's life had meaning and needed to be acknowledged in a formal manner.

Peer Support Groups

Administrators are aware that staff members have death in their personal lives. Through such programs as an employee assistance program, peer group support could be offered to staff during this period. These groups may be open-ended or scheduled for a discrete time frame.

Memorial Services and Bereavement Follow-up

Some departments in the hospital, such as AIDS centers and hospice, may have, as part of their operations, memorial services and bereavement follow up. These services may be available to all staff, as well as to families. On a timely basis, the hospital may also have a memorial service for all who have died in the institution, and invite families and significant others, along with staff, to express their feelings about the deceased. This time of remembrance can offer the family the opportunity to meet the staff that had taken care of the patient, and express their gratitude for the care and concern that was given during the dying process.

At times, when staff members die, the hospital also needs to acknowledge these deaths in a formal manner. This may be done at a formal memorial service or at the department where the person worked. In one hospital, the director of nursing was killed in an automobile accident. Administrators went to each nursing station to share the news and had follow-up meetings with the staff to encourage them to express their feelings.

During the construction for new facilities, consideration should be given to providing some private areas in the hospital's critical care units that would give family and staff a quiet place to express their feelings during the dying process and the death. The rooms do not have to be large, but should have quiet colors, comfortable furniture, a telephone, and a box of tissues. Those areas should be available in times of crisis, so that interactions of a serious and emotionally painful nature do not have to be held in the hallways or solariums, with others present. Consideration should also be given to having staff available who can address these issues. This can be done by the social workers, chaplains, clinical liaison nurses, or administrators who have skill in dealing with situations such as a death in the emergency room, maternity unit, or any area of the hospital.

Reflections

What has brought the medical community to direct its focus on end-of-life care has been some major studies and reports that have analyzed how terminal care is practiced. Most of these studies were physician-authored, which indicates that the medical community is taking a leadership role in investigating the care of the dying. One of the reasons for these investigations has been the shared discomfort with current practices in care and the growing reality of the need for a better means to serve those who are very ill. Some of these projects have included major medical associations redefining their role in medical practice in delivering care at the end of life (Lynn & Lynch Schuster, 2000).

The use of the term *palliative care* has gained a greater acceptance in the medical community. Even though the hospice movement started the interest in the care of the dying in the United States, the concepts of palliative medicine and palliative care appears to be more acceptable to the medical community than the term *hospice*. Some of the reasons for this may be the restrictiveness of the hospice regulations, the perceived death sentence of the word, the empty beds in acute care hospitals, and/ or the support and continuity of care given to patients and families starting the care approach early in the disease process.

Some other issues influencing the care of the dying are physician-assisted suicide and euthanasia. The medical community must take clear leadership in these areas, or, as has happened in the past, medical decisions will continue to be made in the courts (O'Connor, 1999; Portenoy, 1997).

The questions for hospitals are:

1. How will each hospital respond, based on individual characteristics, to the needs of the patient, family, and caregivers in response to dying and death in their institution (Steinhauser, Christakis, & Clipp, 2000)?
2. How will teaching hospitals integrate end-of-life care into practice patterns for their house staff?
3. How will the government and insurance companies define end-of-life care for reimbursement (Cassel & Vladeck, 1996)?

It will be hoped that palliative care will include all the elements of hospice care. One would hope that time will prove that "palliative," defined as "to ease without curing," is the care provided in hospitals for end-of-life care, and not Webster's second definition of *palliative*, which is "to cover by excuses and apologies" (Webster's, 1997).

Conclusions

Biomedical technology in U.S. health care is rapidly changing, psychosocial aspects are similarly changing, although not as rapidly. A more humanistic approach is apparent at the beginning of life, evidenced in the increased numbers of birthing rooms around the nation, and at the end of life, with the continuing development of palliative care services and the already existing hospice programs. It is becoming clear that individuals are gradually seeking to control more of their own health care. Perhaps the desire for more control over our own lives is a response to a universal threat of death (O'Connor, 1986).

Hospitals, though life-affirming, need to address the fact that patients are dying in the acute care setting. Hospital administrators should choose to address issues concerning dying, and to create an environment for the patient, family, and health care professionals that will foster mutual support in the process of living and dying.

Discussion Questions

1. How do individual hospital characteristics affect the response to dying and death in an institution?
2. How can teaching hospitals integrate end-of-life care into practice patterns for their house staff?
3. How should the government and insurance companies define end-of-life care for reimbursement?

References

Albom, M. (1997). *Tuesdays with Morrie: An old man, a young man, and life's greatest lesson.* New York: Doubleday.

Allen, W. (1972). *Without feathers.* New York: Warner Books.

American Associations of Colleges of Nursing. (2001). End of life nursing education curricula. Retrieved January 23, 2001, from www.master@aacn.mche.edu

American Board of Internal Medicine. (1996). *Care for the dying: Identification and promotion of physician competency.* Philadelphia.

American College of Physicians Ethics Manual (4th ed.). (1998). *Annals of Internal Medicine, 128,* 576–594.

Anershed, B., & Ternestedt, B. (1998). Involvement of relatives in the care of the dying in different cultures. *Cancer Nursing, 21*(2), 106–116.

Barzansky, B., & Veloski, J. (1999). Education in end-of-life care during medical school and residency training. *Academy Medicine, 74*(10 suppl), S102–S104.

Bascom, P., & Tolle, S. (1995). Care of the family when the patient is dying. *Western Journal of Medicine, 163*(3), 292–296.

Billings, J. A., & Block, S. (1997). Palliative care in undergraduate medical education: Status report and future direction. *Journal of the American Medical Association, 278*(9), 733–738.

Blank, L. (1995). Defining and evaluation physician competence in end-of-life care. *Western Journal of Medicine, 163,* 297–310.

Buchman, R. (1999). Communication in palliative care. In D. Doyle & G. Hanks (Eds.), *Oxford textbook of palliative medicine* (2nd ed., pp. 47–61). Oxford, England: Oxford University Press.

Callahan, D. (1990). *What kind of life?* New York: Simon & Schuster.

Cassel, C. (1997). *Approaching death-improving care at the end of life.* Washington, DC: National Academy Press.

Cassel, C., & Omenn, G. (1995). Dimensions of care of the dying patient. *Western Journal of Medicine, 163*(3), 224–225.

Cassel, C., & Vladeck, B. (1996). ICD-9 code for palliative or terminal care. *New England Journal of Medicine, 335*(16), 1232–1233.

Christakis, N. (2000). *Death foretold: Prophecy and prognosis in medical care.* Chicago: University of Chicago Press.

Cloud, J. (2000). A kinder, gentler death. *Time, 156*(12), 60–74.

Corr, C. (1999). Death in modern society. In D. Doyle, G. Hanks, & N. MacDonald (Eds.), *Textbook of palliative care* (pp. 28–36). New York: Oxford University Press.

Covinsky, K. (1994). The impact of serious illness on patients' families. *Journal of the American Medical Association, 272,* 1839–1844.

Cruzan v Director, Missouri Department of Health, 497 U.S.-111 L Ed. 2d 224, 100sCt.:2841 (1990).

Davis, B., Cherkryn Reimer, J., & Materns, N. (1994). Family functioning and its implications for palliative care. *Journal of Palliative Care, 10*(1), 29–36.

Dying Well in the Hospital, [Special supplement]. Editor: Daniel Callahan. (1995). *Hastings Center Report, 25*(6), S1–S36.

Emanuel, E., & Emanuel, L. (1998). The promise of a good death. *Lancet, 251,* 21–29.

Emanuel, L. (1995). Editor: Daniel Callahan. Structured deliberation to improve decision making for the seriously ill. Dying Well in the Hospital [Special supplement]. *Hastings Center Report, 25*(6), S14–S17.

Ferrell, B., & Virami, R. (2000). Analysis of palliative care content in nursing textbooks. *Journal of Palliative Care, 16,* 39–47.

Foley, K. (1996). Palliative medicine, pain control, and symptom assessment. In *Caring for the dying: Identification and promotion of physician competency* (pp. 12–18). Philadelphia: American Board of Internal Medicine.

Frankl, V. (1950). *Man's search for meaning.* New York: Simon & Schuster.

Gilbar, O., & Steiner, M. (1996). When death comes: Where should patients die? *The Hospice Journal, 11*(1), 31–48.

Gostin, L. (1997). Health law and ethics, deciding life and death in the courtroom. *Journal of the American Medical Association, 278*(18), 1523–1528.

Grande, G., Todd., C., & Barclay, S. (1997). Support needs in the last year of patient and care dilemmas. *Palliative Medicine, 13,* 202–209.

Hardwig, J. (1995, December). The SUPPORT project and the invisible family. *Hastings Center Report* [Special Supplement], S23–S25.

Hogan, C., Lynn, J., Gabel, J., Lunney, J., O'Mara, A., & Wilkinson, A. (2000). *Medicare Beneficiaries' Costs and Use of Care in the Last Year of Life: Final Report to the Medicare Payment Advisory Commission.* Washington, DC: Medicare Payment Advisory Commission.

Hunt, M. (1989, March 5). Patients' rights-body and mind. *The New York Times Magazine,* 55–56.

Jacobson, J. A., Francis, L. P., & Battin, M. P. (1997). Dialogue to action: Lessons learned from some family members of deceased patients at an interactive program in seven Utah hospitals. *Journal of Clinical Ethics, 8,* 359–371.

The Jerusalem Bible. (1966). Garden City, New York: Doubleday.

Kennedy Schwarz, J. (1999). Assisted dying and nursing practice. *Image: Journal of Nursing Scholarship, 3*(4), 368.

La Puma, J., Schiedermayer, D., & Sieger, M. (1995). How ethics consultation can help resolve dilemmas about dying patients. *Western Journal of Medicine, 163,* 262–267.

Lynn, J., & Lynch Schuster, J. (2000). *Improving care for the end of life: A sourcebook for health care managers and clinicians.* New York: Oxford University Press.

Lynn, J., Teno, J., & Harrell, F. M. (1995). A controlled trial to improve care for seriously ill hospitalized patients. *Journal of the American Medical Association, 126*(2), 97–106.

Matousek, M. (2000). The last taboo. *Modern Maturity,* Sep–Oct. pp. 49–62.

McCormick, T., & Conley, B. (1995). Patients' perspectives on dying and on the care of dying patients. *Western Journal of Medicine, 163*(3), 236–243.

Meisel, A., Snyder, L., & Quill, T. (2000). Seven legal barriers to end of life care. *Journal of the American Medical Association, 284*(19), 2495–2501.

Moyers, W. (2000). *On our own terms; Moyers on dying.* Discussion Guide, EBC and Public Affairs Television. New York: Thirteen WNET.

O'Connor, P. (Summer 1986). Spiritual elements of hospice care. *Hospice Journal, 2*(2), 99–108.

O'Connor, P. (1999). Hospice vs. palliative care. *Hospice Journal, 14*(3/4), 123–137.

O'Connor, P., & Sendor, V. (1997). *Hospice and palliative care: Questions and answers.* Lanham, MD: Scarecrow Press.

Portenoy, R. (1997). Determinants of the willingness to endorse assisted suicide. *Psychosomatic, 38,* 277–287.

Quill, T. (2000). Initiating end-of-life discussions with seriously ill patients. *Journal of the American Medical Association, 284*(19), 2502–2507.

Quinn, T. (1997). Health, law and ethics: Palliative options of last resort. *Journal of the American Medical Association, 278*(23), 2099–2104.

Rabow, M., & Hardie, G. (2000). End of life care content in 50 textbooks from multiple specialties. *Journal of the American Medical Association, 283,* 771–778.

Silveria, M., & Dipiero, A. (2000). Patients' knowledge of options at the end of life: Ignorance in the face of death. *Journal of the American Medical Association, 282*(19), 2483–2489.

Steinhauser, K., Christakis, N., & Clipp, C. (2000). Factors considered important at the end of life by patients, family, physicians and other care providers. *Journal of the American Medical Association, 282*(19), 2476–2482.

Vachon, M. (2000, April). *Losses and gains.* Presentation at the Calvary Hospital Conference, New York.

Wald, F. (1979, February). Assumptions and principles, underlying standards work group on death and dying. *American Journal of Nursing,* 296–297.

Webster's Dictionary. (1997). Englewood Cliffs, NJ: Prentice-Hall, Inc.

Weissman, A. D. (1972). *On dying and denying.* New York: Behavioral Publications.

Wilson, B., & Richardson, A. (1999). Nursing research and Palliative care. In D. Doyle, G. Hanks, & N. MacDonald (Eds.), *Textbook of palliative care* (pp. 97–102). New York: Oxford University Press.

Worden, W., & Proctor, J. (1982). *Breaking free of fear to live a better life now.* Englewood Cliffs, NJ: Prentice-Hall.

Young, R. (1988). It's Over, Debbie. *Journal of the American Medical Association, 259*(2), 272.

Six

Dying at Home

Barbara B. Germino

Barbara B. Germino is co-editor of this book, and her biography can be found on page ii.

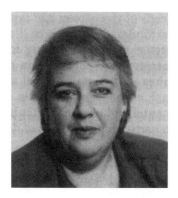

In the United States, the place for dying has continued to change from what occurred before the turn of the century to the present. In the late nineteenth century, death at home was the norm. The twentieth century was a period of time when the majority of dying occurred in hospitals. As late as 1998, a national report indicated that, of the 2 million people in the United States who die every year, 80% were still dying in hospitals (Office of Technology Assessment, 1998). How much of the dying process takes place in hospitals, long-term care settings, freestanding hospices, home, and other settings is another question for which inconsistent and incomplete data exist. Knowing that hospital stays have shortened, the acuity of hospital inpatients has increased, and that people are living longer with some major, common chronic illnesses, including some kinds of cancer, congestive heart failure, and chronic obstructive pulmonary diseases, it is important to examine predictors of dying at home, preferences for dying at home, and consequences for caregivers.

Nationwide, increasing interest in seeking quality end-of-life care has begun to impact on the awareness of consumers about options for shaping the nature and quality of their life at its end. Major media coverage of issues related to the end of life (and particularly issues of pain management), and large funding initiatives supporting community-based demonstration projects involving many segments of the community, have made end-of-life care issues much more visible and salient to the public at large. Federal and other research funding initiatives are supporting long-needed study of issues and interventions around end-of-life care. For health care professionals, especially those in medicine and nursing, national standardization of curricula and training in end-of-life care have begun to develop a large cadre of experts who are training and teaching others. The widespread availability of hospice services, which allow patients and families to choose the place for dying and to influence and shape care at the end of life, has helped many people to have the kind of death they choose. New models for delivery of end-of-life care in the home and less-restrictive reimbursement may emerge in response to consumer and caregiver demand.

There are a number of issues that influence whether a person dies at home. Some factors have been studied systematically; other influences are inductively derived from related research and reported observations and commentaries. Health care system or contextual factors, including, in the United States, health care costs and efforts toward cost containment, as well as third-party reimbursement, including the Medicare hospice benefit, are environmental factors which have seemed to influence the place of death, for many dying persons (McCusker, 1983; Moinpour & Polissar, 1989). Who, if anyone, makes and communicates a decision about the place of death, and the timing of that decision, are factors that may reflect the interaction of environmental, person/family, and illness influences on the probability of dying at home. The availability, ability, and willingness of family or significant others to care for the dying person, and to commit to being with that person in the face of uncertainties about the future, influences individual and family choices about where to live the final period of life. Dying persons' and families' or significant others' experiences, values, and feelings would also seem to be profoundly important in such choices, as would the availability of supportive and care delivery services that meet the needs of the person and family at home. The nature of the illness and its trajectory, particularly the length of illness and the intensity of demands on the ill person and those caring for him/her, may influence the ability of caregivers to persevere in providing care at home. Prolonged and intense caregiving certainly can take its toll on physical and mental health, but, more recently, research has documented the positive aspects of caregiving as well. This chapter will discuss each of these influences, in an effort to clarify those forces, both environmental and personal, which help to shape the events at the end of life, and in particular, the place of death.

Health Care Environment Factors and Predictors of Place of Death

To a great extent, the structure and functioning of the larger health care system has influenced, and will continue to influence, the probability that an individual who is dying will die at home or in a long-term care facility. Studies in the 1980s indicated that home death was associated with the availability of hospice programs and the type of hospice programs (Greer et al., 1986; Moinpour & Polissar, 1989; Mor & Birnbaum, 1983; Mor et al., 1985; Torrens, 1985). It was also suggested that, in the U.S., system factors, such as case mix and federal policies associated with prospective payment and the Medicare hospice benefit, may have influenced not only length of stay in hospitals and hospice, but also may have affected the place of death (Moinpour & Polissar, 1989). Research at that time also indicated that hospice participation was the variable most strongly related to whether or not a cancer patient would die at home. However, whether hospice care is causally related to home death is unclear, as is whether people who prefer to die at home tend to select hospice care (Moinpour & Polissar, 1989). In addition to hospice care, earlier studies indicated that "patients age 85 years and older, and those diagnosed close to death are more likely to die at home than would be predicted by age at death, time from diagnosis to death, and hospice alone" (Moinpour & Polissar, 1989, p. 1550; Greer et al., 1983).

More recently, several studies (Cantwell et al., 2000; Fried, Pollack, Drickamer, & Tinetti, 1999; Izquierdo-Porrera & Trelis-Navarro, 2001; Legg, Kaffenbarger, & Remsburg, 2000) have described predictors of home death in specific populations within the health care system, broadening our understanding of factors that predict the place of death. For a sample of palliative care cancer patients, the desire for a home death by both the patient and the caregiver, support of a family physician, and presence of more than one caregiver were all significantly associated with home death. The major predictive factor was a desire for home death by both the patient and the caregiver. In this study, 47% of the sample died at home (Cantwell et al., 2000).

Taking a slightly different perspective on place of death outside the palliative care system, Izquierdo-Porrera and Trelis-Navarro (2001) explored gender differences with respect to place of death, as well as predictors of place of death by gender. Although there were no significant differences by gender in place, of death in their sample, gender did make a difference in predictors of death in one place—the hospital. For men, digestive comorbidities, vomiting, and weakness predicted a hospital death. Women were more likely to die in a hospital, if they were more functionally dependent or had comorbidities that affected their vision and hearing. In a different population (patients in a community-based, long-term care program), 49% died in the hospital, and only 21% died at home. Among those subjects living at home before death, factors associated with dying at home included being female, having a high level of functional dependence, altered cognitive status, and cancer, chronic lung disease, or coronary artery disease. The investigators suggest that we take a closer look at such factors, in combination with patients' preferences and care needs, in order to understand how to help patients and families make optimal decisions about the site of terminal care (Fried et al., 1999).

In an effort to determine the prevalence, effectiveness, and predictors of planning the place of death, investigators in a study of homebound, community-based elderly, found that, overall, 64% of subjects made a plan to die in a specific place, and the plans were executed successfully in 91% of these situations. The plans, somewhat surprisingly, were made with a median time of 36 days between their formulation and the person's death. Making the plan to die in a specific place was positively associated with a do not resuscitate order, and negatively associated with the lack of an identifiable main medical problem (Legg et al., 2000).

Decisions and Timing of Decisions

Clinicians have observed that, whether a clear personal decision is made about where the terminally ill person wants to die, and whether that decision is communicated to family and professional caregivers, are powerful factors in influencing whether the dying person stays at home or returns home, if hospitalized or admitted to a long-term care or rehabilitation facility, at some point. A number of scenarios characterize such decision processes in the United States of the early twenty-first century. If self-determination is held as the ideal in our culture, the "ideal" scenario is often held to be one in which a person, before ever being identified as terminally ill, formalizes his/her decision to die at home in one or more advance directives—preferably more. After the identity as a dying person is clarified, if that person is still coherent and able, the decision to die at home may still be made, formally or informally, and communicated to family and professional caregivers. In situations in which neither of these scenarios has occurred, when, for instance, the dying trajectory is short and the person, declining too quickly, becomes unable to make such a decision, or when the awareness context is such that the idea of such a decision is not enabled, the opportunity for the dying person to direct his/her final days may be lost.

In the United States, a litiginous society struggling with conflicts between secular and traditional Judeo-Christian values, if a dying person does not make a clear decision and communicate it, decisions about the course of dying, as well as the place of death, may be made as often by institutions and physicians as by those closest to the person who is terminally ill. Ethical dilemmas have become legal battlegrounds, as evidenced by the Cruzan case and others, and the legal precedents being set.

It is commonly stated that more patients wish to die at home than the number able to achieve this goal. However, systematic data about preferences for place of care and place of death are limited in number. In a recent review article (Higginson & Sen-Gupta, 2000), the authors analyze 18 studies determining preferences for place of care and place of death in either the general population or groups, including cancer patients. Preferences for home death ranged from 49 to 100% of respondents, across all but one of the studies. In the exception, only 25–29% of a group of continuing-care patients in London wanted a home death; the remaining preferred death in an inpatient hospice. Among general public respondents in these studies, those who had recent experience of a close friend or family member's dying or death, preferred inpatient hospice care. In a comparison of patients, families, and professionals in a meta-analysis, patients expressed the strongest preferences for dying at home. Despite the methodological limitations of many of the studies, an analysis of only the larger, stronger studies did not alter the finding of a preference for home care at the end of life in over 50% of patients (Higginson & Sen-Gupta, 2000).

Patient and Family or Significant Other Caregivers' Values, Experiences, and Feelings

The dying person's and their family's values, past experiences, and feelings about the past, as well as the current illness, all help to shape their choice of dying at home or elsewhere. For many dying persons and their families, the benefits of being cared for at home outweigh those of being in an institution. These include privacy and control and active family participation in care, which may be part of the separation process and extremely important in the outcome of bereavement for survivors (Amenta & Bohnet, 1987; Craven & Wald, 1979). Wanting to be at home during the dying process does not preclude wanting the place of death to be elsewhere. Consider Woody, a 52-year-old man with esophageal cancer, who, after a year of multiple hospitalizations and treatment regimes, chose to go home for the time remaining. He wanted his wife and daughters, sister and brother, nieces and nephews, and cousins to be around often. His favorite activity, when he was feeling up to it, was reminiscing and telling stories with his large extended family. He spent his days and nights on a large sofa in the living room, and those close to him would come and go, talking and laughing with him until he fell asleep. Home was special to Woody, and that's where he wanted to be living while he was dying. However, in an effort to protect his daughters and his wife, he asked that, when it was clear there was only a few days left in his life, they take him to the hospital to die, so that memories of him dead would not destroy the joy of home to his surviving family. He and his family were able to carry out his plan, and his wife and daughters, years later, tell stories remembering his life and living rather than his death.

For other families, giving care to a dying member may be precluded by their awareness of and response to dying. For family caregivers, developing an awareness of dying does not occur suddenly, but gradually, and is often characterized by uncertainty and anguish (Yates & Stetz, 1999). In addition, there are other factors that may make caregiving difficult, including family members' fears, poor health, limited energy, inability to assume an open-ended responsibility, other family and work demands, or family relationship issues. If the family caregiver or caregivers are elderly or have poor health, they may be willing but unable or fearful of being able to care for a dying member, even though they might wish to do so. Lack of confidence in being able to handle the demands of care may be a factor as well.

Unresolved family relationship issues may be exacerbated by the knowledge that a family member is terminally ill, and may influence the choice of dying at home. An adult child, who might be the only family caregiver, may never have developed an adult relationship with the dying parent, both family members may be aware on some level of that unresolved struggle, and may choose to resolve their unfinished business through the process of caregiving, or to leave it unaddressed. The dying person's and family's choice of where to die may reflect, at least in part, the dynamics of family relationships.

Patient and family value systems are another factor in the complex equation that represents the possibility of dying at home. In some families and in some subcultures, not having a person who is dying in a hospital, where "everything, the best of everything, can be done, right up until the last," is less than what is considered the best care. For others, not caring for one's own goes counter to what is most important and strongly held. In the traditional Appalachian white subculture, for instance, hospice workers may have to struggle to convince people and their families to accept their services before a crisis occurs or symptoms are out of control. The response, "We care for our own," is a common one and calls for understanding of values that include suspicion of outsiders and rejects their intrusion into the home.

Finally, consideration must be given to the patient's and family's attempts to find some meaning in the dying and in their participation in that process. The anticipation of loss of the dying person to the family, and to each family member, is part of the struggle to find some meaning. Much of what occurs for families, either in the decision to care or continue to care for a dying person at home, is a reflection of that family's relationships in the past. Krant's (1974) chapter on families of the dying describes eloquently the dynamics of both mature and ambivalent relationships, and how these relationships continue to be reflected during the dying process. He notes that one key to the problem of continued and ongoing living, and the resolution of grieving, is the manner and meaning of the dying. Although these do not alleviate the pain of loss, there are far greater problems when family conflicts and tensions characterize a family member's dying, and the strains characteristic of such situations can lead to serious problems for surviving family members. The decision to care for a family member at home, and the likelihood that family members can persevere in this decision if the dying is particularly difficult or prolonged, is likely to be influenced by the nature of family relationships and the meaning of caregiving during the dying process.

Research on caregiving has indicated that, in spite of the stresses, demands, and uncertainty of caring for a family member or significant other who is dying, caregivers try to live day to day, and to get satisfaction out of providing comfort for the patient (Hull, 1993). Caregivers find ways, even under difficult circumstances, to create meaning or pleasure in the situation of caregiving, including using customary routines that are comforting and satisfying to both the caregiver and the person being cared for.

Reading together, bedtime rituals, familiar ways of spending time together, like watching a favorite television show or listening to music, have been described by caregivers as ways of maintaining a comforting normalcy. Innovative routine breakers are activities that add some interest or stimulation to the day and often emerge from simple and ordinary activity. Cartwright, Archbold, Stewart, and Limandri (1994) have described such activities as sustaining relationships, enhancing self-esteem and self-worth of the ill person and caregivers, strengthening or renewing relationships, and increasing empathy and mutuality.

Availability and Fit of Support Services

For the person without family and without a significant other willing to support the person's choice to die at home, the choices may not include dying at home, unless their personal resources, including third-party reimbursement, are extraordinary, or unless health care resources can be obtained and coordinated in a continuing manner. Hospices providing home care services have often required that there be a primary caregiver in the home, and other agencies have tended to be hesitant to provide care to those living alone, once they reach a point when constant care and/or monitoring is required. In such situations, especially because hospitalization is no longer always an option, the dying person, if resources are available, may end up in a long-term care facility to live out his or her final days. That may not be a satisfactory solution for the dying person or for those attempting to provide that person services at home, but may be the only option that fits the need of constant observation and care.

Even when family members and significant others are available and willing to provide care at home, those persons often need services that may or may not be available. Specifically, research has indicated that family members often need education related to home care management skills, in particular, related to helping patients move from bed to chair and to ambulate safely, and related to comfort care and symptom management (Grobe, Ilstrup, & Ahmann, 1981; Kirschling, 1986). Other services for which family members commonly feel the need include in-home medical monitoring, equipment to assist in care, transportation, personal care, household upkeep and chores, financial assistance or counseling, and respite care (Grobe, Ahmann, & Ilstrup, 1982).

Services required may or may not be available, depending on where the dying person and family live. In many rural areas of the United States, for instance, the availability of such educative and support services is limited, if available at all. The fit of a person's and family's wishes for care to be provided at home, and the supportive services that might make that possible, may be poor. Options that do tend to be available, such as long-term care (often at a distance), may create problems, such as isolation of the dying person from the family, the demands of adjusting to a new environment at a time when energy to meet such demands is limited, transportation problems, costs, and the difficulty of dealing with feelings of disappointment and guilt that personal and family goals could not be achieved.

Trajectory of the Illness

In a classic and often-quoted study, Glaser and Strauss (1968) introduced the concept of dying trajectory—the length, course, shape, and pattern of the final portion of a dying person's life, as well as the work it requires both of the dying person and those caring for that person. They observed that patients and professionals may have very different perceptions of trajectories, and that different types of trajectories create different kinds of work and different kinds of problems for those involved.

As difficult as sudden, unexpected death may be, the slow, lingering process of dying may be most distressing in our culture, because "dying is the inexorable and visible eradication of culturally stated personal meanings and concepts" (Krant, 1974, p. 340). A prolonged and difficult dying trajectory, with death at an uncertain future time, and with loss of bodily functions, loss of independence, and loss of the ability to do things that are important to the dying person, is a difficult one for many dying persons to accept and for many families to manage, as well. Many dying persons fear becoming a burden to those they love, losing their ability to care for themselves, and having to depend more on others (Krant, 1974). In his poignant discussion of dying and dignity, Krant (1974) notes that, for many, dying is a series of losses of body functions, the control over one's life, of feelings of self-esteem, and of loved and important aspects of life. Such losses bring suffering, and may alter individual behavior in ways that cause family and others in the environment to withdraw, because of the pain of their own losses. Prolonged and difficult dying at home may have the further effect of isolating the family caregivers, as well as the patient, from vital interaction with others and from the support that can be drawn from such relationships. Lack of support, and the physical and emotional demands of caregiving, endanger the health and well-being of even young and healthy family members. Family caregivers who have health problems, and whose age may predispose them to health problems, are at particular risk. Morbidity and mortality rates for widows and widowers have been known to be higher within the year following the spouse's death. Examinations of morbidity and mortality rates for other family caregivers, in relation to the demands of caregiving and to resources for assistance and support, are badly needed.

In contrast, the work of the most difficult and demanding of dying trajectories may in fact be buffered by the opportunity for the dying person to be cared for at home. With the opportunity for continuing contact with a caring professional or team of professionals, and access to support and respite services, the difficulties arising in a prolonged dying trajectory may be anticipated, acknowledged, and addressed. Central to dying at home as an advantage, whatever the dying trajectory, is the opportunity for personalized care and the sense of being in control of one's living while dying.

Conclusion

Clearly, even a brief examination of factors that may influence the opportunity, quality, and outcomes of dying at home, although each focuses our attention on particular issues, all are part of the context for dying, and interact with one another to shape the decisions and experiences related to the place for dying. Social and health care system factors may place powerful constraints on choices about where to be cared for while dying. The availability of specific kinds of information and services fitted to the needs of the person and family cannot be assumed, and may be the most significant factor in situations where services are very limited. The dying person and family's personal experiences, meanings, and resources for facing this situation are crucial, as is the unfolding of the dying trajectory. The choice of a place to be cared for while dying is one of a set of final important choices that may help to bring meaning to a life nearing its end.

Discussion Questions

1. What are some of the factors that predict whether people will die at home or in other settings?

2. According to the available evidence, do most people prefer to die at home? How do these preferences relate to the predictors of where people will actually die?
3. A number of caregiver characteristics and values affect caregiving at home for a loved one at the end of life. Discuss key characteristics and values that help to shape caregiving when someone is dying at home.

References

Amenta, M. O., & Bohnet, N. L. (1987). Communicating with dying patients. *Nursing, 17*(3), 100.

Cantwell, P., Turco, S., Benneis, C., Hanson, J., Neumann, C., & Bruera, E. (2000). Predictors of home death in palliative care cancer patients. *Journal of Palliative Care, 16*(1), 23–28.

Cartwright, J., Archbold, P., Stewart, B., & Limandri, B. (1994). Enrichment processes in family caregiving to frail elders. *Advances in Nursing Science, 17*(1), 31–43.

Craven, J., & Wald, F. (1979). Hospice care for dying patients. In L. Kruse, J. Reese, & L. Hart (Eds.), *Cancer pathophysiology, etiology and management*. St. Louis: Mosby.

Fried, T. R., Pollack, D. M., Drickamer, M. A., & Tinetti, M. E. (1999). Who dies at home? Determinants of site of death for community-based long-term care patients. *Journal of the American Geriatrics Society, 47*(1), 25–29.

Glaser, B. G., & Strauss, A. L. (1968). *Time for dying*. Chicago: Aldine.

Greer, D. S., Mor, V., Morris, J. N., Sherwood, S., Kidder, D., & Birnbaum, H. (1986). An alternative in terminal care: Results of the National Hospice Study. *Journal of Chronic Disease, 39*(9), 9–26.

Grobe, M. E., Ilstrup, D. M., & Ahmann, D. L. (1981). Skills needed by family members to maintain the care of an advanced cancer patient. *Cancer Nursing, 4*(5), 371–375.

Grobe, M. E., Ahmann, D. L., & Ilstrup, D. M. (1982). Needs assessment for advanced cancer patients and their families. *Oncology Nursing Forum, 9*(4), 26–30.

Higginson, I. J., & Sen-Gupta, G. J. (2000). Place of care in advanced cancer: A qualitative systematic literature review of patient preferences. *Journal of Palliative Medicine, 3*(3), 287–300.

Hull, M. M. (1993). Coping strategies of family caregivers in hospice home care. *Caring, 12*(2), 78–88.

Izquierdo-Porrera, A., & Trelis-Navarro, J. (2001). Predicting place of death of elderly cancer patients followed by a palliative care unit. *Journal of Pain and Symptom Management, 21*(6), 481–490.

Kirschling, J. M. (1986). The experience of terminal illness on adult family members. In B. M. Petrosino (Ed.), *Nursing in hospice and terminal care: Research and practice*. New York: Haworth Press.

Krant, M. J. (1974). *Dying and dignity: The meaning and control of a personal death*. Springfield, IL: Charles C Thomas.

Legg, B., Kaffenbarger, K. P., & Remsburg, R. (2000). Prevalence, effectiveness and predictors of planning the place of death among older persons followed in community-based long-term care. *Journal of the American Geriatrics Society, 48*(8), 943–948.

McCusker, J. (1983). Where cancer patients die: An epidemiologic study. *Public Health Reports, 98*(2), 170–175.

Moinpour, C. M., & Polissar, L. (1989). Factors affecting place of death of hospice and non-hospice cancer patients. *American Journal of Public Health, 79*(11), 1549–1551.

Mor, V., & Birnbaum, H. (1983). Data watch. Medicare legislation for hospice care: Implications of National Hospice Study data. *Health Affairs, 2*, 80–90.

Mor, V., Schwartz, R., Laliberte, L., & Hiris, J. (1985). An examination of the effect of reimbursement and organizational structure on the allocation of hospice staff time. *Home Health Services Quarterly, 6*(1), 101–117.

Torrens, P. R. (1985). Hospice care: What have we learned? *Annual Review of Public Health, 6*, 65–83.

Yates, P., & Stetz, K. M. (1999). Families' awareness of and response to dying. *Oncology Nursing Forum, 26*(1), 113–120.

Seven

Stories of the Living Dying: The Hermes Listener

Paula G. Balber

Paula G. Balber received a master's degree in psychiatric nursing in 1970 from New York University. Since that time, she has counseled both individuals and families in outpatient and inpatient clinical settings in psychiatry and oncology. She has been a hospice nurse and clinical director of several hospice programs. Ms. Balber has lectured extensively on family dynamics and individual issues involved with cancer, chronic illness, and death and dying. She has published on care of the dying in Prevention and Treatment of Complications in Oncology for Physicians, *edited by John Laszlo, and* Stories of the Living Dying *in* The Forum, *the newsletter for the Association of Death Education and Counseling. The verbatim story material in this chapter comes from a two part video-tape project she co-directed,* Telling Times: Stories of the Living Dying, *funded by the North Carolina Humanities Council.*

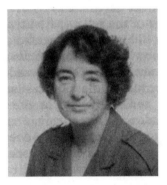

Well, I was born in . . . I was born March 6, 1909; on that same night, there was a little white girl which my mother had worked there in the kitchen. They lived in the house and my daddy run the gin. This old man had a gin and his daughter was born on the same night I was. And, of course, her mother didn't have any milk at all, and she asked the doctor and the doctor asked my mother, or so they told me. Her brother told me, if it hadn't been for my mother, his sister would have died. And I've heard her say, and I've heard so many people say, and of course she did that and this little girl, I seen her, I seen her myself as we grew up and we played together in the yard.

Brian S., 79 years old, 1 month before death

Stories are accounts. They are chronicles, descriptions, statements, narratives, history (Churchill, 1989). Throughout our lives, particularly as we journey through transitions, we tell stories, if only to ourselves, about the experiences that form and shape us. As each of us becomes aware that our known life is ending and that, as Janoff-Bulman notes, our assumptions about ourselves, the world, and what is meaningful often shatter in the face of this knowledge, the need to tell stories, "narrative hunger" named by Reynolds Price (Churchill, 1989), often becomes more compelling as we face the transition to death (Janoff-Bulman, 1992). During this time, in particular, people tell stories about their lives, past, present, and future, to family and friends, and to the health care professionals who work with them. For the listener, personal stories, like that told by Mr. S., evoke powerful images of the "self" of the storyteller and his formative experiences, and in a profound way, reveal the familial, historical, cultural, and religious/spiritual forces that shaped that individual's life and how he approaches death. For a professional working with the living-dying, those with illnesses in which death is certain (Pattison, 1967), it is a privilege and responsibility to hear the stories of a person's life. They are a source of psychic education for the listener and teller both, and a means to enhance the quality of the life of the teller (patient) and the family.

This chapter focuses on people whose stories are stimulated by the knowledge of certain death. The population described was dying from cancer or AIDS. The words of the storytellers you read here are verbatim accounts unless otherwise noted. We will examine the personal stories of several people in the context of the living-dying process as it is traditionally conceived, and as it can be framed within the universal story of the "Hero's Adventure," the monomyth of the archetypal journey to a renewed, transcendent self (Campbell, 1968). This chapter also focuses on ways to facilitate the telling of the stories, to understand the possible meanings of the material for that individual, and to incorporate this information in working therapeutically with those who are living-dying and their families.

To begin, we will review briefly some cultural, familial, and intrapersonal aspects of living-dying:

> When I was in Vietnam, I was a fighter pilot. One day, we were on our third mission into the jungle and my best buddy was navigator. Suddenly, out of nowhere a rocket blew up the back end of my plane; I was on fire when I parachuted out of the burning plane and was rescued by some other guys, Americans. I had third degree burns over half my body and was in the hospital for months. My buddy was blown to Hell.
> (paraphrase) James R., 35 years old, immediately after being told he had weeks to live

Advances in medical technology and shifts in medical ethos mean that most people are told these days when they have a fatal illness. Knowledge that an illness will end in death catapults people and their families into a state in which the world is no longer familiar. Once they are told that their lives are coming to a close, people become aware that both their bodies and the reactions of those around them seem unpredictable and may remain unpredictable. For some, like James R., this information, abruptly delivered, exploded a carefully reconstructed life, blowing buried trauma up to the surface, and served as a harbinger of things to come. For others, the sentence may be shocking, but not surprising, because they have experienced ongoing illness and increasing debilitation. In any case, for all, their lives are never quite the same; each becomes the living-dying, a marginal being.

In our culture the sense of an isolated, marginal state of the living-dying is quite pronounced. As a society, we are so intent on progressing, achieving, and acquiring, that the dying, who are only being and yielding have little place; indeed, many of us fear or feel helpless in the face of this inevitable state. From members of the medical establishment who regard them as treatment failures, to younger relatives who may despair the loss and know that, with this death a buffer against their own deaths disappears, we encourage the dying to fight and hold on, and we support the ongoing lack of awareness that death is approaching. In addition, because so much of the dying takes place unattended in hospital rooms (May, 1989), when we are dying we are deprived of a known path and role models to guide us through this experience. Thus, an important form of psychic education, as well as support, is lost, not only to those now dying, but to all of us who will eventually face the same experience. This lack of education impoverishes us and renders us all the more vulnerable to greater distress.

In a number of cultures, however, by virtue of tradition or historical events, death is held in the individual and community consciousness long before the event, and preparation for it is an important task both for individuals and the community. For example, in Mayan Indian culture, death is a phenomenon for which one carefully prepares, in one way, by living with the coffin to get to know it. In addition, chosen members of the community are gathered around to hear recommendations for future behavior (Price, 1988). In Ireland, elderly villagers look for premonitions that death is coming, and pray that God will grant them "a 'holy death,' a slow, gradual, even painful death, one that is met head on: alert, awake, aware, and with full faculties of sense and reason" (Scheper-Hughes, 1983, p. 140). Lifton describes Hiroshima survivors, although isolated within the larger society, as having an acute awareness that death is within them, the sense of a permanent encounter with death (Lifton, 1976a, p. 23).

Most Americans, by contrast, live their adult lives in the realm of awareness of what might be called "middle knowledge," first described by Avery Weissman and elaborated by Lifton, "where we both know that we will die and resist and fail to act upon that knowledge" (Lifton, 1976b, p. 23). Even if people are aging and have already acknowledged that death is nearing, in reverie, reminiscence, and in the preparations for disposing of belongings, including their bodies, middle knowledge often prevails, in part because of our society's traditional response.

In addition, for most people, even when death is welcome, the disruption of the familiar (both internal and external), the perception and treatment by others that demonstrates we are no longer our familiar selves, and the threat of all the unknowns, provokes a rise in anxiety and fear, both for patients and families. Shneidman (1978) describes this as a dire situation in which the person will behave as he has in response to previous experiences of threat or failure. Loss (past, present, and future) and grief permeates this phase as well (Block, 2001). Depression occurs in 17–50% of cancer patients (Breitbart, Rosenfield, et al., 2000; Goldberg, 1988). Along with depression, fear, and anxiety, patients and families experience other psychic distress. Guilt and shame predominate when people believe that it is their behavior that has caused the disease, when they have many regrets about the past, when they feel responsible for burdening their families financially, or for causing the reprioritizing of family time and the expenditure of physical and emotional energy necessary to meet their needs (Lewis, Haberman, & Wallhagen, 1986; Lewis, 1989; Welch-McCaffrey, 1988). Some also experience guilt for abandoning family members who are dependent on them. In addition, anger, frustration, and exhaustion are equal partners for patients and families, as they all struggle with the "being" that no longer performs, health care providers who may not take into account unique needs and requirements, and a world that moves along without consideration for them and their experience.

> We start dying the moment we are born. Death is woven into life and grows lives toward its own death, and from the death of things it outgrows. But, one day, death, in the real sense, approaches. It means growing through and beyond this literal dying, the ultimate growing beyond self. (Durckheim, 1990, p. 5)

Living-dying, unquestionably, is one of the most difficult stages that people and their families must endure, even if death per se is welcome. This is true, as Durchheim notes above, even as we have experienced the many other preparatory symbolic and literal deaths in our lives. There are, however, other dimensions to the experience. These dimensions may be empowering for those dying and educational for people with whom they are involved. Many people seem to live up to the experience, rather than just accommodate to it or be destroyed by it. They seem to acquire a recurring and thus enduring sense of grace, of being blessed, and honor or personal integrity, in the ongoing process of yielding to death.

In looking for clues as to how this evolves, one can review the literature that describes how people cope and who copes well, delimit the factors that offer support, and detail what it is that helps to give meaning to the experience; it is valuable information and this chapter will do some of that. However, there is that somewhat intangible, transcendent connectedness to the penultimate and enduring that threads the experience, surfaces periodically, and lends itself to the acquisition of attributes necessary for growing beyond the pain of dying. Perhaps, as the hermetic tradition states, "When you are ready to become a stranger to the world, you then receive the final teaching" (Kingsley, 1997, p. 22). Different religions and spiritual traditions would define the teaching as "knowledge of God" (Kingsley, Ibid), access to the divine within us (Atkinson, 1995, p. xii), or awareness of the primal Aum, the infinite sound that is the origin of names and forms, yet is beyond designation (Gangadean, 1999, p. 58). Yet this connectedness may be embodied even in those who disaffirm a personal spiritual/religious belief, and sometimes occurs in those one would never expect to be able to move beyond lifestyle and personal problems. It is inherently present in many acts of creativity, but it is especially evident in the metaphors of myth and literature.

Since in this chapter, we use myth to approach the transcendent relatedness, to encompass the spiritual/religious realm, and to frame the personal stories, it is important to define what we mean by myth. Many believe (especially pre-Joseph Campbell) that myth means tale, as in untruth, apocrypha. In fact, it is defined as, "the expression of the unobservable realities in terms of observable phenomena" (Leach, 1967, p. 1). "Mythology is poetry, metaphorical. It has been well said that mythology is the penultimate truth, penultimate because the ultimate cannot be put into words. Mythology pitches the mind beyond that rim to what can be known but cannot be told" (Campbell, 1988, p. 163). "The aim of myths and symbols was to reach man's higher centers, transmit to him ideas inaccessible to the intellect and to transmit them in such forms as would exclude the possibility of false interpretations" (Ouspensky, 1989, p. 4). Myths provide guiding images about ways to perceive the universe and order our experiences within it. They provide the role models for archetypal human experiences from this, "vast store of our ancestral knowledge and the latent potentialities of the human psyche" (Atkinson, 1995, p. 25). This often occurs without our conscious knowledge of the ways they affect us. Because they aid us to move beyond every day and ordinary constructs, because they connect us to the ubiquitous mystery, myths are particularly prominent in times of momentous personal transitions, such as in the living-dying process, when familiar ways of being and perceiving no longer exist, and what lies ahead is part of the mystery.

> There lived an old priest-magician, Hunnoes, who had identical twin sons, Mo and Ho. According to custom, his elder son should succeed him, but which was the elder? 'To whichever brings back the Bitter-Rose, I shall hand on the great knowledge.' Mo climbed Mount Cloudy to search for this flower of discernment which retreats at the first hint of fear and is like looking for night in broad daylight. Striking a rock with his hammer to place a screw ring, he accidentally kills a hollow man who lives in rock made of emptiness and who eats the void and drinks empty words. The next day they find Mo's empty clothes; he has been killed in revenge by the hollow men. Hunnoes tells Ho that he must kill his now hollow brother. 'Then Mo will live among us again.' Despite his bursting heart, Ho finds and strikes his brother's head and enters his body. With Mo's memories within him, now transformed, Moho finds and retrieves the Bitter-Rose, and Hunnoes was able to leave the world peacefully, having passed on the great knowledge. (Daumal, 1986, pp. 75–78, summary)

At the mythologic level, several (May, 1988; Atkinson, 1995; among others) describe this liminal stage of living dying as a kind of hero's adventure, based in large part on the description by Joseph Campbell. He speaks of the, "basic motif of the universal hero's journey, leaving one condition and finding the source of life to bring you forth into a richer or mature condition" (Campbell, 1988, p. 163). Daumal's myth of the fractured soul bespeaks the rigor of this spiritual journey, which end and begin in the birth of the transcendent being who can surpass surface dualities, and who can command greater wisdom. By necessity, the first step in any hero's journey is taking leave of the familiar (Campbell, 1968). For the living dying, the call to leave the comfortable world often comes from the messenger-physician who reveals the diagnosis and prognosis. Then, or soon after, according to myth, the hero encounters a protective figure, one who is a willing helper at critical times, a symbol of trust and guardianship, the conductor of the soul to the afterworld, a role such as Hermes, the Divine Herald, enacted in Greek mythology (Hamilton, 1942). For the dying, this figure might be a health care professional, clergy, or one who in previous days was simply friend or family; in any case, the guardian is a wise being who lures the hero to the threshold and aids in the crossing. The barrier is formidable, but according to Campbell, it must be overcome in order to reach the next stage of the journey, the descent into confusion, fear, and grief filled darkness.

The darkness may be seen as the unconscious (Campbell, 1968) or as that glide we take backward in time and inward, deep into the psyche, where we meet our personal demons and the demons of our family and culture (Atkinson, 1995). It may also be seen as the confused, frightened state that occurs when internal and external guiding images are destroyed. Temptation arises during this time (Atkinson, 1995), temptation to retreat into old, familiar patterns, temptation to deny the prognosis, temptation to avoid the beauty and harshness of this world and ourselves. For the dying this darkness is evoked by the trials of illness, the overwhelming losses and role transitions, by the unbidden eruption of pain laden past events, and frightened projections onto an unknowable future. This step also involves battling the hollow men, the powerful defenders of inscribed values and personal limitations that keep us from knowing important truths about our living and dying and about that which supports transcendence. Finally, however, if successful, people come to terms with the darkness through transformation of consciousness in which they are held within the enfolding arms of a greater wisdom. This brings with it a tolerable sense of choosing death (Callan, 1989), a measure of peace with the past. and one's altered identity, and a sense of relative ease about what lies ahead. In addition, there are those who may evolve into a more whole, enlarged presence with a greater capacity to guide and teach us from their seat of newly created wisdom.

One way many living-dying people traverse the necessary path of this journey, open to illuminating revelations, and gain grace, integrity, and transcendence, is by weaving personal stories, personal myths. Life review is often the grounding for these stories. Influenced by hopes and wishes for the future, many people interpret and symbolize moments of the past in order to serve present needs and to allay fears (Hulbert, 1988; Molinari & Reichlin, 1985). Much of these stories become the substance of life review, a term designated by Butler (1963), and later described as, "an attempt to come to terms with old guilt, conflicts and defeats, and to find meaning in one's accomplishments" (Lo Gerfo, 1980–1981, p. 42). In particular, people find renewed meaning and a path through the disorienting darkness by remembering the lustrous moments of the past. In this way the living-dying can keep alive treasured images of the self to preserve their sense of a continuous identity (Castelnouvo-Tedesco, 1980), and they can perpetuate important portions of that identity to provide for their symbolic immortality, their families, who will remember them in self defined ways after death (Unruh, 1983). In addition, people denote important memories that preserve family values and traditions. The very first story of this chapter, in which Brian S. reminisces about his mother saving the life of a white child, is a story meant, at least in part, to pass on his family value of color blind generosity and goodness. People also create narratives about the present, especially their illness experience and its impact; they compose stories about the future, and reach outward to others, both past and present, to provide validating and affirming myth and accounts to guide the way. Personal, familial, cultural, and universal myth and symbol, history, and tradition inform each narrative. We know these more personal myths and stories are cloaked in a myriad of forms, each unique to the individual, and each bearing careful attending, but whether they are narrative of past, present, or future, they serve a number of more generalized functions. The functions of the narratives can be delimited as four: (1) to cope with the illness and its sequelae of fear, grief, and loss (2) to mark a path through the darkness to transcendence, to renewed life (3) to chart and verify meaning in life, and (4) to ensure the continuity of the self and valued wiser images for the individual and those left behind. In their completeness and complexity, narratives may serve several of the functions at once; however, affirming the connectedness with the transcendent often forms the leitmotif throughout the stories of those who are living dying. Literature and experience indicate that the healing process begins with the telling of the story (Danforth & Glass, 2001, p. 515).

Given the above, listening well to stories is a complex and fertile encounter. As Boston, Towers, and Barnard point out, we may never entirely understand the entirety of the journey (Boston, Towers, & Barnard, 2001). However, as a health care professional, if one listens and responds empathetically to story, one becomes part of the narrative and merges into the lived experience. Then, to listen with skill is to assume some part of the role of the willing helper, protective guardian, the "Hermes listener." This is the model described in death and dying literature, as well as in myth, as the one who provides safe conduct (Benoliel, 1985). If one wishes to help the traveler surmount the boundaries and mark a path through the darkness, rather than enact the polar opposite (to guard the surface boundaries, support the hollowness, and halt the journey), there is a necessary therapeutic framework within which to enact one's role. First, it is important to join in the journey with constancy, without abandoning it, until the point at which people must proceed alone. One's professional work should be undergirded by the belief that the patient (and family) is the primary expert in understanding his or her needs, in evaluating the responses to intervention, and in making informed decisions about the care.

This structure is also supported by an attitude that embraces the Rogerian attributes of attentiveness, acceptance, and empathy, yet this framework is only an outward manifestation, and is itself powered by a mythic force. The force that lies beneath and beyond is the silence within, "the primal silence in the tumult" (Durckheim, 1989, p. 7). It is "the stillpoint, calm and strength in the face of threat (proceeding from the belief) that one's internal and external environments are predictable and there is a high probability that things will work out as well as can reasonably be expected" (Jevne, 1987, p. 1). From this stillpoint comes the energy to sustain concentrated, unbiased attention, such that the observer disappears and enters wholly into the experience of being with the living-dying moment by moment. This stance, particularly when encouraging and responding to story, "elicits unbidden insights" from the narrator and provides the direction for the listener so that "one becomes attentive simultaneously to multiple layers, the message beneath the words, the histories behind events, the language of gesture and stance, as well as the subtle selectively that must follow, combining the intuitive and the conscious" (Hejamdi, 1990, pp. 70, 73). In the focused process of attending, one's skills in the therapeutic use of story may be applied with apt timing for the most useful psychological moment, and the practitioner will know what will work to achieve the therapeutic end.

In addition, if one assumes that the stories one hears will be enlightening for both teller and listener, and the prevailing attitude is one of receiving as well as giving, then listening and responding, de facto, become an act of genuinely enhancing a vulnerable self. Further, if one honors story as part of the unique journey of an individual and family, the style in which it is told is valuable in and of itself. The process of the telling, with its dips backward and forward, in the end provides much of the coherence and the meaning of the material to the individual and the therapeutic listener. Reifying story into a rigid, structured series of psychological episodes which one must do in order to have a good dying does violence to the narrator and to the coherence and meaning of the story. Finally, one must be aware in listening to story that, "it is our own stories which give shape to what we hear, about the way we look at lives, which matters we choose to emphasize, which details we considered important, the imagery we use as we made our interpretations" (Coles, 1989, p. 18).

Actually, lately, it's been pretty good for the last couple of days. Last week, though, I was having real bad diarrhea, and I had to wear diapers and little panty shields to protect my clothes. I'm real conscious of how I look; I wear shorts a lot. The only thing is with the shields, when I walk, I can hear the plastic kind of crinkle. It's real embarrassing, so I wear them only when I have on jeans, but then it makes me look like I have a big rear end. For the last 6 months, I've had mouth problems. It's the thrush, and something is eating little holes in the back of the palate of my mouth. It's gotten to the point where I brush my teeth with Novocain. (Paul M., 24 years old, diagnosed with AIDS)

As health care professionals, more often than not we are told explanatory accounts of illness. These accounts initiate the journey and the relationship, and occur throughout. Indeed, they frequently form the majority of the stories of the present. They serve the first function of narrative: to cope with the illness and its sequelae. As such, they demand careful attention.

As a health care practitioner, it is vital to respond first to the illness narrative with competent suggestions and care for symptom relief, as well as assurances that the journey is indeed a joint venture. As each new symptom appears or old ones reappear or are not successfully managed, the patient must know that each will be attended to as long and as often as necessary.

As a Hermes listener, one responds to illness accounts with empathetic, reflective listening that matches the storyteller's patterns, that is, responding with words such as "real embarrassing" if the teller (such as Paul) uses those words, and by matching the patterns captured by the major themes. "It's so hard when you want to look good and you're stuck with noisy diapers and panty shields and Novocain." "It sounds as though you are realizing that you are just not looking or feeling like you want to." This captures the primary salient issues, bears witness to the pain, and encourages more reflection. It provides the invitation to explore a deeper understanding of what causes pain and to "cleanse the soul" by experiencing and letting go of the negative emotions that are the inevitable accompaniment of these experiences. If, as caregiver and witness, one attends to the entirety of accounts such as Paul's, week after week and month after month, they will provide the entrée to a number of explicitly difficult issues of living-dying: changes in body image; concerns about sexuality; the effect of loss of potency and self control. By absorbing the whole and the flow, one can gain appreciation of the depth and power of the illness and its unique meaning to each individual. One can then help the storyteller work through the pain and mourn the losses. This is the grief work, the coping with the illness, that Worden so clearly elucidates as necessary for healing (Worden, 1991).

It is equally vital, if one is to help the teller move into the realm of the transcendent (the second function of story), to include responses to these pain-filled accounts with questions such as, "What keeps you going?" or, "What gives you the courage you clearly have to deal with all this?" This balances the account and stimulates the teller to become more conscious of the strengths, the positives, and the possibilities of becoming the hero in his or her own story, the one who can move through and beyond darkness. The listener also seeks to move the relationship beyond these pain filled accounts of physical and emotional difficulty to narratives that evoke more implicit, deeper meaning and to stories of past and future. It is important to do so, for one reason, because these stories of other parts of the narrator's life and the exploration of deeper meanings of the present put the illness in perspective as part of a continuum, as only one segment of a larger whole. Thus the recent past and present, replete with suffering, does not remain imprinted as the entirety of a life, for the patient or the family (Lewis, 1989).

One may ask many traditional questions to stimulate stories that evoke meaning (the third function of storytelling), from past, present, and future, such as, "What was your childhood like?" "Tell me about your family." "What did you do for a living?" "What do you think will happen next?" However, Doris Betts, a short-story writer and teacher, suggests other, creative means to stimulate story, "that shiny trail of words like a snail would leave, all silver" (Betts, 1989). She suggests such questions as, "Do you have any objects that you cannot throw away?" "What were your lucky breaks?" "Where were your life's turning points?" "What is your favorite memory?" "How was your life different from what you expected?" "In what family members do you recognize yourself?" "What would you like to have done instead of the work that you chose?" "How have you coped with the deaths of one's you've loved?" (Betts, 1989).

These questions are only some that open the door to deepening and enriching accounts. As we demonstrate our willingness to listen to people, it helps to let them know that they belong in this experience with us, and that we value their presence. Often, then, stories erupt, unbidden by us.

We waited up for nights to see where the fire would blow next. The fire, it took all the woods behind my house. My neighbor's house burned down. It was amazing; it skipped around; you couldn't predict where it was going to burn next. I got out there, made sure we put a barrier around the lawn. I was out all the time with the fire doing what I could, watching. We weren't sure we would have a house standing until the fire burned out. It was horrifying. Those days, they seemed like they lasted forever.

(paraphrase) David, with a known prognosis of only a few months to live.

If we return briefly to the monomyth of the hero's journey, the first step for the living-dying is the vault from the realm of the ordinary, triggered by the news of impending death. Both David L. and James R., like many others, spontaneously reacted to the peripherally accepted news by employing the common metaphor of fire from which they both escaped, damaged, but alive. This metaphor powerfully captures the experience of hearing the news of one's impending death, and requires the careful attention of the Hermes listener. It bridges the connections with the mystery, and it bespeaks the overwhelming force and unpredictability one feels when enveloped in it. In the eternal language of symbols, fire also represents transformation by destruction, purification, and regeneration. It is the seed from which each successive life is reproduced (Cirlot, 1962). With its symbolic light, one may glimpse the entirety of the journey and the path to be traveled.

Fire also represents a desire to annihilate time (Cirlot, 1962). When embarked on the journey and connected to the mystery, people often describe time as out of joint and at a standstill. Both ways of experiencing time represent the reality and also a desire (for time to be at a standstill) of many of the living-dying, for whom time, from the moment of being told, no longer marches evenly, but instead lurches between everlasting seconds and foreshortened days (Feigenberg & Shneidman, 1979). This alteration of time sense helps impel the crossing of the boundary into the darkness.

Since a sense of one's days following one another in regular rhythm is destroyed with the news, telling stories, particularly stories such as these, in which fire annihilates time, is an act of control. The storyteller creates new beats of time by, "keeping the past available through memory and conquering the future in advance by anticipation" (Hulbert, 1988, p. 297). This act of control or coping involves self-regulation rather than behavior that more actively alters external conditions, a path that is closing to those dying. It is one way to "turn passivity and helplessness into mastery and action" (Kastenbaum, 2000, p. 279). Storymaking also provides a safe way to discharge the painful emotions, which are the constant companions of the darkness of the illness journey, without endangering important social relations. In addition, although it is true that many avenues of active coping are closed to those living-dying, the stories can remind the narrator of active coping used in the past ("I was out all the time doing what I could"), and may stimulate actions which are still feasible. Finally, these allegorical accounts provide a way of soliciting the listener to affirm that the narrator handled events as well as possible. If a part of terminal illness is the responsive feeling of failure and lack of self-confidence, stories like David L's seek in fact, to validate that, "I did the right thing," a theme commonly embedded in illness accounts (Price, 1987). If honored as responses to threat that reaffirms strength in the face of great difficulty, they set the stage for the narrator to remain perceived as a competent human being throughout the darkest times for him or herself and for the family.

When responding to stories such as these, it is often useful to remain within the metaphor, to highlight the active coping behaviors that are still available, and to reinforce the sense of mastery they offer to the individual, without necessarily taking note of the connection with the illness directly. Paradoxically, then, the therapeutic effect often can be achieved when the listener identifies with the narrator in experiencing the horrors of the fire and the awe filled responses it evokes, without either of them ever directly mentioning that these same feelings are engendered by news of impending death and by the illness and sequelae.

The most memorable example of this type of coping and response to the illness and sequelae occurred with a black policeman dying of multiple myeloma. At first, almost devoid of emotion, he would recount very brief illness stories and say little else about himself. However, in time, one could always locate how far he had progressed in his journey and determine just how he was feeling, from his constant, vibrant stories about how he had integrated the upper echelons of the police department of this small southern city. In these symbolic accounts, he related how he had dealt with authority, how he had bested a foe while resisting temptation to openly lash out, how he had dealt with the ongoing stress of hostile undercurrents, and finally, how he had made alliances with old enemies, and achieved a peace in his department. His somewhat unidimensional metaphor-dependent style of storytelling reminds us that the capacity to talk openly about difficulty varies with each person, and that our ways of remembering, talking about, and coping tend to run in grooves; we have a certain repertoire (Castelnuovo-Tedesco, 1980). By allowing and encouraging his narratives (which were, in fact enlightening), by focusing on the emotion they engendered, and by highlighting the coping skills he used to succeed in his department (which involved a great deal of self-regulation), he was able to maintain control throughout his illness, discharge many of his painful feelings, and achieve some sense of a completed journey.

For this policeman, creating these narratives with his nurse also stimulated him to teach his wife what she needed to know in order to handle the finances and plan for the future for her and their 10-year-old son. He also made very explicit funeral plans and engaged promises from several members of his family to look after his wife and son. These activities and others, performed between bouts of extreme disability, proved that he was doing what he could and helped him feel successful in his climb out of his darkness toward death. They also clearly validated for him and for his listeners the value and meaning he attributed to his life. His self described multiple acts of courage, forbearance, and wisdom in knowing when to openly confront his enemies and when to let be, became, in the telling, a source of pride for him and an education in handling ever-present hostility and testing for the listener. As the months progressed, it became clear to both of us that, in his work as a policeman and in his work to negotiate this journey, he had opened into a more fully empowered human being filled with grace, dignity, and wisdom.

Most people are not like this policeman in his unidimensional metaphor-dependent style of storytelling. If one validates their feelings and their unique methods of coping within the symbolic experiences, it frees them to become more direct as needed. This, in turn, can heighten the sense of experience profoundly shared, lessen the common fear of being unable to tolerate what lies ahead, and thus help enable the living-dying to cross the boundaries to, and then through, the darkness.

Telling stories to a skilled, responsive listener provides just one part of the impetus to cross the threshold and negotiate the darkness. Often, however, the illness experience itself, and the reactions of the people around will impel the crossing into darkness and beyond. As those dying are isolated from society and their inhibitions are burned away by that isolation and by the trials of illness, they often gradually develop an honesty that is less tempered than usual by fears of social reprisal. This honesty encourages many to face the fact that they are going to die. In turn, this encourages a freedom people do not usually experience and provides the undergirding for the path through the darkness. The anthropologist, Langness, using Heidegger as his model, describes a person facing death squarely as a "being as whole, who can thus act authentically, not leveled by the average mode which we adopt in order to live as social beings" (Langness & Frank, 1981, p. 94). There are also those in psychiatry who postulate that what is being introduced and exposed is the self as essence, the constant, unique self that resides at the deepest levels of the psyche, and is unchanging despite life's vicissitudes. This is the self that transcends death (Anscombe, 1989). If we take a more spiritual approach, we might think of this as the birthing ground of that spiritually mature being, the expanded self, which encompasses both the local self and that which touches and enfolds part of the divine, God, the primal Aum.

The move toward the expanded realization of this self, complete with anger, fear, and honesty, is difficult work. It is made manifest in one way by Brian S., who, grinding his fist in his hand, can describe to the first white people to enter his house, his anger at being called "Boy" at the age of 60. He can bitterly recount the times he was treated unfairly by a white foreman at his job in a tobacco plant.

> And he put me up there; I was getting on up in age there; he put me with the young men. But somehow or another I had done it so long that it wasn't no bother to me, and I was throwing off the sheets (of tobacco), and I was really tired. So he said, 'All right boys, jump down and get a quick drink of water and hurry back.' I say, 'Well, I wants a drink of water, but I can't do no running.' But I was tired, and I went and got this water, came back, and ever since then it was a push and a shove and something in the path.

Although Brian S.'s ability to recount the story in part, reflects the greater freedom wrought by changes in our society in the 1960s and 1970s, clearly, it also took personal courage and a leave-taking of imprinted culture to relate it to us, a group of seven white people. Many of his angry assertions ended in defensive undoing, "I love everybody, black, white, everybody." Or, "Lord, if I have done wrong, please forgive me," which signified the anxiety engendered by fears of reprisal.

If not censored, the narrator continues to move toward authenticity. When told to the listener who acts to bear witness and who validates the meaning of the experience, it provides, once again, for discharge of painful emotion through which the storyteller can release emotional attachment to past events and then to societally determined interpretations of one's life. For Brian S., it meant being able to partly lay to rest the bitterness and anger inherent in so much of his life and story.

In addition, he was able to move on to stories about his family, and was able to appreciate that for them, the times had changed enough that his sons and daughters had succeeded in their well-paying, higher status jobs. It became a source of pride to him (and to his listening family), through the storytelling, that he had paved the way for his children, his symbolic immortality, with his ability to remain in a hated job and provide for his family, while encouraging them to stay in school, church, scouts, and fight in the civil rights movement. It balanced the account of his life.

It is a therapeutic gift that the listener brings when he or she helps the narrator enlarge and expand the time frame and sense of self to include important others. It helped Mr. S., and in turn, his family, perceive him (and then them), quite rightly, as "hero" instead of just victim. Thus, through the dance all do together, the old embittered images die, a new one is born, and now, as a man, not a boy, he is perceived as someone with courage and wisdom. Brian S.'s family listened to him much more carefully than before over the next few weeks before he died. They heard with new understanding his stories about his failures and successes. To his family and the listeners, on many levels, he emerged from the darkness and "brought back the boon" of courage, fortitude, and perseverance from his adventure (Campbell, 1968, p. 30). This storytelling also functioned to support the continuity past death of this enhanced self of Brian S., as it will appear in his family after his death, both in stories about his life and in the ways they are changed by these new perceptions and wisdom. It also moved him and his family to appreciate themselves more as part of an ongoing whole, no longer just local, sui generis selves. Thus, in the end, paradoxically, the move toward authenticity and greater "is-ness" of the person acts to pave the way for the final dissolution of the individual as such, and to provide the seeds for the assumption of a more universal, transcendent being.

For the listener, ongoing contact with this kind of authenticity has great value. Not only does it illuminate the ways in which historical, cultural, and familial forces operate and affect individuals, but it can also stimulate a responding authenticity in the willing participant. This teaches the professional much that is useful for the continued work with the living-dying, although it may make it somewhat more difficult to live as comfortably in ordinary society.

> The only time I think about religion, I kind of backslide and go back to bargaining when I'm scared and depressed and alone. According to a woman at work, this is Hell; whatever lies beyond must be better. ("Is this what you feel too?" Listener) I'm beginning to. It's been really hard being by myself. I've got my parent's financial support. I've got my friends, but I really have nobody. I've got lots of bodies, but nobody I can count on. When the time comes and I need somebody, I'm afraid there won't be that person. It is hard to be in a hospital bed and fall into a relationship. (Paul M., 24 years old, AIDS patient)

The confusing darkness descends as the living-dying disconnect from society and its imprint, spend more time in withdrawn musings of events gone by and portents of the future, and continue to face momentous shifts and losses. This forces continued reevaluation of one's whole structure of meaning (Benoliel, 1985). For those like Paul, "What was formerly meaningful may become empty of value" (Campbell, 1968, p. 55). In the ongoing upheaval of the world of the living-dying, especially in the time of darkness, value and priority are often reexamined, sometimes perceived to be outworn, and a reordering and redefinition of meaning often takes place, yet again. In addition, when the diagnosis of cancer or AIDS is accompanied by an early death sentence, such as for David L. and for James R., the search for meaning is stimulated by both diagnosis and certain death, and what remains to hold meaning is inevitably different than if death were not ineluctable.

> I barely made it last time. This time, I don't know. I retired right after I got home. Thank God I had the money, and I enjoyed every minute of my last year. I worried some about the leukemia coming back, but each day I did what was important. Sometimes it was just sitting with my wife and fishing; it wasn't anything like I used to do, traveling and selling; I loved my job, but it didn't matter any more.
>
> (Paraphrase) David L., awaiting the results of his bone marrow biopsy after two rounds of induction chemotherapy to treat his relapsed leukemia

Storytelling is one way of reordering priorities and values, and demarking or validating new meaning in experience for one's remaining life. It provides the undergirding for the transformed self, in part by helping people move beyond anxiety and depression (Lewis, 1989; Brady, Peterman, & Fitchett, 1999). For some, there is both time and the ability to create new lifestyles to match the transformed self. For David L., as for most people, success at work loses importance, and primary relationships with caregivers, family, and friends assume new importance, as they must for the journey to be completed. Studies by O'Connor, Wicker, and Germino (1990) and the discussion by Martens and Davies (1990) validate the observations that derived meaning from significant relationship become critically important in the living-dying. For example, one hospice patient frequently reminisced about his early life with his older brother, whom he had not seen for many years after a fight whose details he could not remember. With each story, his regret grew over the loss of the significant relationship. The listener noted (to herself and eventually to him) that, for him, it no longer seemed as important to be right, no matter what the cost, as it had when he was younger, and there was instead a growing importance and value in spending his shortened time with family. As a result of these conversations, the patient decided to call his brother and make amends. A satisfying reunion was the direct outcome of his narratives and the therapeutic intervention. He had, in essence, finished some unfinished business with this reunion, and seemed more content.

The paraphrased story of David L., who retired to be at home with his wife, illustrates narrative's function as a mechanism of validation for the already enacted shifts in consciousness and behavior. By asking for descriptive detail, and by focusing at great length on these newly important experiences, as the psychologists Bandler and Grinder suggest, the listener helps imprint the meaningfulness of the changed behavior (Bandler & Grinder, 1975). "Tell me what your day was like at home with your wife?" "What is your fishing spot like?" Answers to questions such as these make vivid and palpable the satisfaction gained and support the value of the experience. The listener also periodically asks for continued evaluation of the changed behavior and its meaning. "What is it like being home with your wife?" "Are there other ways you need to spend your time as well?"

Paul's story of the Hell of his loneliness points the way for other work. Formerly content to have "many bodies," his consciousness has shifted and his priorities have been reworked. Unfortunately, there is no way to satisfy the new mandate for involvement with one who cares only for him. As the helping guardian, one can grieve the unfulfilled need with Paul and encourage those relationships that supply some measure of succor. In his work as a nursing assistant with AIDS patients, Paul described circumstances in which he gave and received affection. Helping him ascribe value and meaning to these interactions was a helpful interaction. In essence, it enlarged Paul's appreciation of his experiences of relationships, supported his hope of at least partial fulfillment of his needs for loving connectedness, and decreased his sense of despair. Callan's study validates the great value of this kind of hope in the living-dying (Callan, 1989). In addition, it is equally important to encourage and aid Paul to make concrete plans to attend to his stated need for a caregiver when he gets sicker.

For many, there is also a shift to a renewed emphasis on faith, noted by O'Connor, Wickam, and Germino (1990). Paul's open lack of vital belief and fearful uncertainty about an afterlife is a common theme of the stories of the terminally ill. For them, religious beliefs may have little meaning until death approaches. Only then, grounded in desire or fear, do people construct a belief in a benevolent afterlife or condemnation in Hell. Others find that their faith and religious belief provide meaning in the experience, mark the path of connection with the transcendent, and/or ensure the continuity of the self. For those, like Brian S., faith in God provides the ever-present meaning and sense of order in the past, present, and future. It was quite clear he felt he had nothing to fear on his judgment day. His words, which follow, reflect reliance on God's control and ultimate benevolence amidst the painful, meaningless, earthly darkness in which he had lived.

> Sometimes the old devil get busy and do everything he can to turn people against you. He'll do everything he can to turn people against you. You've got to watch

as well as pray. You think you're doing good, and you think you're doing maybe better than you are. Sometimes you have to sit down and have a day's conversation with the Lord. But, in my life, I believe He will make a way for you. The devil and all his people can't do you no harm. The Lord, he suffered for Job to lose everything he had, but after a while he restored all of it back. Elijah was the same way, and I believe if he get ready for me, look for me somewhere in heaven, I'll be there.

It is also apparent that for Mr. S., like many, nearness to death evokes concerns about wrong doing or sin. This is in part a response to the distress and losses inherent in the illness journey which re-evoke images of other losses and failures. However, equally for many, there is a religious-spiritual power that fuels the fear, the shame, and the guilt they experience. The darkness becomes a time when, as the Talmud states, "Reflect upon three things: from whence you come; to where you are going; and before whom you are destined to give an account" (Spero, 1981–1982, p. 39).

At times, when listening to story, it is not immediately obvious that it is guilt, shame, and religious-spiritual angst that are in fact being exposed. One must often hear countless versions of the same story, themes with variation, "as every aspect of the past is recalled and examined in detail" (Brown & Stroudmire, 1983, p. 380). The reward for doing so is to access both the painful emotions and their source. These rise slowly to the surface in small bits that can be psychically tolerated. Then, the task for the guardian aspect of the Hermes listener is to symbolically hold the storyteller with more frequent visits and increased closeness to help him or her tolerate the inevitable despair, for one must face the despair and travel through it to achieve integrity (Rosel, 1988) and transcendence. The search for atonement becomes a frequent theme in stories (Atkinson, 1995, p. 97). It becomes important to help the storyteller forgive him or herself, to find God's forgiveness, if appropriate, and make reparations, even symbolically. The story of Anne Marie, below, as it evolves, becomes one of great pain and grief about her perceived "sins" and illustrated the evolution of meaning in the repetition of stories.

At first, the story of Anne Marie, a middle-aged woman dying of lung cancer, evokes a sense of self quite opposite from that of Brian S. The ex-wife of a minister, she had always lived a determinedly independent lifestyle even when, in her own words, discretion might have been more prudent. She preserved her image of self-sufficiency in the face of the dependence of illness and dying by recounting many incidents citing her breaks with tradition. Anne Marie reached out for validation of her confrontive independence to the novels of Ayn Rand, whose narrations celebrate unique and self sufficient achievement.

> The first thing he (her husband) came home with, they (his congregation) wanted me to wear a hat to church. He thought this was kind of trivial. There was no reason why, if they wanted me to wear a hat to church, I wouldn't wear a hat to church. I more or less told them, "Hell No!" No way would I let someone else control my life to that extent.

In this episode, Anne Marie appears to be celebrating and preserving her triumphs. She told endless symbolic versions of the account above. "I didn't want to have my baby shower with church women, and I didn't." "I refused to let my husband go to such and such seminary." "I plugged in the church phone only when he was home." "He was a minister. I was not a minister's wife." Each was described as an episode of triumph, but all impelled the inevitable trajectory to divorce, ambivalently wished for, and in the end, actually sought by her husband, who refused to continue counseling despite her pleas to do so. As each variation emerged, her sadness and pain deepened and feelings of guilt and shame arose. Her fear about dying became quite pronounced. At one point, she said that she felt as if she were paying with her life for her past sins related to the church and her marriage. Clearly, she was describing sins of breaking church societal rules, as well as violating the moral values of her religious tradition that frowned upon divorce in the 1950s. This brings to mind Satterly's statements about religious pain, "In most people, guilt asks for and always receives (or perceives) punishment (and spiritual pain). Rooted in shame, spiritual pain sees only an unmasking by God, an occurrence that coincides with death. It is virtually impossible to accept the unconditional love of God while at the same time imposing self judgments of the most severe kind" (Satterly, 2001, p. 32 and p. 36).

To begin to help, the Hermes listener responds with the love inherent in the ever present nonjudgmental attending and validation of feelings. As Anne Marie began to speak more often of God and the church family, she became aware as she talked, that in many instances, church members had been attempting merely to reach out to her. She had originally perceived their contacts as intrusive and abusive. At the listener's suggestion, she sent the remaining elders of the church a thank you letter, an act of contrition, as it were.

The shame and guilt she felt having separated her children from a willing church family was harder to resolve. Again, at the listener's suggestion, which she fearfully but quite willingly embraced, she invited her somewhat estranged children to visit and talk about the past. Anne Marie was able to express her sorrow to them and to ask their forgiveness. They did, in fact, forgive her on some levels, but strain among them was still obvious even as she was actively dying. However, they very clearly acknowledged to her the great gift she gave them in the strengths she role modeled for them which helped make them successful women. Her fierce independence was well noted by all as a strength she relied on to help her create a happier life for herself after the divorce. The family kept in contact until she died. She had declined to write a letter to her ex-husband, which she could send or not as she pleased, but she did keep a journal in which she recorded her feelings about their marriage.

Anne Marie's unfinished business. She said she felt more at peace, her fear about death lessened, and she seemed somewhat renewed and lighter in spirit. One might believe that on some level she forgave herself and believed God had forgiven her as well. "God's forgiveness does not undo the past but helps instead heal the brokenness of the past so as to enable new and renewed community in the future" (Jones, 1993, p. 356).

As we have seen with Anne Marie, and with Mr. S., as his life story melts from sadness and grief into triumph, the phenomenon of triumphal episodes reversing into tragedy over time or tragedy into triumph, is not unusual, as storyteller and listener contemplate the patterns in a life review. Noting the patterns and shifts at the psychologically apt moment helps the narrator perceive discrete events (especially the tragic/triumphal ones) with a new perspective. This ultimately aids the work of evaluation and synthesis. In fact, in the end, the narrator may come to appreciate when the flow of discrete events merges into a whole, each event contains seeds of the dualities of triumph and tragedy, sadness and joy.

The new synthesis provides the wisdom that helps people let go and feel as if their life's work is done. Further, it releases energy previously bound up in old patterns and despair, so that they can live more comfortable lives as they are dying. It makes it possible for them to live more fully in the present, to enjoy the moment's silence, the image of a loved one, a cup to tea, or the sadness and grief more deeply, clearly felt. With this release of energy, and from within the new wisdom, some storytellers begin to emerge into a transcendent, more universal, less local being. This reborn hero is then free to offer to family and other listeners the gift of wisdom and enlarged presence, "the boon," as Campbell names it.

There are times in some lives when too many losses or too much tragedy can overwhelm a storyteller. The Hermes listener must use clinical judgment and skill to attempt to prevent this and/or deal with the ensuing crisis. He or she works to prevent crisis by partializing fears and grief, so that some form of resolution comes with each new episode that circles around the intense memories. Each successful, even if symbolic, resolution (such as sending the thank you letter for Anne Marie) serves to guide and strengthen the sense of creative action, puts some closure to the intense experience, and provides a strengthening role model for the next episode. When handled in this manner, even if the storyteller never finishes all the work that may be apparent to the therapeutic listener, there is a sense of completeness to the journey for the teller and those important to him or her, no matter when the death occurs.

> I love him and I'm ready to go meet him at any time. I think about it a whole lot, most specially when you're laying in there by yourself and half dreaming and wishing, wishing I was with you right now or you were with me. Maybe it won't be too long now. As far as places I see him, it's places we've always been. It's not no strange place at all. I think I'll meet him just like he left me, remembering everything, and I can't help but feel that way. Some people may think, 'Well, she's crazy,' and I don't deny that, but when I know a thing, I know it. Fran said when I was in the hospital and she was holding me, they were trying to do something, and she said I looked right straight at her, and I said, "Would you please let me go; there is somebody waiting for me." I hope the children won't grieve and carry on. I hope they'll be just as happy in my death as I've been in life and expecting in death. So far, I've shedded no tears over it, and I don't think I will. (Ellen C., 65 years old, 2 weeks before her death)

The reunion myths may be perceived not only as a means to cope with catastrophic loss of all that is known or beloved, but also as a revitalizing vision of what lies ahead, apocrypha or not. As people near death, many, not just Ellen C., from the haven of a happy marriage, experience visions of older family or friends who have already died, or of infinite God, beckoning to a world of light. These may be creative acts or biologically driven responses, but as others, such as Atkinson say, "These archetypal experiences lift us out of the realm of the occasional and transitory and into the realm of the ultimate and ever enduring" (Atkinson, 1995, p. 39), or as Campbell notes, "The hero ventures forth from the world of the common day into a region of supernatural wonder" (Campbell, 1968, p. 30). The familial guides are one manifestation of the continued belief in the unbroken line of the human family (Pattison, 1967) or connection with the eternal. For others, such as one older man who had been newly diagnosed with widely metastatic lung cancer 6 months before, visions of approaching death are less literally linked to people or to God. He, who had been silent for days, sat up minutes before his last breath, and in awe, described approaching death as a wondrous opening, a doorway. Most people, of course, yield quietly with no words of description.

We leave this life richer for the journey, even those of us one would not ordinarily note as transformed. None of us ever really negotiates this journey and remains a "common man." This can be true of those we perceive as the least of us. To grieve and rejoice in the inheritance of the past (acknowledged to oneself or another), to live most fully through the pain and bittersweet pleasures of the present, and finally, to confront and release all of known future is, indeed, transformative. According to Campbell (1968, p. 84), this occurs, in part, because:

> The unconscious brings forth life potentialities that we never managed to bring to adult realization. Those other portions of ourselves are there; those golden seeds do not die. If only a portion of that lost totality could be dredged up into light of day, we should experience a marvelous expansion of our powers, a vivid renewal of life.

Flawed as he was (and as we all are) and remains, yet spurred by impending death, Paul M. exemplifies the metamorphosing power of mastering the darkness; he achieved a kind of integrity. Born to the super-rich and status-conscious, he had been neglected and sometimes abused as a child. He left home at 17 years old to join the Navy, from which he received a dishonorable discharge. From then on, he lived with whomever would provide a bed and some semblance of concern for him. His drifter life style (supported financially by his parents) stopped when he was diagnosed with AIDS. Although he had many upsetting quarrels and upheavals with others in the AIDS community, he endured, to doing work with dying AIDS patients. He began as a volunteer, but then successfully completed the nursing assistant certification program and, with pride, maintained a job in the local hospital, working with AIDS patients. He started psychotherapy when he began his volunteer work and spent many hours telling his story, attempting to come to terms with his demons from the past and ingrained habits that continued to haunt him. The following is his story about his work as a volunteer. The narrative reflects his newly developed awareness of the needs of others, although the listener and Paul himself cannot help but be acutely mindful of his projections in the face of the coming role-reversal. It also reflects again the idea of bringing back the boon, the new wisdom, and either living it and/or passing it on in stories told to family and others.

> I think a positive attitude helps. I give support; I stay with the patient when the families go out, like for groceries. I like it to be comfortable and smooth for the patient. If they're scared, it's going to be a miserable death. If you have really

close friends, and you know they care for you, then I don't think the transition to the acceptance stage is so hard. This is why I throw myself into work and going out and making friends, and I've just started crocheting, to keep my time occupied, so I don't keep thinking about it. I know it's there; I'll always know it's there. You know, but I wanted to do what I could, and I guess it's my own guarantee that they'd be there for me when I needed it. I usually run away, except for this; when it comes to this, I think it's because of such a personal effect. If I were to run away from it, I would be denying it.

Although Paul will never be the embodiment of what one might usually think of is the hero, a fully transcendent being, few people actually are. He is, however, very much a hero of his own life story and to others in the AIDS community who marveled at his transformation. Like many of us, however, he matured throughout his illness, and he gained both grace and honor in the process. His ability to give and receive "universal love" with his patients was a gift he gave and received. In part, telling and reworking his story with a Hermes listener (exploring new meaning in his life; creating a budding self that he could treasure and from which would continue his symbolic existence; dealing with his past griefs and losses) was invaluable in helping him to create a new being who found some peace in the past and in the inevitable future. He became an enlarged, more completely whole presence throughout his remaining life. From whence he came, he was transformed. In his unique fashion, as well as he could, he lived to represent the following wisdom from Ellen C., her reply when asked what she thought important to pass on to the next generation:

> Keep on living to the best of your ability and love everybody. Live a happy life and be kind to each other. Take care of each other and live for each other, not just for self. Love them and let them know you love them.

What emerges from the storytelling, for Paul or Ellen, or for any of us, is the hero, "at peace with death, who has died not as the modern man, but as eternal man—perfected, unspecific, universal man—he has been reborn" (Campbell, 1968, p. 20).

> Whatever can be Created can be Annihilated: Forms cannot:
> The Oak is cut down by the Ax, the Lamb fall by the knife,
> But their Forms Eternal Exist Forever. Amen. Hallelujah!
> William Blake (as cited in Powell, 1982)

Discussion Questions

1. List the four functions of the stories of those who are terminally ill. From your own experience, give an example of each.

2. List ten ways to elicit story that are not already mentioned in the chapter.
3. If you were told you only had six months to live, what would you want to tell people important to you?

References

Anscombe, R. (1989). The myth of the true self. *Psychiatry, 52,* 209–217.

Atkinson, R. (1995). *The gift of stories.* London: Bergin and Garvey.

Bandler, R., & Grinder, J. (1975). *The structure of magic.* Palo Alto: Science and Behavior Books.

Benoliel, J. (1985). Loss and terminal illness. *Nursing Clinics of North America, 20*(2), 439–448.

Betts, D. (1989). *Life Stories in Literary Perspective.* Paper presented at the conference: Telling Times: Stories of the Living-Dying, Chapel Hill, N.C.

Blake, W. (1982). Jerusalem. In J. Powell, *The Tao of symbols.* New York: Quill.

Block, S. (2001, June 13). Psychological considerations, growth, and transcendence at the end of life: The art of the possible. *Journal of the American Medical Association, 285*(2), 2898–2905.

Boston, P., Towers, A., & Barnard, D. (2001). Embracing vulnerability: Risk and empathy in palliative care. *Journal of Palliative Care, 17*(4), 248–253.

Brady, M. G., Peterman, A. H., Fitchett, G., et al. (1999). A case for including spirituality in quality of life measurements in oncology. *PsychoOncology, 8,* 417–428.

Breitbart, W., Rosenfield, B., et al. (2000). Depression, hopelessness and desire for hastened death in terminally ill patients with cancer. *Journal of the American Medical Association, 284,* 2907–2911.

Brown, J. T., & Stoudmire, G. A. (1983). Normal and pathological grief. *Journal of the American Medical Association, 250*(3), 378–382.

Butler, R. (1963). The life review: An interpretation of reminiscence in the aged. *Psychiatry, 26,* 65–76.

Callan, D. (1989). Hope as a clinical issue in oncology social work. *Journal of Psychosocial Oncology, 7*(3), 31–46.

Campbell, J. (1968). *The hero with a thousand faces.* Princeton: Princeton University Press.

Campbell, J. (1988). *The power of myth.* New York: Doubleday.

Castelnuovo-Tedesco, P. (1980). Reminiscence and nostalgia: The pleasure and pain of remembering. In S. J. Greenspan & G. H. Pollak (Eds.), *The course of life: Psychoanalytic contributions toward personality development.*

Churchill, L. (1989). Overview: Life stories and terminal illness. Paper presented at the conference: *Telling Times: Stories of the Living-Dying.* Chapel Hill, N.C.

Cirlot, J. E. (1962). *Dictionary of symbols.* New York: Philosophical Library.

Coles, R. (1989). *The call of stories.* Boston: Houghton Mifflin.

Danforth, M., & Glass, Jr., J. (2001). Listen to my words; give meaning to my sorrow: A study in cognitive constructs in middle age bereaved widows. *Death Studies, 25*(6), 513–521.

Daumal, R. (1986). The mountain. *Parabola, 13*(4), 75–78.

Durckheim, K. (1989). The call for the master. *Parabola, 14*(1), 4–14.

Durckheim, K. (1990). The voice of the master. *Parabola, 15*(3), 4–13.

Feigenberg, L., & Schneidman, E. (1979). Clinical thanatology and psychotherapy: Some reflections on caring for the dying person. *Omega, 10,* 1–84.

Gangadean, A. (1997). The awakening of primal knowledge. *Parabola, 22*(1), 56–59.

Goldberg, R. (1988). Psychiatric aspects of psychosocial distress in cancer patients. *Journal of Psychosocial Oncology, 6*(1/2), 139–162.

Hamilton, E. (1942). *Mythology.* New York: New American Library.

Hejmadi, P. (1990). Dhyana: The long, pure look. *Parabola, 15*(2), 70–76.

Hulbert, R., & Lens, W. (1988). Time and self-identity in later life. *International Journal of Aging and Human Development, 27*(4), 293–302.

Janoff-Bulman, R. (1992). *Shattered assumptions: Toward a new psychology of trauma.* New York: Free Press.

Jevne, R. (1987). Creating stillpoints: Beyond a rational approach to counseling cancer patients. *Journal of Psychosocial Oncology, 5*(3), 1–15.

Jones, L. G. (1993). The craft of forgiveness. *Theology Today, 50,* 345–357.

Kastenbaum, R. (2001). Riding the tiger: The challenge in later years. In M. Bloom & T. Gullotta (Eds.), *Promoting creativity across the life span.* Washington, DC: CWCA Press.

Kingsley, P. (1997). Knowing beyond knowing. *Parabola, 22*(1), 21–26.

Langness, L. L., & Frank, G. (1981). *Lives: An anthropological approach to biography.* Novato, CA: Chandler and Sharp.

Leach, E. (1967). Genesis as myth. In J. Middleton (Ed.), *Myth and cosmos* (p. 1). Garden City, NY: Natural History Press.

Lewis, F. (1989). Attributions of control, experienced meaning, and psychosocial well being in patients with advanced cancer. *Journal of Psychosocial Oncology, 7*(1/2), 105–119.

Lewis, F., Haberman, M., & Wallhagen, M. (1986). How adults experience personal control. *Journal of Psychosocial Oncology, 4*(4), 27–41.

Lifton, R. (1976a). Psychological effects of the atomic bomb in hiroshima: The theme of death. In R. Fulton (Ed.), *Death and identity.* Baltimore, MD: Charles Press.

Lifton, R. (1976b). The sense of immortality: On death and the continuity of life. In R. Fulton (Ed.), *Death and identity* (p. 23). Baltimore: Charles Press.

LoGerfo, M. (1980–1981). Three ways of reminiscence in theory and practice. *International Journal of Aging and Human Development, 12*(1), 39–46.

Martens, N., & Davies, B. (1990). The work of patients and spouses in managing advanced cancer at home. *Hospice Journal, 6*(2), 55–73.

May, W. (1989). *Sacred image in narrative.* Paper presented at conference: Telling Times: Stories of the Living-Dying, Chapel Hill, North Carolina.

Molinari, V., & Reichlin, R. (1984–1985). Life review reminiscence in the elderly: A review of the literature. *International Journal of Aging and Human Development, 20*(2), 81–91.

O'Connor, A., Wicker, C., & Germino, B. (1990). Understanding the cancer patient's search for meaning. *Cancer Nursing, 13*(3), 167–175.

Ouspensky, P. D. (1989). The transparent veil of symbolism. *Parabola, 14*(2), 4/8.

Pattison, M. (1967). The experience of dying. *American Journal of Psychotherapy, 21,* 32–43.

Powell, J. (1982). *The Tao of symbols.* New York: Quill.

Price, L. (1987). Ecuadorian illness stories: Cultural knowledge. In D. Holland & N. Quinn (Eds.), *Natural discourse in cultural models in language and thought.* Cambridge, England: Cambridge University Press.

Price, L. (1989). *Life review as a window on culture.* Paper presented at conference: Telling Times: Stories of the Living-Dying, Chapel Hill, North Carolina.

Rosel, N. (1988). Clarification and application of Erik Erikson's eighth stage of man. *International Journal of Aging and Human Development, 27*(1), 11–23.

Satterly, V. (2001). Guilt, shame, and religious pain. *Holistic Nursing Practice, 15*(2), 30–38.

Scheper-Hughes, N. (1983). Deposed kings: The demise of the rural Irish gerontocracy. In J. Sokolovsky (Ed.), *Growing old in different societies* (p. 140). Belmont, CA: Wadsworth.

Schneidman, E. (1978). Some aspects of psychotherapy with dying persons. *Psychosocial care of the dying patient.* New York: McGraw-Hill.

Spero, M. (1981–1982). Confronting death and the concept of life review: The Talmudic approach. *Omega, 12*(1), 37–43.

Tillich, P. (1987). To whom much was forgiven. *Parabola, 12*(3), 38–46.

Unruh, D. (1983). Death: Strategies of identity preservation. *Social Problems, 30*(3), 340–351.

Welch-McCaffrey, D. (1988). Family issues in cancer care: current dilemmas and future directions. *Journal of Psychosocial Oncology, 6*(1/2), 199–211.

Weissman, A., & Worden, W. (1976). The existential plight in cancer: Significance of the first hundred days. *International Journal of Psychiatry in Medicine, 7,* 1–15.

Worden, W. (1982 & 1991, 2nd ed.). *Counseling and grief therapy: A handbook for mental health practitioners.* New York: Springer-Verlag.

Eight

Symptom Management for the Terminally Ill

Fredrica A. Preston, Siew Tzuh Tang, and Ruth McCorkle

Fredrica A. Preston, RNC, AOCN, is an oncology nurse practitioner at North Shore Cancer Center in Peabody, Massachusetts. She received her BSN from Georgetown University and her MSN from New York University. Ms. Preston is an active member of the Oncology Nursing Society and has practiced oncology nursing since 1975, in clinical, administrative, and educational roles.

Siew Tzuh Tang, RN, DNSc, is an assistant professor of School of Nursing, National Yang-Ming University, Taiwan. Dr. Tang was a former deputy director of the Department of nursing at Sun Yat-sen Cancer Center in Taiwan. She established the first oncology home care program in Taiwan, to provide primary hospice home care service to cancer patients.

Ruth McCorkle, PhD, FAAN, is a professor and chair of the doctoral program at the Yale University School of Nursing, where she is director of the Center for Excellence in Chronic Illness Care. Her career began as an oncology clinical nurse specialist in Iowa. Subsequently, she established at the University of Washington and at the University of Pennsylvania nationally recognized graduate programs in cancer nursing. She is internationally known for her research with patients with progressive cancer and for the measurement of patient and family outcomes to improve the quality of their lives.

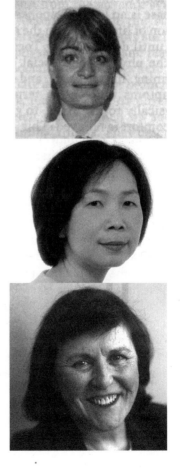

Living with a terminal illness is a challenging life experience, for the person, family members, and professional caregivers. To enhance the quality of the person's experience, within the context of continuing medical treatment and supportive services, requires a coordinated effort among the parties involved. The prevention and management of symptom distress in terminal illness are essential parts of palliative care. For purposes of this chapter, cancer is used as a prototype to illustrate the essential components of symptom management. We discuss factors that directly and indirectly affect the health professional's ability to manage symptoms of terminally ill patients. Included is a discussion of the philosophy, principles, and politics of symptom management.

Curative versus Palliative Approaches

Scanlon (1989) defines the goals of palliative care as "the amelioration of symptoms and disease-related problems and the promotion of the patient's well being and comfort" (p. 492). *Palliative care*, as used here, is defined as the active, compassionate care of terminally ill patients at a time when their disease is no longer responsive to the traditional aims of cure and prolongation of life, and when the emphasis of care is on comfort, quality of life, and fulfillment of psychological, social, and spiritual needs until death (Caring Together, 1987; World Health Organization, 1990). Palliative care embraces principles founded in the physical and social sciences, and requires ongoing assessment, planning, intervention, and evaluation of the physical and psychosocial symptoms inherent in terminal illness. Ministering physically to the dying is not enough—to give a pill or injection and feel confident the discomfort is relieved. Such action supports the belief that patient care is a unidimensional phenomenon, requiring treatment of physical symptoms only. If the focus of palliative care is to be on the person and not the symptom, a multidimensional approach is mandated. Benoliel (1976) has advocated that a balanced perspective on care and cure requires that health care providers be attentive to the impact of disease on the person as well as the body.

Although palliation seems the obvious treatment of choice in terminal illness, there are some diseases in which the choice is not clear-cut. For example, in situations in which the goal of treatment for cancer is not well defined, the individual's goals should direct the focus of care. Cure is a realistic treatment goal for many people with cancer. Hodgkin's disease, testicular cancer, and childhood leukemias are only a few of the cancers considered curable with aggressive, multimodality therapy. The emergence and continued growth of cancer survivorship groups are testament to the fact that, with earlier diagnosis and multimodal therapy, cancer is a curable disease in many cases.

However, cure is not always a realistic goal. The American Cancer Society (2001) predicted 553,400 people would die of cancer in 2001—more than 1,500 people a day. For these patients, treatment and care goals need to be shifted from cure to palliation. Benoliel and McCorkle (1977) have defined quality of life in palliative care as having to do with the opportunities available to the ill person for the achievement of personal goals during whatever period of time the individual has available. The Institute of Medicine (IOM) (1997) Committee on Palliative Care suggested that high-quality end-of-life care should free patients and their families from avoidable distress and suffering; provide care in accord with the patients' and families' wishes; convey that dignity resides in people, not their physical attributes; and help people preserve their integrity while coping with unavoidable physical insults and losses.

Symptom Management: Broadening the Scope

Traditionally, the management of symptoms has been restricted to the physical dimensions of the ill person's problems. With the development of palliative care as a subspecialty of all health-related disciplines, the field has broadened to include the emotional and family dimensions, as well as the physical ones.

Physical Dimensions

We know from clinical experience that some of the major personal problems associated with terminal illness result from the physical symptoms of disease and from the progressive deterioration of the body. Terminal illness is often accompanied by distressing symptoms, such as nausea, anorexia, dyspnea, and pain. These physical changes and resultant functional limitations lead to a state of social dependency, in which the person becomes literally dependent for intimate activities not ordinarily performed by other people (bathing, toileting, feeding, etc.). As physical deterioration occurs, terminal illness is often accompanied by social isolation, a feeling reported by people as they decline. Patients describe people withdrawing from them, and information is controlled that may have implications for the ill person's future (Holland, 1982).

Emotional Dimensions

When family members and health care providers withhold information about the disease and treatment, patients are effectively cut off from talking about their fears and other concerns (Quint, 1966). Terminally ill patients are confronted with multiple fears, including fear of pain and suffering, increased dependency, loss of identity, the unknown future, and death (Buckman, 1998; Seravalli, 1988; Wortman & Dunkel-Schetter, 1979). Patients with cancer often feel as if their own bodies are out of control (Buckman, 1998; Fiore, 1979). They feel helpless because they are unable to affect the course of their own disease. Yet talking with receptive family members and health providers about the person's prognosis, the future, concerns, and fears may not be easy to do, even when full information is provided about the illness and its predictable future. Among the reasons frequently reported by professionals for not talking to patients about their condition is the concern that patients will become depressed and unduly concerned (Buckman, 1998; Dubler & Post, 1998; Vachon, 1995). Not talking with patients about the meaning of their experiences and their understandings of what is happening only adds to their sense of help-lessness, psychological tension, and fear of abandonment (Krant, 1976; Vachon, 1998a).

Family Dimensions

In addition to the patient, family members experience the stressors imposed by terminal illness and the multiple, difficult problems it introduces (Maguire, 1981; Oberst & James, 1985; Schachter & Coyle, 1998). Family communication patterns may change as family members try to protect themselves and others from painful feelings. Hiding feelings is a process many families go through, to withhold their emotional concerns from one another. As a result, many family members often bear their emotional pain alone (Northouse & Northouse, 1987; Stajduhar & Davies, 1998).

Living with terminal illness means restructuring family styles to deal with the demands of medical treatment and the impingement of the disease on usual roles and relationships (Stetz, 1987). Caregiving responsibilities generate competing demands that make family caregivers vulnerable to a host of physical and psychiatric symptoms and disorders (Lederberg, 1998; Stajduhar & Davies, 1998; Vachon, 1998b). In return, the inability of caregivers to meet patients' needs for practical assistance may compromise patients' physical well-being, and unnecessary hospitalization of patients may result (De Conno et al., 1996; Emanuel et al., 1999). If terminal illness is prolonged, it puts extreme pressure on existing social support systems within the family, including depletion of financial and social support resources. Results from the national Study to Understand Patient Prognoses and Preferences for Outcomes and Risks of Treatments (SUPPORT) showed that, by the time the patient had died, in more than 40% of cases, a family member had to quit work or make another major life change to provide care for the patient. Nearly one third of families lost a major source of income, and 25% of families lost most or all of their family savings. Such economic impact of terminal disease occurs 3–6 months before patients' deaths (McCarthy, Phillips, Zhong, Drews, & Lynn, 2000). Extended illness may cause further breakdown in patient and family relationships (Germino, 1991; Kristjanson, 1989; Northouse, 1984; Vachon, 1998b).

Philosophy of Symptom Management

We believe that the ultimate goal in palliative care is to help individuals maintain their integrity, by giving attention to that person's stated goals, wishes, and needs. We believe that the person and family must be informed about what is happening, who is involved, and the range of services available to assist them. We believe the family in which the ill person is a member is the unit of care. Family means one or more persons identified as important by the ill person. The persons identified may or may not be related by birth or marriage. All members of the family require information and ongoing opportunities for questions and discussion of alternatives to facilitate their understanding and participation. Patients and family members need access to information and emergency services on a 24-hours-a-day basis. Services recommended to patients need to be coordinated and planned through the cooperative efforts of all parties involved. Successful management is best achieved when there is congruence of expectations among patient, family, and provider, and mutually understood and accepted goals.

Diagnosis of a terminal illness can be conceived as catastrophic in nature, because it produces major changes in living for the individual and the family. Since the late 1960s, reports describing the degree of symptoms and pain experienced by patients with terminal illness have varied widely. Certainly not all patients who are terminally ill have symptoms that require management. We believe symptoms that the person perceives as distressing can and should be managed. Death, in itself, is unavoidable, but we believe that death without pain is surely the right of every human being. We believe that, if patients are denied opportunities to make choices about the management of their care, health care providers have failed to meet their professional responsibilities in helping the patient achieve a good death. We also recognize that some patients' goals, such as mental alertness, may be incongruent with the goals of symptom relief, if large doses of analgesics are needed. We believe that management decisions must always be guided by the patient's wishes.

Principles of Symptom Management

Symptom management is based on several principles that guide clinicians in the delivery of holistic, palliative care.

Symptom Management Is an Ongoing Process of Assessment, Intervention, and Evaluation

Symptoms vary in their etiology, intensity, duration, and response to treatment. Variations occur not only among persons, but also for individuals over time. Many people experience changes in their symptoms as their disease progresses. Ongoing thorough assessment is needed to identify the etiology of the symptom, and to achieve efficacy of treatment. For example, constipation can be caused by opioids, diet, bowel obstruction, or chemotherapy, each requiring a different management strategy. Administering a laxative, without further assessment, could be harmful to the patient with a bowel obstruction. Pain that was once controlled with MS Contin, 30 mg every 12 hours, may require a dose escalation to achieve the same effect. Assessment and intervention alone, without evaluating their effects, will lead to ineffective symptom management.

The Patient Has the Ultimate Choice in What Symptom Management Strategies Will Be Utilized

We can explain the reasons for the symptoms, offer suggestions about how they might be managed, and teach patients and families how to implement these management strategies. However, if patients believe that treatment of the symptom would further disrupt their lives, it is their right to reject or accept our suggestions. An example is those patients who, despite having been instructed on the importance of, and rationale for, a round-the-clock analgesic schedule to prevent the recurrence of pain, will not take medication when they do not have pain, and only take it when the pain escalates to the point of incapacitating them. The analgesic effect of the medication takes longer to be achieved, and the patient is at greater risk for the nonanalgesic effects of narcotics on demand, such as nausea and sedation. The obvious frustration this can cause caregivers can be tempered by the realization that the patient's autonomy and sense of control have priority.

Symptoms Are Best Managed Using an Anticipatory Approach

Both didactic and experiential lessons provide us two bases upon which the course of a disease or the effects of a treatment can be generally predicted with a reasonable margin of error. We know that the majority of patients on round-the-clock opioid therapy will develop constipation if a bowel regimen is not instituted at initiation of narcotic therapy. We know that a patient with end-stage esophageal cancer may soon develop dysphagia, and will need parenteral pain medication available for that time when the patient is unable to tolerate the oral medication. Anticipation of patients' needs, and provision of resources to meet them prior to their actual occurrence, maximize patients' comfort, with minimal interruptions in care.

We also recognize that end-of-life care is enhanced if problems are addressed at the earliest possible moment. Preventing pain is easier and more beneficial than reacting to established pain. Pain and other physical symptoms are not unique in this regard; emotional, psychosocial, or even spiritual suffering, not addressed during the early stages of an illness, will be more difficult to deal with during the final days of life. The focus of palliative care should be the weeks and months before death when symptoms and needs increase, and interventions can have a significant impact on the well-being of patients and families. The goal is to make the last weeks—not only the last minutes—of life valuable and meaningful.

Symptom Management Requires a Multimodality Approach

Symptoms are multidimensional composites of physical, emotional, and social dimensions. Adopting the traditional unidimensional disease-oriented approach to symptom management negates the interdependence of these dimensions. The first priority in symptom management is to relieve the physical discomfort. Patients who are not beset by physical problems have more free energy to deal with the myriad psychosocial issues commonly encountered as disease advances (MacDonald, 1998). Relief of persistent symptoms is best achieved through concomitant use of pharmacological and nonpharmacological measures. For example, anti-anxiety medications and opioids may be ordered for treatment of dyspnea, in conjunction with oxygen therapy and positioning. These interventions treat the symptoms, but not necessarily the person experiencing the symptoms. For this, the focus must shift to the emotional and social sequelae the symptom has for the patient and family. Are they fearful the patient may suffocate? What are their coping mechanisms for dealing with an obvious deterioration in the patient? Do they feel more assured when someone is with them? Do they have someone with whom to express their existential and spiritual concerns? These are but a few of the questions that demand further exploration and the utilization of a multidisciplinary approach that includes nurses, physicians, pharmacists, social workers, and clergy.

Common Symptoms

Symptoms may not always be directly related to a terminal illness, such as cancer. Symptom etiology must be established, because management is related to etiology, and routinely attributing other symptoms to the cancer can result in inappropriate treatment. Symptoms can be caused by direct tumor involvement, resulting in compression of nerves, blood vessels, and lymphatics (parasthesias, edema, hemorrhage), obstruction of vital organs (pain, constipation, nausea, dysphagia, choking), or invasion into any body part, as evidenced by site-specific symptomatology. For example, tumor invasion of the femur could produce symptoms of pain, decreased mobility, deformity, and edema. Symptoms may be also related to the secondary effects of treatment. Palliative radiation therapy to relieve an esophageal obstruction can cause gastrointestinal-related alterations, such as nausea, esophagitis, and dysphagia. Metabolic imbalances secondary to poor nutrition can lead to nausea, drowsiness, and parasthesias. Correction of the imbalance with supplements often leads to some relief of the symptom. See Table 8.1 for a list of common symptoms experienced in terminal illness, their prevalence, etiology, and potential pharmacological and

TABLE 8.1 Common Symptoms, Their Prevalence, Etiology, and Management Strategies

Symptom	Prevalence	Etiology	Pharmacological	Nonpharmacological
Anorexia	50–85%	1. Pain 2. Nausea and vomiting 3. Mucositis 4. Changes in taste and smell 5. Endogenous mediators (tumor necrosis factor, interleukin-1) 6. Emotional concerns	1. Corticosteroids 2. Antiemetics (if nausea is a problem) 3. Megace (megastrol acetate) 4. Periactin (cyproheptadine HCl) 5. Alcohol	1. Frequent small meals 2. Do not force foods. 3. Frequent oral hygiene 4. Supplemental feedings
Constipation	40–65%	1. Tumor-induced mechanical intestinal obstruction 2. Drugs: opioids, antacids, anticholinergics, diuretics, antidepressants, anticonvulsants, antihypertensive agents, etc. 3. Electrolytes imbalance: hypercalcemia, hypokalemia 4. Neurogenic: spinal cord compression 5. Physiologic: age, immobility, weakness, dehydration, low-fiber diet, poor intake 6. Concurrent disease: diabetes, anal fissure and hemorrhoids	1. Stool softeners 2. Laxatives 3. Senna	1. Establish prophylactic bowel regimen. 2. Discontinue nonessential, potentially constipating medication. 3. Increase dietary bulk. 4. Increase fluid intake. 5. Increase activity as tolerated. 6. Disimpaction

(continued)

153

TABLE 8.1 (*continued*)

Symptom	Prevalence	Etiology	Pharmacological	Nonpharmacological

Diarrhea	7–10%	1. Tumor-induced malabsorption or obstruction: pancreatic carcinoma, pancretic islet cell tumors, colon or rectal cancer
		2. Drugs: laxatives, antacids, antibiotics, NSAIDs, digitalis
		3. Fecal impaction
		4. Gastrointestinal infections
		5. Radiation
		6. Diet: bran, fruit, alcohol
		7. Concurrent disease: diabetes, hyperthyroidism, etc.
			1. Antidiarrheals
			2. Opioids
			3. Steroid enemas
			4. Cause-specific treatment:
			  a. Fat malabsorption: pancreatin
			  b. Radiation-induced: cholestyramine
			  c. Carcinoid syndrome: cyproheptadine
			  d. Pseudomembraneous colitis: vancomycin, metronidazole
				1. Increase fluid intake.
				2. Dietary modifications
				3. Meticulous perianal care
				4. Sitz bath

Dysphagia	Nonhead/neck cancer: 12–23% Head/neck cancer: over 80%	1. Tumor-induced obstruction or external compression: mouth, pharynx, esophagus, mediastinal tumor 2. Motor or sensory cranial nerve damage: brain metastases, cerebral tumor 3. Dry mouth 4. Mucosal infection: candidiasis, herpes simplex, herpes zoster, cytomegalovirus 5. Drowsiness or conscious disturbance	1. Antifungals 2. Steroids 3. Lidocain hydrochloride 4. Magnesium hydroxide 5. Change route of medication to liquid or parenteral	1. Good mouth care 2. Frequent small meals of soft food 3. Room-temperature food 4. Dietary supplements 5. Esophageal dilation 6. Radiation therapy (if caused by tumor compression)

TABLE 8.1 (continued)

Symptom	Prevalence	Etiology	Pharmacological	Nonpharmacological
Dyspnea	30–70%	1. Lung cancer or lung metastasis 2. Tumor-induced airway obstruction 3. Carcinomatous lymphangitis 4. Pleural or pericardial effusion, ascites 5. Pulmonary embolism 6. Pain 7. Anemia 8. Infection 9. Concurrent disease: congestive heart failure, chronic obstructive pulmonary disease 10. Psychological distress: anxiety 11. Metabolic acidosis	1. Opioids 2. Antianxiety medications 3. Diuretics 4. Steroids 5. Bronchodilators	1. Thoracentesis 2. Correct acidosis 3. Position of comfort 4. Oxygen 5. Reassurance 6. Radiation therapy (if caused by tumor compression)

(continued)

TABLE 8.1 (*continued*)

Symptom	Prevalence	Etiology	Pharmacological	Nonpharmacological
Fatigue	50–90%	1. Tumor-induced products: cytokine or tumor degradation products 2. Cachexia/malnutrition 3. Dehydration and electrolyte imbalance 4. Infection 5. Anemia 6. Pain 7. Psychological distress: depression, anxiety, sleep disorders 8. Drugs: opioids, sedatives, etc.	1. Corticosteroids 2. Antidepressants 3. Amphetamines	1. Modify activities of daily living. 2. Rearrange time schedules during the day to assure sleep at night and rest periods during the day.
Fungating growths (usually breast or neck area)	NR	1. Anaerobic infections 2. Necrosis	1. Cleocin rinses 2. Silvadine ointment 3. Dakins solution 4. Flagyl generic (metronidazole hydrochloride) 5. Chemotherapy	1. Frequent dressing changes 2. Odor control 3. Keep area dry.

TABLE 8.1 (*continued*)

Symptom	Prevalence	Etiology	Pharmacological	Nonpharmacological
Hiccup	9%	1. Irritation of vagus nerve: hepatomegaly, bowel obstruction, esophageal obstruction, etc. 2. Irritation of phrenic nerve: Intracranial tumors, tumor infiltration of diaphragm 3. Uremia 4. Infection: subphrenic abscess 5. Psychogenic	1. Chlorpromazine 2. Haloperidol 3. Metocloproamide 4. Midazolam 5. Amitriptyline	1. Rebreathe into paper bag. 2. Relaxation 3. Oropharyngeal stimulation with *safe ureter catheter*
Nausea and Vomiting	40–70%	1. Drugs: opioids, NSAIDs, etc. 2. Intestinal obstruction or constipation 3. Gastric carcinoma 4. Increased intracranial pressure 5. Metabolic disorders 6. Psychological factors: anxiety	1. Anticholinergics: scopolamine 2. Antihistamines: cyclizine 3. Benzodiazepine: lorazepam 4. Butyprophenones: haloperidol 5. Corticosteroids: dexamethasone 6. Phenothiazine: chlorpromazine 7. Metoclopramide 8. 5-H_3 receptor antagonists: ondansetron	1. Small, frequent meals at room temperature 2. Assess and treat underlying causes. 3. Discontinue any precipitant drug, or take it after food. 4. Provide adequate hydration.

(*continued*)

TABLE 8.1 (*continued*)

Symptom	Prevalence	Etiology	Pharmacological	Nonpharmacological
Airway secretions	NR	Fluid accumulation in lungs	1. Anticholinergics: scopolamine, buscopan 2. Morphine 3. Atropine	1. Reassurance to family 2. Suctioning 3. Position of comfort
Seizure	15–25% in patients with brain metastases	1. Tumor 2. Cerebral edema 3. Metabolic disorders 4. Hemorrhage	1. Steroids 2. Anticonvulsants 3. Diazepam	1. Assure open airway. 2. Protect patient from harm. 3. Correct metabolic disorders.
Sore mouth	NR	1. Monilial infection 2. Poor dentition 3. Malnutrition	1. Antifungal agents 2. Viscous xylocaine and diphenhydramine rinses	1. Frequent oral hygiene 2. Oral irrigations 3. Avoid alcohol or mouth rinses containing alcohol. 4. Dietary modifications

NR: Not reported.

nonpharmacological management strategies (Bruera, 1998; Bruera & Neumann, 1998; Komurcu et al., 2000; Turnbull, 1986; Twycross & Lack, 1984; Yasko, 1983). Since the 1970s, cancer pain has been extensively studied, and, subsequently, state-of-the-science knowledge and principles of cancer pain management have been established. In this chapter, cancer pain management is used as a prototype of symptom management for terminally ill patients; we recognize that knowledge and experiences gained from cancer pain management may be successfully transferred to other symptoms.

Pain

Pain is a mutifaceted phenomenon that affects a person's total being—physical, emotional, social, and spiritual. An estimated 70–90% of patients with advanced cancer experience pain at some point in their illness (Bruera & Neumann, 1998; Foley, 1998; Portenoy & Lesage, 1999). The actual or potential relief of pain is a major concern for patients and their families. Unfortunately, this concern is not warranted. Several large-scale and well-known studies showed that, among dying patients, pain remains inadequately treated, with a reported frequency ranging from 20% to more than 70% (Desbiens & Wu, 2000; Hanson, Danis, & Garrett, 1997; Lynn et al., 1997; McCarthy et al., 2000). For example, evidence from the SUPPORT study showed that more than one fourth of patients with cancer experienced serious pain 3–6 months before death, and more than 40% were in serious pain during their last 3 days of life (McCarthy et al., 2000). When cancer pain persists, when it appears not to improve, or when the patient begins to believe that there is no pain relief available, patients feel helpless and hopeless. Cancer pain threatens relationships with the outer world at the same time as it weakens the inner structure, pushing the person toward suffering. Cancer pain becomes patients' central focus and dominates their lives (Breitbart, 1989; Portenoy, Thaler, Kornblith, Lepore, Friedlander-Klar, Foley, et al., 1994). However, pharmacological and non-pharmacological treatments, based on available well-established treatment guidelines (Agency for Health Care Policy and Research, 1994; WHO, 1990), should ensure adequate pain relief in 95% of cases (Portenoy & Lesage, 1999). The primary reasons for this insufficient management of cancer pain result from the fact that voids still exist in understanding and application of existing knowledge of cancer pain management and in the individualization of pain assessment and management. Many clinicians have become too comfortable with a "cookbook" approach to pain management, so diligently looking at equianalgesic tables and drug dose escalation charts that they can lose sight of the person experiencing the pain and a basic tenet of pain management: Pain is a subjective, multidimensional experience, and patients are unique in their pharmacological and nonpharmacological needs, tolerance, and effects.

Successful pain management begins with the belief that the person has pain. Obvious as this statement may be, patients are often challenged to "prove" their pain exists before appropriate interventions are initiated. Assessment of pain is best conducted using a methodological approach. The American Pain Society and the AHCPR (1994) recommend that regular measures of pain be incorporated into routine health care and the patient medical record, such as the "fifth-vital sign." Major critical pain assessment criteria should include (Miaskowski, 1988; Portenoy & Lesage, 1999):

1. description of the pain: onset, pattern, quality, and course;
2. location and radiation;
3. severity (numerical scales are often utilized for rating pain, that is, 0 = no pain, 5 = worst pain, to allow the individual to rate his or her own pain, while providing consistency in criteria for comparison);
4. aggravating and relieving factors;
5. previous treatment modalities and their effects; and
6. meaning and impact of the pain: It is useful to ascertain how patients view their own symptoms. It has been recognized that the degree of perceived distress or suffering from a given symptom, and the physiological disturbance from a given disease, may not perfectly correlate (WHO, 1998).

Pharmacological Management

Along with effective communication skills, pharmacological management remains the keystone to successful pain control. Multidrug regimens utilizing opioids and nonopioids are employed to enhance pain control. Opioids work on the central nervous system, altering the perception of pain; nonopioids directly affect the peripheral nervous system. Factors to be considered in the choice of analgesics include age, route of administration, type and severity of pain, and clinical status. Elderly patients metabolize medications more slowly, and may need a dose modification to prevent drug accumulation and resultant toxicities. The other end of this age-related spectrum is the younger patient who may require increased doses or increased frequency of analgesics, because of a higher metabolism (Hanks & Cherny, 1998; Walsh, 2000).

The preferred route for analgesics is oral, and scheduling is around the clock, not simply on demand. The trend is to utilize sustained-release opioids (MS Contin, Roxanol), available in the oral form and administered every 8 or 12 hours. Patients on these long-acting opioids should also have immediate-release analgesics available for treatment of breakthrough pain. When the oral route is contraindicated, analgesic patches and suppositories are also useful, if large doses of opioids are not indicated. Parenteral opioids provide another alternative for optimal pain relief. Continuous parenteral infusions of opioids provide effective pain control and fewer side effects, and eliminate the "peaks and valleys" of bolus injections (Portenoy & Lesage, 1999; Walsh, 2000).

Opioids have the potential for contributing to the development of side effects, which usually diminish with continued administration and are responsive to interventions. The management of side effects of opioids is essential to cancer pain control, and can widen the therapeutic window by permitting the use of higher, more effective doses. The common side effects of opioid treatment include sedation, nausea and vomiting, constipation, and respiratory distress. See Table 8.2 for a list of commonly used opioids. Naloxone is a drug used routinely for opioid-induced respiratory distress, but it is usually contraindicated in terminal care. Naloxone is suggested only for life-threatening respiratory depression and/or severe sedation or coma (Hanks & Cherny, 1998; Walsh, 2000).

Fear of addiction remains a prime factor for undertreatment of pain. This fear is expressed by patients, family members, nurses, and physicians. Understanding the differences between addiction (psychological dependence), tolerance, and physical dependence are essential. Tolerance is a pharmacologic property defined by the need to increase doses to maintain the same effects (Passik, Portenoy, & Ricketis, 1998; Portenoy & Lesage, 1999). However, there is no maximum or ceiling dose for opioids. The right dose is the dose that controls pain without excessive or intolerable adverse side effects and that can be achieved through gradual adjustment of the dose (MacDonald, 1998; Portenoy & Lesage, 1999). In addition, tolerance to the analgesic effect of narcotics usually occurs in tandem with tolerance to the nonanalgesic effects (nausea, sedation, respiratory depression), offering little risk of increasing toxicity with increased dosage.

Physical dependence is defined as the occurrence of an abstinence syndrome (withdrawal) following abrupt dose reduction or administration of

TABLE 8.2 Opioids Commonly Used for Pain Management

Drug	Dose (mg) equi-analgesic to 10 mg morphine IM		Onset in minutes		Duration in hours	Side Effects	Comments
	IM/SC	PO	IM/SC	PO			
Meperidine (Demerol)	75–100	300	10	30–60	2–4	1. Nausea and vomiting 2. Constipation 3. Respiratory depression 4. CNS disturbance 5. Orthostatic hypotension	1. Poor PO:IM ratio and ineffective 2. May cause accumulation of toxic metabolites (Normeperedine), resulting CNS excitation (tremors, myoclonus, and seizures), especially in elderly or kidney failure patients 3. Not recommended for chronic pain management

TABLE 8.2 (continued)

Drug	Dose (mg) equi-analgesic to 10 mg morphine IM		Onset in minutes		Duration in hours	Side Effects	Comments
	IM/SC	PO	IM/SC	PO			
Morphine: Immediate release	10	20–30 60*	10–20	30–60	3–6	1. Nausea and vomiting 2. Constipation 3. Respiratory depression 4. CNS disturbance: sedation, confusion, hallucinations 5. Orthostatic hypotension 6. Urinary retention	1. Morphine is the drug of choice for routine management of moderate to severe opioid-responsive pain. 2. Special precautions for patients with severe respiratory impairments, asthma, hepatic failure or increased intracranial pressure 3. Doses need to be adjusted for patients with renal failure, to avoid opioid toxicity. 4. Because of the delayed onset of sustained-release morphine, an immediate-release morphine is recommended in the dose titration period.

(continued)

TABLE 8.2 (continued)

Drug	Dose (mg) equi-analgesic to 10 mg morphine IM		Onset in minutes		Duration in hours	Side Effects	Comments
	IM/SC	PO	IM/SC	PO			
Oxycodone	15	20–30	15–45		2–4	1. Nausea and vomiting 2. Constipation 3. CNS disturbance: Limited data suggest a lower likelihood of hallucinations than morphine.	1. Oral oxycodone combined with ASA (Percodan) or acetaminophen (Percocet), which provides 5 mg of oxycodone, is a useful drug for moderate pain in step 2 of the analgesic ladder. 2. Doses of pure oxycodone can be escalated for the effective management of severe pain in step 3 of the analgesic ladder.

TABLE 8.2 (continued)

Drug	Dose (mg) equi-analgesic to 10 mg morphine IM		Onset in minutes		Duration in hours	Side Effects	Comments
	IM/SC	PO	IM/SC	PO			
Codeine	130	200	15–30	30–60	2–4	1. Nausea and vomiting 2. Constipation 3. Respiratory depression 4. CNS disturbance: dysphoric 5. Orthostatic hypotension	1. Codeine is the most commonly use opioid for the management of mild-to-moderate pain. 2. Generally combined with aspirin or acetaminophen 3. Ineffective in those patients who lack a specific hepatic enzyme that converts codeine to morphine, or who are taking drugs that inhibit the enzyme's function, such as cimetidine

(continued)

TABLE 8.2 *(continued)*

Drug	Dose (mg) equianalgesic to 10 mg morphine IM		Onset in minutes		Duration in hours	Side Effects	Comments
	IM/SC	PO	IM/SC	PO			
Methadone (Dolophine)	10	20	10–20	30–60	4–8	1. Nausea and vomiting 2. CNS disturbance 3. Urinary retention	1. High mean oral bioavailability 2. Long plasma half-life, averaging approximately 24 hours. Therefore, there is greater likelihood of cumulative toxicity. 3. Methadone is not recommended for use in patients who: a. are elderly or demented; b. are delirious or confused; c. have raised intracranial pressure; d. are in respiratory, hepatic, or renal failure.

TABLE 8.2 (continued)

Drug	Dose (mg) equi-analgesic to 10 mg morphine IM		Onset in minutes		Duration in hours	Side Effects	Comments
	IM/SC	PO	IM/SC	PO			
Hydromorphine (Dilaudid)	1.5	7.5	15–30	15–30	2–4	1. Respiratory depression 2. CNS disturbance 3. Orthostatic hypotension 4. Urinary retention 5. Circulatory depression 6. Suppression of cough reflex	High solubility, the availability of a high-concentration preparation (10 mg/ml), and high bioavailability by continuous subcutaneous infusion, make hydromrphone suitable for subcutaneous infusion.

(continued)

TABLE 8.2 (*continued*)

Drug	Dose (mg) equi-analgesic to 10 mg morphine IM		Onset in minutes		Duration in hours	Side Effects	Comments
	IM/SC	PO	IM/SC	PO			
Levophanol (Levodromoran)	2	4	unknown	60–90	4–8	1. Respiratory depression 2. CNS disturbance 3. Orthostatic hypotension	1. Levorphanol is used as a second-line agent in patients with chronic pain who cannot tolerate morphine. 2. Discrepancy between plasma half-life and duration of analgesia may predispose to drug accumulation following the initiation of therapy or dose escalation. However, problems with drug accumulation is less than those produced by methadone. 3. Less GI toxicity than morphine

Note: The intramuscular and intravenous routes are usually recognized to be equivalent. The intramuscular route is not recommended for care of terminally ill patients.

*From single-dose study, however, for prolonged treatment with oral morphine, oral to parenteral relative potency ratios will be 1:2 or 1:3.

References: Cherny, N. I. (2000). The management of cancer pain. *CA—A Cancer Journal for Clinicians, 50*, 70–116.

Hanks, G., & Cherny, N. (1998). Opioid analgesiac therapy. In D. Doyle, G. W. C. Hanks, & N. MacDonald (Eds.), *Oxford Textbook of Palliative Medicine* (pp. 331–355). New York: Oxford University Press.

Walsh, D. (2000). Pharmacological management of cancer pain. *Seminars in Oncology, 27, 45–63*.

an antagonist (Passik et al., 1998). Gradually tapering doses of opioids can prevent the occurrence of withdrawal syndrome. Addiction is recognized as a psychological and behavioral syndrome, and is defined as the compulsive use of a substance, resulting in physical, psychological, or social harm to the user, and in continued use, despite that harm (Passik et al., 1998). Suboptimal dosing may in fact produce this psychological craving for opioids—pseudoaddiction—thereby creating a situation it intended to prevent (Passik et al., 1998). When effective analgesia is administered and pain relief is achieved, the aberrant behaviors of pseudoaddiction usually cease. Evidence from studies showed that psychological dependence to opioids, caused by pain treatment, is rare in individuals with no history of addictive disorders. The reported incidence of psychological dependence ranged from 0 to 5% (Dellemijn, Duijn, & Vanneste, 1998; Derogatis et al., 1983; Passik et al., 1998; Perry & Heidrich, 1982; Porter & Jick, 1980; Schug et al., 1992).

Adjuvant treatment of pain includes the use of medications traditionally utilized for other purposes. These include the tricyclic antidepressants, steroids, phenothiazines, and antihistamines. Nonpharmacological methods of pain control include radiation therapy, heat/cold massage, positioning, transcutaneous electrical nerve stimulation (TENS), distraction, relaxation, Reiki, acupuncture, and hypnosis. Selection of one or more of these methods must be individualized.

Politics of Symptom Management

The term *politics* is used here to mean the connections related to the health care system and its administration. Politics in the context of symptom management has to do with the operations of the members of the health care team in systems, the policies and philosophies of the institution, and the competency of health professionals in the science of terminal care and art of symptom management. Health professionals need to recognize the mission of their individual institutions, because palliative care is not always a priority. Professionals must balance their palliative care approaches with the goals of medical treatment. Unless professionals keep in mind the politics of their organizations, it is difficult to meet patient and family needs systematically. Political issues related to symptom management must be approached with "savvy" and thoughtfulness, especially since the issues are highly charged and emotionally laden.

Educational Directives for Symptom Management

Overall, the evidence suggests that the majority of health professionals have not been adequately trained to manage patient symptoms in palliative care (Ferrell, Virani, Grant, Coyne, & Uman, 2000; Goodell, Donohue, & Benoliel, 1982; Scott, MacDonald, & Mount, 1998). A study conducted by the IOM (1997) reported one of the key barriers to high quality of end-of-life care is health care professionals' inadequate knowledge of pain management, symptom relief, and other dimensions of terminal illness care. Until now, medical or nursing education, in general, still emphasizes traditional roles organized around a hierarchical model of acute medical care. Curricula for health professionals fail to include the special clinical skills and knowledge associated with palliative care and the preparation of teamwork in the context of complex organizations. Recently, Ferrell, Virani, and Grant (1999) conducted an analysis of end-of-life content in nursing textbooks, and reported that only 2% of the overall content, and 1.4% of chapters, in nursing texts were related to end-of-life care. Another survey, from 2,333 oncology nurses, showed that less than 13% of the subjects rated their basic nursing education in the end-of-life care as very adequate (Ferrell et al., 2000). Benoliel (1987–1988) states that death education for health professionals requires more than introduction of new content into already crowded courses or curricula on palliative care, it requires ongoing opportunities to grapple with the complexities of choice and decision making affecting the lives of others in profound ways. A number of individuals and groups have systematically introduced courses or programs in death education into their schools and continuing inservice education (Benoliel, 1982; Bertman, Greene, & Wyatt, 1982; Danis et al., 1999; Degner & Gow, 1988; Ferrell et al., 1999; Goodell et al., 1982), but, clearly, educational standards are needed, so that all professionals are exposed to essential palliative care content, especially pain and symptom management.

Congruency of Goals

A major task of palliative care is the establishment and communication of mutually acceptable goals for the patient, family members, and professional caregivers. Ultimately, the patient's goals can and should shape the care they receive, establishing parameters of aggressiveness (i.e., medical intervention), and providing caregivers a basis upon which to formulate interventions. Although the patient's goals remain paramount, consideration must also be given to the other members of the care triad: the family and care providers.

Goals must be clearly stated, and never assumed. Goals may also change over time. For example, initially, patients may want to receive aggressive therapy, even though there may be little chance of controlling their cancer. With the continued growth of their cancers and the deterioration of their bodies, patients' goals may shift toward a peaceful death with no heroics. However, if this shift has never been communicated, life support measures may be initiated and families and health care providers subsequently may be left to make decisions without knowledge of the patients' wishes.

A Supportive Environment

Resources to provide support for patients and families have not evolved in tandem with the changing care environment for the terminally ill. We have discharged patients to home, assuming continuity and even improvements in care, yet we cannot ensure the availability of adequate services to manage symptoms on a 24-hour basis. Family members are placed in a dual position of provider and recipient of care. Their new role of care provider may exacerbate the disequilibrium experienced with the role changes that accompany a family member's terminal illness. A balance must exist between relieving the patient's physical and emotional distress and equal attention to the family's psychosocial needs and concerns. Interventions that help the family achieve a sense of control over the environment may decrease their sense of helplessness, prepare them to meet the challenges inherent in caregiving (Jepson, McCorkle, Adler, Nuamah, & Lusk, 1999; McGuinnis, 1986), and even reduce family caregivers' psychological distress after the patient's death (McCorkle, Robinson, Nuamah, Lev, & Benoliel, 1998). These interventions include the provision of concrete care instructions in conjunction with ongoing guidance and support.

Value and Cost of Terminal Care

The present financial climate of health care has shifted the care of terminally ill patients away from the hospital. No longer are dying patients admitted to hospitals, where care is delegated to professional caregivers, and families maintain a silent vigil with little or no direct care involvement. Many terminally ill patients are now cared for in their homes, where their families and community health nurses assume the role of primary caregivers. This transition from hospital to home offers obvious benefits to patients, such as personal comforts, maintenance of autonomy, and increased presence of family and friends, but the care can be overwhelming for families and for community nurses.

In the past, community nurses focused on health maintenance and education. Patients with complex care requirements were admitted to hospitals, where they were cared for by the hospital staff until they stabilized or died. This scenario has changed with the implementation of diagnostic related groupings, an increase in consumer awareness, and the institutional turmoil many hospitals are experiencing. Patients are not only discharged "sicker and quicker," but some are not even admitted, thereby requiring that complex levels of care be instituted in the home. There is undeniable evidence that cost factors are dictating the type of care received, by whom, and for what period of time (Baird & Mortenson, 1990; Hughes et al., 1997; Sager, Easterling, Kindig, & Anderson, 1989).

Ideally, patients with complex problems are referred to a home health agency or hospice for provision of professional care, a large component of which is nursing. As a result, the acuity of home care clienteles has increased dramatically (Hughes et al., 1997; Mulhern, 1987; Sager et al., 1989). Community nurses are now administering opioid infusions, managing complex symptoms, and providing a range of physical and psychological support to patients and families. Insurance reimbursement for these home nursing visits is based primarily on skilled nursing care (such as wound care, infusions, ostomies, nutritional feedings, etc.), and often is limited to a specific number of visits. This process has changed the focus of community nursing from maintenance and education to crisis intervention, and nurses are often faced with juggling complex patient care needs with everchanging reimbursement regulations. Government cost-containment efforts have also put pressure on home health agencies to discharge patients as quickly as possible (Coleman, 1988). Current eligibility and benefit structures are so restrictive that only a narrow range of services will be paid for, with significant constraints placed on the intensity and duration of care (Johnson, 1998; Kaplan & O'Connor, 1987; Reif, 1987).

Given these financial and nursing constraints, management of the physical distress of the symptoms may become the only goal that appears financially compensated. The challenge is to maintain a holistic patient management focus, when extrinsic forces limit the level of professional involvement.

One way to achieve the successful management of patient symptoms at home is the provision of continuous support to family members. If mechanisms for communication are ongoing and well-established between the primary caregiver in the home and the home health nurse, problems can be anticipated and crises prevented. Often, nurses avert complications by monitoring patient's symptoms over the telephone, reporting changes in patient status to the physician, and securing treatments, such as medications, before symptoms become incapacitating (McCorkle et al., 1989; McCorkle, Hughes, Robinson, Levine, & Nuamah, 1998).

Concerted efforts are needed to expand reimbursement regulations to include telephone calls and case management activities, rather than limiting them to fee-per-visit schedules. In addition, a reevaluation of payment of services is needed for patients whose conditions are changing. Patients are frequently discharged from home health agencies once their condition becomes stabilized. Alternative, cost-effective programs need to be developed to monitor the maintenance of their status.

A Model of Care for Successful Symptom Management

Innovations in palliative care are needed that will facilitate shared decision making among patients, family members, and health professionals. We propose a model of care that ensures quality of life, by assisting members of the patient's support network to maximize the capacity of living day to day. The model's major feature includes a focus on management of symptoms, provision of continuity of care, and the formation of partnerships with patients and their support networks (Saunders & McCorkle, 1985; McCorkle et al., 1998). Patients and family members manifest multiple physical, emotional, and social problems, which are best resolved through a collaborative, multidisciplinary team effort. The most commonly identified team members in palliative care include physicians, nurses, and social workers. We propose that the nurse is in an ideal position to coordinate and manage services, as the patient's needs change from acute to chronic and progressive within end-of-life situations.

There is tremendous potential among nurses for leadership in the creation and maintenance of palliative care services for patients and families. Nurses, as a collective, must be willing to engage in the politics of negotiation for reallocation of health care resources toward individualized services. Nurses must be able to establish a power base for influencing decisions with various organizations offering health care benefits, such as the American

Association for Retired Persons, at the local, state, and national levels of government. As individualized services are established, nurses must also move toward formalizing emergent practices into standards of care (Bookbinder et al., 1996). In keeping with the adoption of standards of practice is the need to develop a consistent, universal nomenclature for assessing, monitoring, and evaluating patients' symptoms. Standardized methods for assessing symptoms need to be incorporated routinely into the patient's plan of care (McCorkle, 1988).

We believe that the successful development and implementation of palliative care services depends on the support of administrators in all disciplines and across all settings. Administrators and key leaders in their individual practice disciplines need to recognize the complexity of problems, and lead the way to breaking down the barriers to successful symptom management. See Table 8.3 for a list of potential barriers.

Once the problems are recognized, palliative care services may be fostered through skilled negotiations with those in positions of power (Benoliel, 1987–1988). To promote interdisciplinary teamwork, social mechanisms need to be created within organizations. The inclusion of palliative care within mainstream health care requires a radical reordering of priorities and a strong commitment to collaborative practice. At the very heart of the matter, health professionals must be willing to confront, continuously, the demands of the conflicting goals of cure versus palliative

TABLE 8.3   Barriers to Successful Symptom Management

1. Fear of addiction to medications
2. Fear of untoward side effects from medications
3. Lack of ongoing consistent evaluation of symptoms
4. Incomplete assessment of etiology of symptoms
5. Lack of individualized treatment plans
6. Knowledge deficit regarding pharmacological and nonpharmacological strategies for symptom management
7. Ineffective communication among patients, families, and members of the health care team
8. Incongruent goals among patients, families, and members of the health care team
9. Lack of institutional policies to ensure a balance of priorities between cure and palliative care
10. Lack of administrative support within institutions to develop palliative care practice standards
11. Restrictive interpretation of reimbursement regulations
12. Lack of reimbursement for a variety of palliative care services

care. Mechanisms that support the patient's right to participate in care, and to make the final decisions about treatment, are essential. As demands for services increase and resources become scarce, it is imperative that health professionals keep pace and develop systems and regulations that ensure the continued development of the subspecialty of palliative care. Patients, family members, and potential consumers may be the most powerful group to safeguard the future of palliative care, by insisting that the quality of their living is as important or more important than aggressive therapies to prolong their lives.

Discussion Questions

1. Mrs. Morgan, a 45-year-old woman with ovarian cancer, currently receives morphine continually by infusion (2 mg/hr and 0.5 mg for breakthrough pain) for her bone pain. Over the past 24 hours, she complained that when she changed her position, that is, gets out of bed, her bone pain became intolerable. As her primary home care nurse, what nursing interventions will you take in order to help Mrs. Morgan restore her previous satisfactory level of pain control?

2. Mr. Brown, an 88-year-old man with colon cancer that had metastasized to lung and bone, was admitted because of bowel obstruction. Initially, Mr. Brown's primary physician, Dr. Smith, planned to conduct palliative surgery to relieve Mr. Brown's bowel obstruction. However, the surgery was cancelled after the radiographic diagnosis revealed that Mr. Brown's colon cancer had extensive peritoneal involvement and there were multiple bowel obstructions. Dr. Smith suggested total parenteral nutrition (TPN) to meet Mr. Brown's nutritional needs. However, Mr. Brown refused surgery for intravenous access placement to receive intravenous supplements. He told the nurse that he is happy with his life and he is not suffering right now. He sometimes experiences thirst, but that is relieved by sucking on a piece of small ice cube. He has no appetite. He understands that, without TPN or intravenous supplements, he may die with dehydration. However, he does not want to live longer with "tubes" connected to him. The only thing that he wants is to let nature take its course. He has asked his physician to order his favored Jewish wine and ice cream. As his primary nurse, how will you deal with this situation?

References

Agency for Health Care Policy and Research (AHCPR). (1994). *Clinical practice guideline number 9: Management of cancer pain.* Rockville, MD: AHCPR Publication.

American Cancer Society. (2001). Cancer Statistics, 2001. *Ca: A Cancer Journal for Clinicians, 51,* 15–36.

Baird, S. B., & Mortenson, L. E. (1990). Economic concerns in the changing health care delivery system. *Cancer, 65*(3, Suppl.), 766–769.

Benoliel, J. Q. (1976). Overview: Care, cure and the challenge of choice. In A. Earle (Ed.), *The nurse as caregiver for the terminal patient and his family* (pp. 9–30). New York: Columbia University Press.

Benoliel, J. Q. (Ed.). (1982). Death influence in clinical practice: A course for graduate students. In *Death education for the health professional.* Washington, DC: Hemisphere.

Benoliel, J. Q. (1987–1988). Health care providers and dying patients: Critical issues in terminal care. *Omega, 18,* 341–363.

Benoliel, J. Q., & McCorkle, R. (1977, May). Ethical considerations in treatment. In *Proceedings of the Second National Conference on Cancer Nursing* (pp. 63–68). New York: American Cancer Society.

Bertman, S. K., Greene, J., & Wyatt, C. A. (1982). Humanistic health career education in a hospice/palliative care setting. In J. Q. Benoliel (Ed.), *Death education for the health professional* (pp. 143–152). Washington, DC: Hemisphere.

Bookbinder, M., Coyle, N., Kiss, M., Goldstein, M. L., Holritz, K., Thaler, H., et al. (1996). Implementing national standards for cancer pain management: Program model and evaluation. *Journal of Pain and Symptom Management, 12,* 334–347.

Breitbart, W. (1989). Psychiatric management of cancer pain. *Cancer, 76,* 2336–2342.

Bruera, E. (1998). Research into symptoms other than pain. In D. Doyle, G. W. C. Hanks, & N. MacDonald (Eds.), *Oxford textbook of palliative medicine* (pp. 179–185). New York: Oxford University Press.

Bruera, E., & Neumann, C. M. (1998). Management of specific symptom complexes in patients receiving palliative care. *Canadian Medical Association Journal, 158,* 1717–1726.

Buckman, R. (1998). Communication in palliative care: A practical guide. In D. Doyle, G. W. C. Hanks, & N. MacDonald (Eds.), *Oxford textbook of palliative medicine* (pp. 141–156). New York: Oxford University Press.

"Caring Together." (December, 1987). *The report of the expert working group on integrated palliative care for persons with AIDS.* Ottawa, Ontario: Health and Welfare Canada.

Coleman, S. (1988). Discharge planning from the home health agency. In P. O'Hare & M. Terry (Eds.), *Discharge planning: Strategies for assuring continuing of care* (pp. 175–180). Rockville, MD: Aspect.

Danis, M., Federman, D., Fins, J. J., Fox, E., Kastenbaum, B., Lanken, P. N., et al. (1999). Incorporating palliative care into critical care education: principles, challenges, and opportunities. *Critical Care Medicine, 27,* 2005–2013.

De Conno, F., Caraceni, A., Groff, L., Brunelli, C., Donati, I., Tamburini, M., et al. (1996). Effect of home care on the place of death of advanced cancer patients. *European Journal of Cancer, 32,* 1142–1147.

Degner, L. F., & Gow, C. M. (1988). Preparing nurses for care of the dying: A longitudinal study. *Cancer Nursing, 11,* 160–169.

Dellemijn, H., Duijn, H. V., & Vanneste, J. A. L. (1998). Prolonged treatment with transdermal fentanyl in neuropathic pain. *Journal of Pain and Symptom Management, 16,* 220–229.

Derogatis, L. R., Morrow, G. R., Fetting, J., Penman, D., Piasetsky, S., Schmale, A. M., et al. (1983). The prevalence of psychiatric disorders among cancer patients. *Journal of the American Medical Association, 249,* 751–757.

Desbiens, N. A., & Wu, A. W. (2000). Pain and suffering in seriously ill hospitalized patients. *Journal of American Geriatrics Society, 48,* S183–S186.

Dubler, N. N., & Post, L. F. (1998). Truth telling and informed consent. In J. C. Holland (Ed.), *Psycho-oncology* (pp. 1085–1095). New York: Oxford University Press.

Emanuel, E. J., Fairclough, D. L., Slutsman, J., Alpert, H., Baldwin, D., & Emanuel, L. L. (1999). Assistance from family members, friends, paid care givers, and volunteers in the care of terminally ill patients. *New England Journal of Medicine, 341,* 956–963.

Ferrell, B., Virani, R., & Grant, M. (1999). Analysis of end-of-life content in nursing textbooks. *Oncology Nursing Forum, 26,* 869–876.

Ferrell, B., Virani, R., Grant, M., Coyne, P., & Uman, G. (2000). Beyond the supreme court decision: Nursing perspectives on end-of-life care. *Oncology Nursing Forum, 27,* 445–455.

Fiore, N. (1979). Fighting cancer—one patient's perspective. *New England Journal of Medicine, 300,* 284–289.

Foley, K. M. (1998). Pain assessment and cancer pain syndromes. In D. Doyle, G. W. C. Hanks, & N. MacDonald (Eds.), *Oxford textbook of palliative medicine* (pp. 310–331). New York: Oxford University Press.

Germino, B. (1991). Cancer and the family. In R. McCorkle, M. Grant, M. Frank-Stromborg, & E. S. Barid (Eds.), *Cancer nursing: A comprehensive textbook* (2nd ed., pp. 81–92). Philadelphia: W. B. Saunders.

Goodell, B. W., Donohue, J. I., & Benoliel, J. Q. (1982). Death education in medical school: A seminar on terminal illness. In J. Q. Benoliel (Ed.), *Death education for the health professional* (pp. 43–58). Washington, DC: Hemisphere.

Hanks, G., & Cherny, N. (1998). Opioid analgesic therapy. In D. Doyle, G. W. C. Hanks, & N. MacDonald (Eds.), *Oxford textbook of palliative medicine* (pp. 331–355). New York: Oxford University Press.

Hanson, L. C., Danis, M., & Garrett, J. (1997). What is wrong with end-of-life care? Opinions of bereaved family members. *Journal of American Geriatrics Society, 45,* 1339–1344.

Holland, J. C. (1982). Psychological aspects of cancer. In J. F. Holland & E. M. Frei (Eds.), *Cancer medicine* (pp. 1175–1184). Philadelphia: Lea & Febiger.

Hughes, S. L., Ulasevich, A., Weaver, F. M., Henderson, W., Manheim, L., Kubal, J. D., et al. (1997). Impact of home care on hospital days: A meta-analysis. *Health Services Research, 32,* 415–432.

Institute of Medicine (IOM). (1997). In M. J. Field & C. Cassell (Eds.), *Approach death: Improving care at the end of life* (p. 4). Washington, DC: National Academy Press.

Jepson, C., McCorkle, R., Adler, D., Nuamah, I., & Lusk, E. (1999). Effects of home care on caregivers' psychosocial status. *Image: Journal of Nursing Scholarship, 31*, 115–120.

Johnson, C. N. (1998). Hospice: What gets in the way of appropriate and timely access. *Holistic Nursing Practice, 13*, 8–12.

Kaplan, M. P., & O'Connor, P. M. (1987). The effect of Medicare on access to hospice care: Patterns of eligibility requiring the availability of a primary care person. *The American Journal of Hospice Care, 4*(4), 34–42.

Komurcu, S., Nelson, K. A., Walsh, D., Donnelly, S. M., Homsi, J., & Abdullah, O. (2000). Common symptoms in advanced cancer. *Seminars in Oncology, 27*, 24–33.

Krant, M. J. (1976). Problems of the physicians in presenting the patient with the diagnosis. In J. W. Cullen, B. H. Fox, & R. N. Isom (Eds.), *Cancer: The behavioral dimensions* (pp. 269–274). New York: Raven Press.

Kristjanson, L. J. (1989). Quality of terminal care: Salient indicators identified by families. *Journal of Palliative Care, 5*(1), 21–28.

Lederberg, M. S. (1998). The family of the cancer patient. In J. C. Holland (Ed.), *Psycho-oncology* (pp. 981–993). New York: Oxford University Press.

Lynn, J., Teno, J. M., Phillips, R. S., Wu, A. W., Desbiens, N., Harrold, J., et al. (1997). Perceptions by family members of the dying experience of older and seriously ill patients. *Annals of Internal Medicine, 126*, 97–106.

MacDonald, N. (1998). Palliative care—an essential component of cancer control. *Canadian Medical Association Journal, 158*, 1709–1716.

Maguire, P. (1981). Repercussions of mastectomy on the family. *International Journal of Psychiatry, 1*, 485–503.

McCarthy, E. P., Phillips, R. S., Zhong, Z., Drews, R. E., & Lynn, J. (2000). Dying with cancer: Patients' function, symptoms, and care preferences as death approaches. *Journal of American Geriatrics Society, 48*, S110–S121.

McCorkle, R. (1988). Measure of symptom distress. *Seminars in Oncology, 3*, 248–256.

McCorkle, R., Benoliel, J. Q., Donaldson, G., Georgiadou, F., Moinpour, C., & Goodell, B. (1989). Randomized clinical trial of home nursing care for long cancer patients. *Cancer, 64*, 199–206.

McCorkle, R., Hughes, L., Robinson, L., Levine, B., & Nuamah, I. (1998). Nursing interventions for newly diagnosed older cancer patients facing terminal illness. *Journal of Palliative Care, 14*, 39–45.

McCorkle, R., Robinson, L., Nuamah, I., Lev, E., & Benoliel, J. Q. (1998). Effects of home nursing care for patients during terminal illness on the bereaved's psychological distress. *Nursing Research, 47*, 2–10.

McGuinnis, S. (1986). How can nurses improve the quality of life of the hospice client and family. *Hospice Journal, 2*, 23–33.

Miskowski, C. (1988). *Supportive care for the cancer patient*. Valley Cottage, NY: A. H. Robbins.

Mulhern, P. J. (1987, May). High-tech nursing in the home and community. *Proceedings of Fifth National Conference on Cancer Nursing*. Atlanta, GA: American Cancer Society.

Northouse, L. (1984). Preventive intervention with the recently bereaved. *Archives of General Psychiatry, 34*, 1450–1454.

Northouse, P. G., & Northouse, L. (1987). Communication and cancer: Issues confronting patients, health professionals and family members. *Journal of Psychosocial Oncology, 5*, 17–46.

Oberst, M., & James, R. H. (1985). Going home: Patient and spouse adjustment following cancer surgery. *Topics in Clinical Nursing, 1,* 46–57.

Passik, S. D., Portenoy, R., & Ricketts, P. L. (1998). Substance abuse issues in cancer patients: Part 1: Prevalence and diagnosis. *Oncology, 12,* 517–521.

Perry, S., & Heidrich, G. (1982). Management of pain during debridement: A survey of U.S. burn units. *Pain, 13,* 267–280.

Portenoy, R., & Lesage, P. (1999). Management of cancer pain. *Lancet, 353,* 1695–1700.

Portenoy, R. K., Thaler, H. T., Kornblith, A. B., Lepore, J. M., Friedlander-Klar, H., Foley, K., et al. (1994). The Memorial Symptom Assessment Scale: An instrument for the evaluation of symptom prevalence, characteristics and distress. *European Journal of Clinical Oncology, 30,* 1326–1336.

Porter, J., & Jick, H. (1980). Addiction rare in patients treated with narcotics [Letter to the Editor]. *New England Journal of Medicine, 302,* 123.

Quint, J. C. (1966). Communication problems affecting patient care in hospitals. *Journal of American Medical Association, 195,* 126–127.

Reif, L. (1987). The real victims of the crisis in home care: Patients and their families. *Home Health Care Services Quarterly, 8,* 1–4.

Sager, M. A., Easterling, D. V., Kindig, D. A., & Anderson, O. W. (1989). Changes in the location of death after passage of Medicare's prospective payment system: A national study. *New England Journal of Medicine, 320,* 433–439.

Saunders, J. M., & McCorkle, R. (1985). Models of care for persons with progressive cancer. *Nursing Clinics of North America, 20,* 365–377.

Scanlon, C. (1989). Creating a vision of hope: The challenge of palliative care. *Oncology Nursing Forum, 16,* 491–499.

Schachter, S. R., & Coyle, N. (1998). Palliative home care—Impact on families. In J. C. Holland (Ed.), *Psycho-oncology* (pp. 1004–1015). New York: Oxford University Press.

Schug, S. A., Zech, D., Grond, S., & Dorr, U. (1992). Long-term survey of morphine in cancer pain patients. *Journal of Pain and Symptom Management, 7,* 259–266.

Scott, J. F., MacDonald, N., & Mount, B. M. (1998). Palliative medicine education. In D. Doyle, G. W. C. Hanks, & N. MacDonald (Eds.), *Oxford textbook of palliative medicine* (pp. 1169–1199). New York: Oxford University Press.

Seravalli, E. P. (1988). The dying patient, the physician and the fear of death. *New England Journal of Medicine, 319,* 1728–1730.

Stajduhar, K. I., & Davies, B. (1998). Death at home: Challenges for families and directions for the future. *Journal of Palliative Care, 14*(3), 8–14.

Turnbull, R. (1986). (Ed). *Terminal care.* Washington, DC: Hemisphere.

Twycross, R. C., & Lack, S. A. (1984). *Therapeutics in terminal cancer.* London: Churchill Livingstone.

Vachon, M. L. S. (1998a). The emotional problems of the patient. In D. Doyle, G. W. C. Hanks, & N. MacDonald (Eds.), *Oxford textbook of palliative medicine* (pp. 883–907). New York: Oxford University Press.

Vachon, M. L. S. (1998b). Psychosocial needs of patients and families. *Journal of Palliative Care, 14*(3), 49–56.

Vachon, M. L. S. (1995). Staff stress in hospice/palliative care: A review. *Palliative Medicine, 9,* 91–122.

Walsh, D. (2000). Pharmacological management of cancer pain. *Seminars in Oncology,* *27,* 45–63.

World Health Organization. (1990, April). *Cancer pain relief and palliative care: Report of a WHO expert committee.* (Technical Report Series No. 804). Geneva, Switzerland: World Health Organization.

World Health Organization. (1998). *Symptom relief in terminal illness.* Geneva, Switzerland: World Health Organization.

Wortman, C. B., & Dunkel-Schetter, C. (1979). Interpersonal relationships and cancer: A theoretical analysis. *Journal of Social Issues, 35,* 120–155.

Yasko, J. M. (Ed.). (1983). *Guidelines for cancer care symptom management.* Reston, VA: Reston.

Nine

Hospice and Palliative Care: A Legacy in the Making

Inge B. Corless and Patrice K. Nicholas

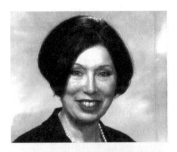

Inge Baer Corless is co-editor of this book, and her biography can be found on page ii.

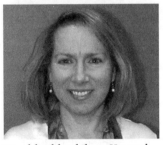

Patrice Kenneally Nicholas graduated from Fitchburg State College, Fitchburg, Massachusetts, with a bachelor's of science in nursing, and received a master of science degree in nursing and a doctor of nursing science degree from Boston University School of Nursing. She completed a certificate of advanced study in primary care at the Massachusetts General Hospital Institute of Health Professions Graduate Program in Nursing, and is certified as an adult nurse practitioner. Dr. Nicholas was a postdoctoral fellow at the Harvard School of Public Health, focusing her research on quality of life in chronic illness. She received a master of public health degree in international health while at Harvard. Dr. Nicholas is currently associate professor in the graduate program at the MGH Institute of Health Professions.

The modern hospice movement arose when the concern that something more should be done for terminally ill persons was transformed into the conviction that something more could be done. Supporters of the movement perceived that fragmented, isolated activities might be organized into coordinated, comprehensive care provided by an interdisciplinary team whose focus was the patient and the family (Lack, 1977). Crucial to this transformation has been the work of Dame Cicely Saunders and Dr. Elisabeth Kübler-Ross, the former in symptom management and spiritual care, and the latter in the psychosocial sphere (Kübler-Ross, 1969; Saunders, 1960, 1979). Saunders, in particular, with her clinically oriented studies, has led the movement of science in the service of terminal illness care. Thus, the choice became not one of cure versus care, nor of care devoid of scientific underpinnings, but a recognition of the current limitations of scientifically based cure and an emphasis on scientifically based care (Melzack, Ofiesh, & Mount, 1976; Twycross, 1983).

The choice to participate in hospice care has become an option for those who have access to a program for which they meet the admission criteria. Not every terminally ill person has such access, however, even though a publication by the National Hospice Organization (1991, p. 3) stated: "If you receive Medicare benefits, you're entitled to hospice care." Furthermore, even if a program is geographically accessible, an individual may not be deemed eligible by the hospice program.

The question of access to palliative care services is dependent largely on the availability of such programs. Moreover, following the work of Ferris and Cummings (1995), who proposed that access to palliative care services begin with the onset of symptomatology, the question of eligibility is no longer framed in the number of days, weeks, or months of life remaining. Access to palliative care services is provided for all with potentially life-limiting diseases, early in the disease trajectory. Thus, the conundrum of entitlement facing potential hospice recipients—access and eligibility—is not applicable to palliative medicine recipients. These issues are explored in this chapter, which examines some of the questions currently facing hospice and palliative care services in the United States.

In this chapter, the term *palliative care program* will be used interchangeably with *hospice* as a form of end-of-life care. Palliative care programs were developed in England and Canada at the same time that hospices emerged in England and the United States. Balfour Mount used the term to refer to his new program at the Royal Victoria Hospital in Montreal. This program, which opened shortly after St. Christopher's Hospice was established by Dame Cicely Saunders, attempted to incorporate hospice principles in a tertiary care facility.

The term *palliative care* is also used to refer to the renewed organizational attempt to change the manner in which the dying are treated in hospitals (Billings, 1998). Palliative medicine is the new medical specialty whose practitioners provide palliative care. Palliative care services in tertiary care facilities use a consultation model not unlike that established by the hospice team at Roosevelt-St. Luke's Hospice. These services are often requested for patients who are terminally ill, although theoretically they should be provided to anyone with a life-shortening disease. While the terms palliative care program and hospice will be used interchangeably, the term *palliative care service* is reserved for the latest iteration of holistic care for those facing a life-threatening or chronic disease. The relationship of hospice and palliative care services is examined later in this chapter.

Background

The rapid development of hospice and palliative care programs in the United States, as well as throughout different countries of the world, has occurred, for the most part, in the last two decades. *Hospice* has been described as a concept of care, a program of care, and a place for care (Corless, 1984). As a concept of care, hospice was inextricably bound to the activities of the death awareness movement (Feifel, 1959). Changing attitudes legitimizing death and dying as a subject for scholarly inquiry have brought into sharp relief the contrast between dying in a hospital enshrouded in technology, and dying at home surrounded by those one loves (Feifel, 1994). Hospice as a concept of care provides a mechanism to span the chasm of the modern and traditional visions of dying. In particular, hospice espouses: choice with regard to the place of one's dying; attention to the comfort of the individual; a consideration of spiritual, social, and psychological concerns, as well as the physiological and functional manifestations of the disease process; a focus on the family, as well as on the patient; an emphasis on dying, death, and the bereavement that follows; the provision of interdisciplinary care (not simply the attention of professionals from multiple disciplines); and the implementation of coordinated care across care settings.

These attributes are incorporated into hospice as a program of care. Wald (1994) described the foundational steps that led to the program of care in the United States, known as the Connecticut Hospice. The history of this period has been depicted by Cohen (1979), Corless (1983a, 1983b, 1985), Davidson (1978), Foster, Wald, and Wald (1987), Hillier (1983), Lack and Buckingham, (1978), Mount (1976), Osterweis and Champagne (1979), Saunders (1978, 1986), Stoddard (1978), Wald (1994), and Walter (1979).

Hospice as a program of care is not setting-bound, and may be independent or affiliated with another organization, such as a hospital or home care agency. Care is provided to the individual in the home, hospital, or extended care facility. Hospice as a place for care is *the* place for care, and is setting-oriented, whether as a freestanding structure or as part of another facility.

Beyond such conceptualizations, however, most definitions of hospice fail to capture the sense of mission of what has taken on many of the attributes of a social reform movement in health care. As with the early days of any such movements, there were moments of excess. The passion for hospice began in a decade marked with hopes for social reform and racial equality, the elimination of poverty, the despair over the assassination of political leaders, and protracted civil and military conflict. The hope for social transformation yielded to the denial of a generation torn between choices of Vietnam or Canada, and a reifying of the choice between cure and care. The battle cry of the foot soldiers of the hospice movement—"we care"—was hurled against the stalwarts of cure-oriented therapy, thus dichotomizing approaches that should be complementary rather than alternative, a vision not expounded until the groundbreaking work of the Canadian Palliative Care Association and, in particular, Ferris and Cummings (1995). The hospice movement also needlessly impugned the motives of many health care practitioners, creating enmity toward hospice.

The failure of hospice to change how people died in hospitals was amply demonstrated by the SUPPORT study (1995), wherein 4,301 hospitalized patients were, on average, expected to live 6 months or less. Doctors were mostly unaware or did not adhere to their patients' wishes for end-of-life care. Further, almost one half of the do-not-resuscitate orders were written in the last day or two of life. The implementation of an intervention failed to change these patterns of behavior. As a result, major foundations, notably the Robert Wood Johnson Foundation and the Soros Foundation, made a commitment to changing this pattern, by a massive program of professional and community research and education.

The introduction of palliative medicine as a medical specialty may have a more profound impact on care of the dying than was the case with hospice. As a medical specialty, palliative medicine will be a legitimate subject for study in the nation's medical schools. Palliative medicine, led by physicians, and secondary- and tertiary-care-focused, is more professionally insular, however, than is true of hospice. The latter was a community-based movement led by nurses, together with notable physicians, other professionals, and volunteers, as a more holistic approach to end-of-life care. Palliative care services are physician-dominated, with variable input from other professionals. Indeed, concern has been expressed that these services will lack the holistic approach of hospice (O'Connor, 1999). Part of the reason for this may be the question of compensation for services.

Physician services are billable. Constraints on reimbursement for professional services may have an impact on the composition of departments of palliative care. Compensation has also been a problem for hospice programs.

The hospice movement, in striving to change approaches to care of the dying, was itself changed, when efforts to secure reimbursement for care emphasized the potential for cost savings. However, this attempt to secure a firmer financial foundation for hospice programs was made at the cost of limiting the mandate of hospice to those with the resources to remain at home. More significant, the price of becoming part of the system was to lose the charismatic elements of a social movement and become tamed, albeit legitimized, by the system. The hospice movement was co-opted by the federal establishment. The cost of such bureaucratization was to limit access to hospice to those who might have been sustained at home by traditional home care agencies (Corless, 1984; Rhymes, 1990).

Traditional home care compensation is provided on a per visit basis, with reimbursement limited to "skilled" nursing care (including teaching and assessment), physician's visits, and other prescribed and circumscribed modalities, such as physical therapy. Psychosocial concerns and other nonphysically oriented care and support are not reimbursable in traditional home care. Hospice funding, on the other hand, provided reimbursement on a capitation basis, incorporating such levels of care as routine home care, continuous home care, inpatient respite care, and general inpatient care. The importance of capitation, from a federal standpoint, was as a means of controlling the costs of care. From a hospice perspective, the new approach to funding provided reimbursement for the aspects of terminal illness care not captured by traditional home care funding mechanisms, aspects such as psychosocial visits, family care, medications, and out-of-pocket expenses. However, the boon of stability of funding was purchased at a cost of restricted access to care (Corless, 1983c). McCann (1988) notes: "Without national support of a definition of hospice care which goes beyond the parameters of reimbursement and addresses access to quality care for patients and families, we fail to support the right of any patient in America to have equitable access to hospice services and high quality care" (p. 18). A similar statement might be made about palliative care services.

A Question of Access

McCann's (1988) statement about hospice addresses the heart of the argument about hospice and palliative care services, that is, the right of any citizen to have access. The structure of the Medicare hospice benefit assumes that a lay caregiver will be present for the recipient of the hospice benefit. The reimbursement schedule was originally calculated on that assumption (Corless, 1985). It is amazing, therefore, that the hospice benefit has not been challenged in the courts as being discriminatory to terminally ill individuals without the requisite caregiver. This argument has been propounded previously, notably that single persons, those with a partner in frail health, or individuals from a family where there are multiple problems all are disenfranchised (Corless, 1987–1988).

No discrete benefit provides compensation for palliative care services. Given that palliative care services are rendered over the course of an illness, and are an add-on rather than a substitute for other care, there has been some caution in confronting financial issues. It is likely that bottom-line issues will need to be addressed, particularly if financial shortfall is a problem confronting the larger institution. On the other hand, appropriate palliative care may facilitate discharge and thus provide cost savings.

Questions of access to palliative care services are greatly dependent on the availability of specially trained personnel who offer such services in secondary and tertiary care facilities. Patients from a variety of backgrounds are hospitalized with referral to palliative care services not contingent on family constellation, namely, the presence of a caregiver.

The question of access, however, is of paramount concern to hospice programs across the United States (Beresford & Connor, 1999; Corless, 1990). Specifically, is the access being contemplated one of access by individuals representing a greater spectrum of society, or is it access by more of the individuals and families who meet the characteristics assumed by the Medicare model?

If access implies attracting individuals with the requisite support structure, then the question of access is one of advertising. The subtext of the Medicare message to the disenfranchised (those without a caregiver) is that they are not eligible for a premium product. The difference in access is between a system designed for the care of the terminally ill that is the standard of care and one, for lack of an alternative, that is standard care. The introduction of palliative care services, however, may transform standard care into the standard of care at least in tertiary care facilities.

The question of access for minorities and other underserved populations, in most institutions, is in part one of marketing, when individuals with social support are sought as the potential recipients of care (Harper, 1990). Clearly, however, access involves more than marketing. It involves sensitivity to the cultural values of potential recipients of care (Beresford, 1990a;

Crawley et al., 2000), and it involves care provided with respect and concern for the lives of those affected. It is culturally sensitive, and, better yet, it is humanly sensitive. It is what hospice care purports to be.

Access for minorities and all underserved populations is limited further by a benefit structured to ensure care at home. Inpatient care, in the Medicare hospice benefit, serves as a backup and not as an alternative to home care. Beresford (1989) speaks to this distinction: "Residential hospice care should be differentiated from inpatient hospice care which is intended primarily for the short-term acute medical needs of hospice patients or for brief periods of respite for exhausted family members" (p. 12). Residential care, a new setting inspired largely by the acquired immunodeficiency syndrome (AIDS) epidemic, was the missing setting for which inpatient care was substituted in New York City's hospitals, in an effort to maintain access to hospice care for diverse populations (Corless, 1987–1988).

Although the hospice benefit's financing is viable for serving the needs of the "haves," it is inadequate for the provision of service to the "have-nots." Furthermore, regulatory constraints placed on hospice programs that sought to serve their clients by providing inpatient care in hospitals to individuals without other resources, and in the last stages of their lives, no longer could call themselves hospices given the lack of emphasis on home care. As a result, their clients could not avail themselves of the hospice benefit, and were restricted to the provision of care as outlined in traditional reimbursement mechanisms. And, although hospice or palliative care programs could provide nonreimbursed care, financial supplementation from other sources was required for a program to continue its services. Does the Health Care Financing Administration (HCFA) have a responsibility to either revise its regulations or provide federal dispensation, so as to make hospice benefits available to all Medicare recipients?

The inability to provide inpatient hospice care to individuals dying in hospitals is directly related to the Medicare hospice benefit, which includes a constraint on the percentage of total care to be provided on an inpatient basis. And, although the constraint applies to the program and not the individual patient, programs have been hesitant to endanger fiscal viability. This constraint has modulated the impact of the hospice movement, and led to the findings of the SUPPORT investigators and to the emergence of palliative medicine and palliative care services. While access is dependent on the availability of palliative care services and physician referral, it is available to hospitalized individuals.

Access to hospice involved outreach. Stoddard (1990) pleaded for attention to the ghettos in the United States, stating that it is there that "hospice international outreach ought to begin. This is where the hospice concept is most desperately needed today with its attitudes, its skills, and its extraordinary power to rebuild fractured communities" (p. 30). She suggested placing demonstration hospice teams in storefronts or abandoned warehouses in New York and Los Angeles, bringing hospice to those in need of such care. Whether such individuals could be maintained at home or not, the presence of hospice teams near their clients would enhance outreach programs and access to care.

Hospice programs in rural areas incur the costs of travel over great distances (Beresford, 1990b). The economies of aggregating clients in an easily negotiated area, usually within 30 minutes of the hospice program, are lost when clients are located at significant distances from one another, and from the hospice office. Without the presence of a hospice program, however distant, the individual is deprived of access to the hospice benefit. Hospice programs that provide such access at a cost to their own financial probity have received special consideration by funding agencies. To the degree that federal or state regulations inhibit access to hospice programs, these regulations subvert the congressional mandate of legislation designed to enhance such access. As Congressman Leon Panetta stated (1981) in introducing hospice legislation: "The legislation that will be before the Congress is a beginning, a good solid beginning. . . . We can make the hospice story a reality—a fulfillment of the moral test of a nation dedicated to serving those in need. That is our bond. That is our pledge. That is our commitment" (p. 8542).

This good solid beginning was constrained by governmental regulation. Palliative care services are constrained by lack of financing, about which more is said shortly. Palliative care services, which are institutionally focused, need partners in the community. Hospice programs have demonstrated their ability to maintain dying persons in the community. An approach that encompasses palliative care services and hospice, not as alternatives but as complementary, is required. How this might be accomplished is discussed later in this chapter.

Access to Hospice Care for Those with AIDS

The strictures of hospice reimbursement also had an impact on access to services for those infected with the human immunodeficiency virus (HIV) (Shietinger, 1986). Such limitations could have been predicted, given the assumption of the presence of a caregiver by the regulations and the problematic availability of such an individual for the HIV-infected person.

The resultant financial considerations may not have been as significant as other factors in the failure to assume responsibility for the care of terminally ill persons with AIDS. Some hospice programs failed to provide care, as a result of fear related to the infectiousness of the disease, concern about stigma, and prejudice against those infected with HIV. All of these factors have been noted in the responses of other health care providers (van Servellen, Lewis, & Leake, 1988, pp. 6–8). A hospice program's financial concerns, however, can serve as a convenient screen to shield exploration of the real reasons for failure to provide care to HIV-infected persons.

Prejudice against HIV-infected individuals related to their life-styles, whether sexual orientation or substance use, may result in inadequate and inappropriate care. Fortunately, a number of hospice programs rose to the challenge, and provided exquisite care to their terminally ill clients infected with HIV/AIDS. The availability of new treatment regimens has had such a dramatic impact on the health of HIV-infected persons that most hospice programs dedicated solely to HIV-infected persons have closed. The good news is that such programs are no longer needed. The bad news is that hospice providers with HIV/AIDS expertise may not be available for those dying of this disease. And, although theoretically, one would expect hospice providers to care for terminally ill persons whatever the problem, sadly, such is not always the case. Fortunately, such situations of lack of willingness to care are, now, not common.

Although not all hospice programs readily accepted clients with AIDS, not all failure to do so was a result of prejudice. The illness trajectories of the person with cancer and the person with AIDS are different, with the latter requiring the use of expensive medications (Corless & Nicholas, 2000). As previously noted, the advent of new therapeutic regimens has transformed HIV/AIDS care in the United States. Such is not the case in developing countries that cannot afford the costs of these expensive regimens. And, while lack of affordable medications is a question that must be addressed by countries, drug companies, charitable foundations, and humanity as a whole, even a solution to this problem would not eliminate the need for palliative care. The problems in developing countries are compounded by a delay in the identification of infected individuals. This delay has implications not only for the spread of disease, but also for the degradation of an infected person's immune system, making him or her a sicker person, if and when he or she is ultimately identified. For any number of reasons, hospice and palliative care services are important for the care of the terminally ill in such countries. The presence of help provides hope. And hope is part of the spiritual environment for hospice care.

A Question of Spiritual Care

The hospice approach purports to encompass the physical, psychological, social, and spiritual needs of the patient. Saunders (1986), Wald (1986), and others have expressed concern that the spiritual aspects of care have been neglected. This neglect is not surprising, given the perception by many caregivers that the spiritual concerns of a patient more properly belong to the patient and his or her religious counselors. Publication of the *Assumptions and Principles of Spiritual Care for the Terminally Ill* provides a new and different perspective (Corless et al., 1990): "Caregivers should be aware that they each have the potential for providing spiritual care, as do all human beings, and should be encouraged to offer spiritual care to dying patients and their families as needed" (p. 80). The obvious danger is that an overzealous caregiver will attempt to impose his or her religious precepts or beliefs on a patient. The authors of *Assumptions and Principles of Spiritual Care for the Terminally Ill* considered this possibility, and state, in Principle 18: "Caregivers should guard against proselytizing for particular types of beliefs and practices" (p. 79).

A more recent concern of hospice providers is that the spiritual and psychosocial components will be omitted by palliative care services, or, at the least, be given a back seat to the "medical" issues. A referral for chaplaincy services connotes multidisciplinary awareness, but not necessarily interdisciplinary teamwork. A physician-dominated team is not in keeping with the spirit of care envisaged by hospice providers. It is likely to be characteristic of hospital-based palliative care services, however.

As significant as spiritual care is for patients and families, it is also important for caregivers (Ley & Corless, 1988). A spiritual environment is an important resource for health care workers confronted on a continual basis with the deaths of patients. Staff sessions with a psychiatrist, no matter how empathetic, locate the difficulty within the individual, rather than as a characteristic of a stressful situation in which much is demanded of the professional. That is not to say that work with a psychiatrist may not be beneficial. It is, however, to situate the problem in the caregiving environment. Palliative care service providers have given insufficient attention to the spiritual aspects of the caregiving environment.

Spirituality adds a dimension to life that connects an individual to a sphere beyond himself or herself. An environment that allows for spiritual expressions changes the way in which interactions occur to one of greater acceptance of the other, regardless of individual beliefs. In such an environment, the loss of another can be acknowledged, and in so doing an individual's life is affirmed (Corless, 1986). Finding hospice profession-als to be more spiritual in their personal lives than in their work, Millison and Dudley (1990) speculate: "Perhaps there are deterrents or obstacles within hospice programs that prevent professionals from freely expressing their spirituality with patients" (p. 76). This is likely also to be the case for the providers of palliative care services. Precepts regarding separation of church and state may have influenced hospice workers, in the Millison and Dudley study, in subtle ways, to maintain a distinction between work and spirituality. Equating religion with spirituality may compound the difficulties. Spirituality may also be perceived as solely a personal attribute, rather than as a component of the environment.

Although hospice programs profess to provide spiritual care, the sub-stance of such care may be illusory. Noting a patient's religious practice on an intake sheet is not equivalent to providing spiritual care; nor is the presence of a chaplain as a member of the team, although each may contribute to a positive outcome. Spiritual care implies integration, not separation. Spiritual care is not the work of any one individual. It is the culmination of the efforts of all involved in care, to provide an environment in which reflection on life and death and other issues is encouraged.

Saunders, as noted previously, was a pioneer in her insistence on both effective symptom control and the presence of a religious-spiritual environ-ment at St. Christopher's Hospice (Daaleman & Vander Creek, 2000). The incorporation of the arts at the Connecticut Hospice, as described by Bailey (1994), is a secular expression of some of these same felt needs. The challenge of integrating the sacred with the scientific, though acknowledged to be important, may be viewed as secondary to the more pragmatic issues of program survival in an increasingly financially constricted environment, or may be denied in a highly technological curative atmosphere. Thus, spiritual care may be neglected because it is not seen as fitting into the paradigm of cure-oriented patient care, or because of the priority given to physical and psychosocial patient care and the emphasis on financial con-cerns as the "life or death" of a program.

A Question of Finances

The health of hospice programs and palliative care services departments are dependent, in large part, on finances. The impact of third-party payers is significant. Decisions by hospice care providers are being countermanded by third-party intermediaries who determine the appropriateness of care and the level of reimbursement for a given patient. Clearly, hospice teams are free to provide the care that is deemed appropriate. Reimbursement, however, is determined by the fiscal intermediary. This situation seems incongruous, given the "cap" of dollars (for the total number of patients) already in place in order to curb governmental expenditures for hospice patients. The issue for palliative care services is reimbursement for services (Foubister, 2001). Using traditional billing mechanisms, physicians and advanced practice nurses are billed for consultation. Billing for team conferences is not available.

The problem of finances encompasses still other issues, including those of the cost of "outliers," the need for acute inpatient care or continuous home care, and the responsibility of hospice programs for therapies. Outliers are patients who use a disproportionate share of resources. Often this occurs as a result of a longer-than-expected stay in the hospice program. Such individuals may skew the calculations (and expenses), particularly of small hospice programs, which by nature of their size do not possess the financial resilience to provide a counterweight to the intensive or extensive use of resources. Recognition of the outlier problem has resulted in modifications to compensate hospice programs more adequately.

The need for acute care or the provision of continuous care at home are decisions made by hospice care providers, which, unless adequately documented, may be open to rejection by the fiscal intermediary. Such determinations are similar to those made in traditional home care, in which the need for the service must be documented painstakingly if fee-for-service reimbursement is to occur. Initially, per diem rates were thought to obviate the need for creative writing exercises in patient charts. Unfortunately, such is not the case.

Responsibility for the provision of medications and therapies has been a potentially explosive issue, since palliative radiation, chemotherapy, surgery, and other palliative procedures have become the financial responsibility of the hospice program. Developments such as total parenteral nutrition (TPN), a method of providing nutritional sustenance via a surgically implanted tube, are now incorporated into the care of persons at home. Such approaches may require careful monitoring, as, for example, with TPN, to prevent metabolic imbalance (Newman & Capozza, 1991). The cost of one day of TPN exceeds the hospice home care per diem rate, making such therapies prohibitive, if required for a lengthy period of time and/or for multiple patients.

The financial issues for palliative care services are in part those of the secondary and tertiary care facility. Given that reimbursement is governed by diagnostic-related groups, a patient remaining in hospital for longer than the average time becomes an expense for the hospital, if patient and family are unable to pay. The push to make palliative care a separate diagnosis may alleviate some of this problem.

It doesn't resolve the problem, however, of what outpatient or community services will support the patient discharged to home. Given that palliative care services are available to patients from diagnosis to death in hospital, and hospice programs are largely focused on care in the community for the last 6 months of life, it behooves both types of programs to coordinate their services for the benefit of patients. There is a need for creativity to enhance such program-to-program collaboration.

A Question of Innovation

Innovative approaches to the provision of hospice care have entailed establishment of satellite hospice centers or teams, to provide care to people living in large geographic areas, hospice arrangements with nursing homes, and mega-hospice programs such as Hospice Care, Inc. (HCI), which operates "comprehensive inpatient and home-care hospices in Boston, Chicago, Dallas, Fort Lauderdale, Fort Worth, Houston, and Miami" (HCI, 1990, p. 1). The key to the success of HCI is, in part, expert and centralized management. In addition to other economies, HCI participates in an electronic media claims hook-up between HCI and Medicare. The result is a "cost turnaround of less [sic] than 30 days from date of service" (HCI, 1990, p. 6). Delays in reimbursement can spell financial gloom, if not doom, for hospice programs. And many programs with less electronic sophistication experience such delays.

Expansion of services to nursing homes, by a hospice team whose members work with the patient, family, and nursing home staff, is reflective of the model of hospice as a consultation team whose members go to the patient, wherever he or she is located. The consultative approach was exemplified first by the palliative care team at the Royal Victoria Hospital in Montreal, and the Hospice of Marin in California. Such a model, particularly when the collaboration is with a nursing home or group home, obviates the concern about a caregiver.

Hospice care may become available to a greater number of individuals, when society and discrete communities solve the question of the financing of residential care for debilitated individuals who lack the necessary support to remain at home, whether such care is given in a group home, by a host family, in a nursing home, or some other type of residence for care. Such innovative solutions will enhance access to hospice care.

Access to palliative care services is important, given that nearly one half of all deaths still take place in hospitals. In part, this may occur as a result of unanticipated deaths, the technological requirement of the care situation, or the lack of another site for care. The challenge for palliative care services is to change the way care is rendered for life-threatening and death-ensuing illnesses. The emphasis on comfort care need not be restricted to the terminal phase of illness. And, although this seems obvious, the practice of medical care has not incorporated this precept until recently. Further, the patient needs to be central in the decision making, that is, the patient or, if he or she is unable, designated others, make the decisions regarding the mode of dying, and not the physician. The palliative care provider is present to facilitate the comfort of the patient, and to help the dying person and family complete relevant activities.

A Question of Choice

Hospice as a holistic concept of care, providing attention to the physical, psychological, social, and spiritual needs of a patient, has been perceived by its adherents as a countervailing force to those espousing the "right to die." Palliative care providers share this holistic philosophy of care.

The goals of hospice and palliative care services concern enhancing the quality of life of patients and their families. The usual methodology is to control troublesome symptoms, to allow the person to live comfortably until he or she dies. But what of the small residual of patients for whom symptoms cannot be managed adequately? Is it part of the hospice and palliative care mandate that patients live in suffering until they die? Are there instances in which suffering continues unabated despite the best efforts of all concerned? Further, do some team members abandon these "treatment failures"?

And what of the individuals who find themselves in such circumstances? What are their rights? What are their options? If hospice and palliative care services are concerned with giving clients control, as Tuohey (1988) states, what are the parameters of such control? The very notion of "giving control," a notion applied to "patients" in a variety of settings, implies an inequity of power (Corless, 1991). The terms *patient* and *giving control* require further examination.

The term *client* implies a greater parity among the parties in the relationship than does the term *patient*, with its historic denotation of a dependent relationship in which the roles are superordinate and subordinate. Perhaps the time has come for a consideration of the implications of such labeling.

Giving control, in hospital parlance, usually refers to such things as choice of foods, when to engage in morning ablutions, whether to engage in "social" activities, and, more recently, within a defined range, patients having control of analgesia for pain management. Patients who selected hospice as a caregiving option have exhibited *choice*, if not *control*, by selecting hospice as their caregiving option. The term *giving control*, in this context, has an uncomfortable connotation. Perhaps it is a result of the aforementioned inequity of power implied between caregiver and care recipient and the ability of one party in the relationship to determine if and when control is to be shared. It is clearly also a consequence of the increasing physical dependence of the patient on the caregiver. This inequality is all the more apparent in hospitals in which the social structure is emblematic of this power differential.

A more congenial term is *choice*, not as in giving someone a choice, but as in choice inherent in the individual. Under such circumstances, the expectation is one of the hospice and palliative care services client making choices about all aspects of his or her care. Not all persons will welcome the opportunities of such a model, but that too would be the client's choice, rather than one that is imposed. Clients would determine the degree to which decision-making is shared, rather than automatically being the recipients of professional decision-making.

The obvious question that follows such deliberations is, Does choice include whether to maintain or relinquish life? Note that questions of sustaining life are those of caregivers. The question addressed here is, does the individual have the right to determine when to die? Care must be taken not to phrase this question as one of a determination of when an individual has suffered enough. Phrased in this manner, the issue becomes one of "earning" the right to make a choice.

If hospice and palliative care programs presume to give clients control, should that control be limited to the trivial, or does it concern reinforcing an individual's right to make choices regarding living and dying? Although the hope for adequate symptom control will be for a life fully lived, what approaches will be used when those hopes are not fulfilled and the patient concludes that enough is enough? The current discussions of living wills in acute care facilities also apply to hospice programs. Specifications about not suffering may result in drug dosages that reduce the level of consciousness, when suffering cannot otherwise be alleviated (Wanzer et al., 1989). The use of terminal sedation is being discussed as a practice in palliative care services (Quill, 2000; Sulmasy, 2000). The availability of various professionals in hospital may account for the discussion of this option by palliative care professionals, rather than as a hospice practice.

Choices about life and death should not entail activities contrary to health care workers' commitments to preserving life (Singer & Siegler, 1990), nor should they entail actions that create liability for criminal prosecution—that is, a patient's right to choice does not include asking the care provider to engage in actions for which the provider may be penalized. Unassisted self-termination may be possible in a minority of cases. What if those individuals wishing to bring their lives to a close are too weak to implement their wishes? Hospice professionals perceive such a demand as in conflict with the ethos of hospice care, and would therefore focus on comfort care. Palliative care providers, on the other hand, have been engaged in an active debate on these issues. This distinction may result from the active choice for hospice and the hospice philosophy of care espoused by the providers of such care. Referrals for palliative care services may be for the control of various symptoms. The recipients of such care may find they are terminally ill when they are too weak or "ill"-prepared to take their own lives. And, although palliative care professionals also eschew participation in or assistance with self-termination, the practice of terminal sedation may alleviate awareness of a life soon to end that the care recipient finds too intolerable to bear.

Removal of life-sustaining technology that has become burdensome is another question more likely to face palliative care professionals than those engaged in hospice care. The removal of such technology when requested is in keeping with the question "Whose life is it, anyway?" The answer to this question clarifies the issue of unwanted life-sustaining technology. Clearly, hospice and palliative care services will need to reconsider other such issues in light of changing case law, state statutes, and values about living and dying.

End-of-Life Care: An Answer

The concept of hospice, emboldened by the imperative that something more should be done for the dying person, was created when health care providers determined something more could be done. Although much of the foregoing discussion concerns issues currently facing hospice and palliative care services, this chapter would not be complete without a consideration of the role of the family in hospice and palliative care. Saunders and McCorkle (1985) are correct in observing that families are partners in the provision of care. Unless a family assessment and family plan of care are developed, it is arguable whether the family is part of the unit of care prior to bereavement (Saunders, 1993). Families facilitate care at home, which is why individuals without such support may not receive hospice care.

Palliative care services are provided largely in the hospital. The role of the family as caregiver is not prominent in this setting. Here, family as part of the unit of care is more straightforward. In hospice, as noted, family is both recipient of and provider of care. This has created a complex relationship with the family. This difficult situation has resulted in a unit of care, part of which is also part of the caregiving team. The impact of caregiving on the family and the adequacy of family care under these circumstances needs to be addressed (Raveis & Siegel, 1991).

Indeed, the quality of end-of-life care is currently being examined by a number of organizations and researchers. How to measure quality of care, as perceived by someone with diminished consciousness, is a major challenge. The approach of having family members evaluate such care, and their perception of its quality, is a pragmatic approach. However, if the evaluator also participated in the caregiving, what is being measured? There may be no easy answer.

Hospice programs have given a clear answer to the question of the potential for terminally ill persons to remain at home to die. The response is dramatically in the affirmative. Palliative care services have taken up the challenge of transforming dying in hospitals to the quality achieved by hospice programs in the home or in specially designated hospice units. If palliative care services succeed in accomplishing in hospitals what has been achieved by hospice programs in the home, then their combined contribution may be to facilitate a greater appreciation for living as the humane possibilities for dying are actualized. What a legacy!

Discussion Questions

1. How are hospice and palliative care services portrayed in the media?
2. Which of the issues discussed in this chapter will have the greatest impact on the viability of hospice and pallliative care services?
3. Are the issues the same?

References

Bailey, S. (1994). Creativity and the close of life. In I. Corless, B. Germino, & M. Pittman (Eds.), *Dying, death, and bereavement: Theoretical perspectives and other ways of knowing* (pp. 327–335). Boston: Jones & Bartlett.

Beresford, L. (1989). Alternative, outpatient settings of care for people with AIDS. *Quality Review Bulletin, 15,* 9–16.

Beresford, L. (1990a). Creative approaches to minority outreach. *NHO Hospice News, 10*(3), 6, 11–12.

Beresford, L. (1990b). Hospice leader Jack Lee advises small rural hospices on issues of growth. *NHO Hospice News, 10*(9), 4–5.

Beresford, L., & Connor, S. (1999). History of the National Hospice Organization. *The Hospice Journal, 14*(3/4), 15–31.

Billings, J. A. (1998). What is palliative care? *Journal of Palliative Care, 1*(1), 73–81.

Cohen, K. P. (1979). *Hospice prescription for terminal care.* Germantown, MD: Aspen Systems.

Corless, I. B. (1983a). Models of hospice care. In N. Chaska (Ed.), *The nursing profession: A time to speak* (pp. 540–550). New York: McGraw-Hill.

Corless, I. B. (1983b). The hospice movement in North America. In C. Corr & D. Corr (Eds.), *Hospice care principles and practice* (pp. 335–351). New York: Springer.

Corless, I. B. (1983c). A response to the evaluation of the NYS Hospice Demonstration Project. *Journal of the New York State Nurses Association, 14,* 6–9.

Corless, I. B. (1984). Hospice: The state of the art. *Proceedings of the Fourth National Conference on Cancer Nursing, 1983* (pp. 29–35). New York: American Cancer Society.

Corless, I. B. (1985). Implications of the new hospice legislation and the accompanying regulations. *Nursing Clinics of North America, 20,* 281–298.

Corless, I. B. (1986). Spirituality for whom? In F. Wald (Ed.), *In quest of the spiritual component of care for the terminally ill* (pp. 87–96). New Haven: Yale University.

Corless, I. B. (1987–1988). Settings for terminal care. *Omega, 18,* 319–340.

Corless, I. B. (1990, September). The death, dying and hospice movement: The past and the coming decade (keynote address). *Tenth Annual Interdisciplinary Seminar Ten and Then.* Albany: New York State Hospice Association.

Corless, I. B. (1991). Review of Tuohey, caring for persons with AIDS and cancer: Ethical reflections in palliative care for the terminally ill. *Journal of Palliative Care, 7,* 1.

Corless, I. B., & Nicholas, P. K. (2000). Long-term continuum of care for people living with HIV/AIDS. *Journal of Urban Health, 77*(2), 176–186.

Corless, I. B., Wald, F., Autton, N., Bailey, S., Cockburn, M., Cosh, R., et al. (1990). Assumptions and principles of spiritual care, developed by the Spiritual Work Group of the International Work Group on Death, Dying and Bereavement. *Death Studies, 14,* 75–81.

Crawley, L. C., Payne, R., Bolden, J., Payne, T., Washington, P., & Williams, S., for the Institute to Improve Palliative and End-of-Life Care in the African American Community. (2000). *Journal of the American Medical Association, 284*(19), 2518–2521.

Daaleman, T. P., & Vander Creek, L. (2000). Placing religions and spirituality in end-of-life care. *Journal of the American Medical Association, 284*(19), 2514–2517.

Davidson, G. W. (1978). *The hospice—development and administration.* Washington, DC: Hemisphere.

Feifel, H. (Ed.). (1959). *The meaning of death.* New York: McGraw-Hill.

Feifel, H. (1994). Attitudes toward death: A personal perspective. In I. Corless, B. Germino, & M. Pittman (Eds.), *Dying death, and bereavement: Theoretical perspectives and other ways of knowing* (pp. 49–60). Boston: Jones & Bartlett.

Ferris, F. D., & Cummings, I. (Eds.). (1995). *Palliative care: Towards a consensus in standardized principles of practice.* Toronto, Canada: Canadian Palliative Care Association.

Foster, Z., Wald, F. S., & Wald, H. J. (1978). The hospice movement: A backward glance of its first two decades. *The New Physician, 27,* 21–24.

Foubister, V. (2001, February 26). Palliative care: Mainstream model. Amednews.com. Retrieved ___, from http:www.AMA-assn.org/sci-pubs/amnews/puk_01/ prsa0226.htm

Hospice Care, Inc. (1990). *Introducing Hospice Care, Incorporated, to Dr. Inge B. Corless.* Document.

Harper, B. C. (1990). Doing the right thing. *Hospice, Spring,* 14–15.

Hillier, R. (1983). Terminal care in the United Kingdom. In C. Corr & D. Corr (Eds.), *Hospice care: Principles and practice* (pp. 319–334). New York: Springer.

Kübler-Ross, E. (1969). *On death and dying.* New York: Macmillan.

Lack, S. A. (1977). The hospice concept-the adult with advanced cancer. In *Proceedings of the American Cancer Society Second National Conference on Human Values and Cancer* (pp. 160–166). Chicago: American Cancer Society.

Lack, S. A., & Buckingham, R. W., III (1978). *First American hospice.* New Haven: Hospice, Inc.

Ley, D. C. H., & Corless, I. B. (1988). Spirituality and hospice care. *Death Studies, 12,* 101–110.

McCann, B. A. (1988). Hospice care in the United States: The struggle for definition and survival. *Journal of Palliative Care, 4,* 16–18.

Melzack, R., Ofiesh, J. G., & Mount, B. M. (1976). The Brompton mixture: Effects on pain in cancer patients. *Canadian Medical Association Journal, 115,* 125–128.

Millison, M. B., & Dudley, J. R. (1990). The importance of spirituality in hospice work: A study of hospice professionals. *Hospice Journal, 6,* 63–78.

Mount, B. M. (1976). *Palliative care service: October 1976 report.* Montreal: Royal Victoria Hospital/McGill University.

National Hospice Organization. (1991). *About hospice under Medicare.* South Deerfield, MA: Channing L. Bete.

Newman, C. F., & Capozza, C. M. (1991). Home nutrition support in HIV disease. *Journal of Home Health Care Practice, 3,* 25–51.

O'Connor, P. (1999). Hospice vs. palliative care. *Hospice Journal, 15*(3/4), 123–137.

Osterweis, M., & Champagne, D. S. (1979). The U.S. hospice movement: Issues in development. *American Journal of Public Health, 69,* 492–496.

Panetta, L. E. (1981). Presentation for National Hospice Organization, November 12, 1981. St. Louis, MO. Published in the *Congressional Record-House* (November 18, 1981) 8541–8542.

Quill, T. E., & Byock, I. R. (2000). Responding to intractable terminal suffering: The role of terminal sedation and voluntary refusal of food and fluids. ACP-ASIM End of Life Care Consensus Panel. *Annals of Internal Medicine, 132,* 408–414.

Raveis, V. H., & Siegel, K. (1991, February). The impact of care giving on informal or familial caregivers. *AIDS Patient Care,* 39–43.

Rhymes, J. (1990). Hospice care in America. *Journal of the American Medical Association, 264,* 369–372.

Saunders, C. M. (1960). *Care of the dying.* London: MacMillan.

Saunders, C. M. (1978). Evolution of the hospices. In R. Mann (Ed.), *The history of the management of pain: From early principles to present practice* (pp. 167–178). Cameforth, England: Parthenon.

Saunders, C. M. (1979). Nature and management of terminal pain and the hospice concept. In J. J. Bonica & V. Ventafridda (Eds.), *Advances in pain research and therapy* (pp. 635–651). New York: Raven.

Saunders, C. M. (1986). Modern hospice. In F. Wald (Ed.), *In quest of the spiritual component of care for the terminally ill* (pp. 41–48). New Haven: Yale University.

Saunders, J. M. (1993). Personal communication.

Saunders, J. M., & McCorkle, R. (1985). Models of care for persons with progressive cancer. *Nursing Clinics of North America, 20,* 365–377.

Shietinger, H. (1986). Hospice care needs of the person with AIDS. *Journal of Palliative Care, 2,* 31–32.

Singer, P. A., & Siegler, M. (1990). Euthanasia: A critique. *New England Journal of Medicine, 322,* 1881–1883.

Stoddard, S. (1978). *The hospice movement.* New York: Stein & Day.

Stoddard, S. (1990). Hospice: Approaching the 21st century. *The American Journal of Hospice and Palliative Care, 7,* 27–30.

Sulmasy, D. P., Ury, W. A., Ahronheim, J. C., Siegler, M., Kass, L., Lantos, J., et al. (2000). Responding to intractable terminal suffering. *Annals of Internal Medicine, 133*(7), 560–561.

The SUPPORT Principal Investigators. (1995). Controlled trial to improve care for seriously ill hospitalized patients: The Study to Understand Prognoses and Preferences for Outcomes and Risks of Treatments (SUPPORT). *Journal of the American Medical Association, 274,* 591–1598.

Tuohey, J. F. (1988). *Caring for persons with AIDS and cancer: Ethical reflections on palliative care for the terminally ill.* St. Louis, MO: Catholic Health Association of the United States.

Twycross, R. G. (1983). Principles and practices of pain relief in terminal cancer. In C. Corr & D. Corr (Eds.), *Hospice care: Principles and practice* (pp. 55–72). New York: Springer.

van Servellen, G. M., Lewis, C. E., & Leake, B. (1988). Nurses' responses to the AIDS crisis: Implication for continuing education programs. *Journal of Continuing Education in Nursing, 19,* 6–8.

Wald, F. (1986). In search of the spiritual component of hospice care. In F. Wald (Ed.), *In quest of the spiritual component of care for the terminally ill* (pp. 25–33). New Haven: Yale University.

Wald, F. (1994). Finding a way to give hospice care. In I. Corless, B. Germino, & M. Pittman (Eds.), *Dying, death and bereavement: Theoretical perspectives and other ways of knowing* (pp. 31–47). Boston: Jones & Bartlett.

Walter, N. T. (1979). *Hospice pilot project report.* Haywood, CA: Kaiser Permanente Medical Center.

Wanzer, S. H., Federman, D. D., Adelstein, S. J., Cassel, C. K., Cassem, E. H., Cranford, R. E., et al. (1989). The physician's responsibility toward hopelessly patients: A second look. *New England Journal of Medicine, 320,* 844–849.

Ten

Regulatory Issues in the Care of Dying

Judi Lund Person

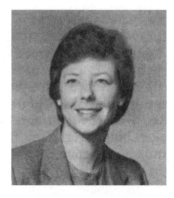

Judi Lund Person graduated with honors with a BSW from the University of North Carolina at Greensboro and a masters degree in public health from the University of North Carolina at Chapel Hill. She has been Executive Director of Hospice for the Carolinas (HFC)—formerly Hospice of North Carolina—since 1980. Hospice for the Carolinas is the state hospice organization, serving North Carolina since 1977 and North and South Carolina since 1993. The organization provides technical assistance, legislative and regulatory advocacy, and educational services to the 100 hospice programs in the two states.

Lund Person served for six years on the board of directors of the National Hospice Organization (NHO). She has both chaired and served on numerous national committees including the legislative task force and the AIDS resource committee. A winner of the prestigious Peter Keese Award for the advancement of hospice care in North Carolina, she has led Hospice for the Carolinas to four national awards, including the 1993 NHO President's Award for Excellence in Educational Programming.

A recognized national leader in the field of hospice care, Lund Person consults across the country with state hospice organizations and local hospice providers, specifically relating to statewide data collection and legislative and regulatory advocacy.

Lund Person has served on the boards of several statewide nonprofit health and volunteer organizations. She is a founding member, and also served as president, of the recently created North Carolina Center for Nonprofits.

Introduction

In the past few years, the complications of increased medical technology and the emphasis of the medical community on "treating at all costs" has created a growing awareness of the legal and regulatory issues that face health care providers who care for terminally ill patients.

This chapter will provide an overview of the key legal and regulatory issues that are part of the field of death and dying. While not intended to be a detailed analysis, and limited by issues pertinent to the United States, the concepts will help to focus this discussion and give the reader additional resources to pursue.

Patients' Rights

Patient rights is not a new concept. As early as 1901, the New York courts ruled that "every human being of adult years and sound mind has a right to determine what shall be done with his own body" (Kelly, 1981). Continued concentration on the topic over the last two decades has brought it to the attention of the health care community and the courts as well as the public.

In 1973, the American Hospital Association approved a "Patient's Bill of Rights," which included the competent adult patient's right of informed consent and the right to refuse treatment (Siner, 1989). In that same year, the judicial council of the American Medical Association recognized the "reciprocal rights and duties of physicians and terminally ill patients. It was recognized that physicians had a moral obligation to share the burden of responsibility with their competent, terminal patients as to what life-prolonging measures might be used" (Siner, 1989). In the summer of 2001, Congress passed a Patient Bill of Rights, that allows for limited lawsuits against HMOs. The Senate adopted new patients' rights legislation late last week. Will the proposal improve health care in America? (7/02/01) More recently, the Patient Bill of Rights has been approved by Congress which gives patients.

In the summer of 2001, the US Senate passed a Patient Bill of Rights which allowed for limited lawsuits against HMOs. The US House passed an amended version of a Patient Bill of Rights and the bill was sent to conference committee. The issue died in conference committee. Much attention has been given to the rights of patients in the managed care setting, and new internal and external reviews have been implemented by managed care organizations to provide appropriate reviews of coverage and claims.

At this writing, states are also considering adopting patient rights statutes to allow patients to sue their managed care plan.

Two Landmark Cases for Patient Rights

The case of Karen Ann Quinlan in 1976 was the first case involving the withdrawal of life-sustaining medical care from a permanently incompetent adult. She was the first modern icon of the right-to-die debate. The 21-year-old Quinlan collapsed after swallowing alcohol and tranquilizers at a party in 1975. Her friends attempted resuscitation. In the emergency room, she was resuscitated and placed on a respirator. One year later, she was in a chronic persistent vegetative state, ventilator dependent and receiving nutrition through a nasogastric tube (Emmanuel, 1988). Her family waged a much-publicized legal battle for the right to remove her life support machinery. Their wishes conflicted with the attending physician's opinion that discontinuation of the respirator was a violation of medical ethics (Emanuel, 1988). The case went to the New Jersey Supreme Court, where the court established the following framework for reviewing this and future cases:

1. Is there a right to terminate medical care?
2. What types of care can be terminated?
3. From what types of patients can care be terminated?
4. Who should act as the decision maker?
5. What are appropriate criteria for justifying the termination of medical care? (Emanuel, 1988)

In their decision, the NJ Supreme Court decided that an individual's constitutional right to privacy included a right to refuse medical care and recognized this right for incompetent patients (Siner, 1989). The respirator was removed, but Quinlan kept breathing after the respirator was unplugged. She remained in a coma for almost 10 years in a New Jersey nursing home until her 1985 death. After the Quinlan case, many state courts have ruled that the individual's right to refuse medical care is permissible.

As a result of the attention given to the Quinlan case, and to increasing questions and pressures from the medical community and the public, the President's Commission on the Study of Ethical Problems in Medicine and Biomedical and Behavioral Research issued its final report "Deciding to Forego Life-Sustaining Treatment," in 1983. This landmark report clearly recognized patient autonomy in issues concerning terminal care and pointed out the need for an appropriate surrogate to act in accordance with the patient's wishes (Siner, 1989). One of the guidelines with far-reaching implications recommended by the President's Commission was the "Physician's Responsibility toward Hopelessly Ill Patients," which included the withdrawal of artificial feeding (Wanzer, Adelstein, Cranford, et al., 1985).

Another landmark court test of patient rights was the decision by the U.S. Supreme Court in June, 1990, in the case Cruzan v. Director, Missouri Health Department. On June 25, 1990, the United States Supreme Court issued an opinion in the case of Cruzan v. Director, Missouri Department of Health, the first right-to-die case to be heard by the US Supreme Court. Nancy Cruzan, 26, was in a car accident in 1983. When paramedics arrived at the scene they could not detect any respiratory or cardiac function. With cardiopulmonary resuscitation, her breathing was restored, but permanent brain damage was sustained. From 1983 until her death, she existed in a persistent vegetative state, where she was oblivious to her surroundings without voluntary movements. She had reflex actions and could breath on her own, but was unable to receive adequate nutrition without a feeding tube. A gastrostomy tube was surgically implanted four weeks after the accident.

In 1987, when there was no longer any hope for her recovery, Nancy Cruzan's parents requested that the gastrostomy tube be removed. Cruzan did not have a signed living will, but had verbally expressed to a roommate her desires not to live "like a vegetable." When the hospital staff would not allow the removal of the tube unless there was a court order, Nancy's parents sued. In the Missouri trial courts, the judge concluded that Cruzan had a fundamental right to liberty both in the federal and state constitutions, to be free from further treatment. He ordered the tube removed.

An appeal by state officials to the Missouri Supreme Court overruled the trial judge, stating that "there was no state or federal constitutional right retained by an incompetent person to override the state's 'unqualified' interest in life." The Missouri living will law allowed for the removal of life-sustaining treatment only when death is inevitable "within a short time"; it does not allow for the removal of artificial feeding tubes (Kamen, 1989).

The Supreme Court, in its opinion, focused on a limited portion of the case: whether Missouri could require a clear and convincing standard of proof to allow the withdrawal of a life-sustaining treatment from an incompetent patient. The Constitution permits a state to require the provision of life-sustaining treatment to an incompetent patient unless there is "clear and convincing" evidence that the patient authorized the withholding of treatment while still competent. The decision was based on the due process clause of the Fourteenth Amendment (no State shall deprive any person of life, liberty or property without due process of law), different from the lower courts which based their decisions on the patient's right to privacy. Of note in the Supreme Court decision is the assumption made by the Court that artificial nutrition and hydration are considered medical treatment. Justice O'Connor wrote a concurring opinion which expressed her support for appointed proxies to make health care decisions as a safeguard to failing to honor a patient's wishes (Pearlman, 1991).

The Supreme Court decision is limited in scope and gives Missouri alone guidance in this case. No other state is required by this decision to change state law or ethical standards which allow the withdrawal of life-sustaining treatments. It continues to underscore the importance of written, advance directives, and the communication which should occur between patient and physician while the patient is competent and able to make health care decisions. At the same time, a significant education process will be required if the use of written advance directives is to be widely accepted, since at this writing, only 9% of Americans have living wills.

Advance Directives

Advance directives is the name given to the two types of directives to medical personnel in which patients may maintain control over the care that is provided, in the event they lack the capacity to do so at the time treatment decisions need to be made. The advance directive is also based on the assumption that health care providers will prefer to make decisions for patients in a way that reflects as closely as possible the patient's own views. The two types of advance directives are the living will and the durable power of attorney, also called a health care power of attorney or a health care proxy.

Living Wills

The living will was originally proposed in 1967 by Louis Kutner as a way for "a patient with a terminal illness to document and specify the nature of future medical care in the event of incapacitation" (Siner, 1989). The legal principle of the living will is the right of a competent adult to refuse treatment. California enacted the first Natural Death Act in January 1977, specifying that the living will would be used in the case of a terminal condition. Living will statutes were originally adopted by states to allow patients to make decisions about their care before they become hospitalized or incompetent. Since 1976, every state has enacted one or more health care advance directive statutes. Most states have at least two statutes, "one establishing a living will type of directive; the other establishing a proxy or durable power of attorney for health care" (Sabatino, 1999). States have been moving toward a simplified approach to the statute, combining existing advance directive statutes into one flexible advance directive act. By 1998, 15 states had comprehensive statutes: AL, AZ, CT, DE, FL, KY, ME, MD, MN, MS, NJ, NM, OK, OR, VA (Sabatino, 1999).

The National Conference of Commissioners on Uniform State Laws developed a Uniform Health Care Decisions Act in 1993. The model Act establishes simple requirements for recognizing nearly any type of written or oral statement as an advance directive. Five states have now adopted a version of this Act: MS, AL, DE, ME, and NM (Sabatino, 1999). With the increased attention being given to end of life care issues at the state level, state legislators and policy-makers are encouraged to make advance care planning documents more consumer-friendly.

As living will legislation has been implemented by various states, experts have identified the following problems with the living will statutes:

1. The term *terminally ill* is defined differently in each state, according to Fenella Rouse, executive director of the Society for the Right to Die, New York City (Hudson, 1989). Many states' living will statutes limit the application to "terminal and incurable" conditions. Not all living will statutes include brain death and persistent vegetative state as part of the legal definition of death.

2. Only 9% of all Americans have drafted living wills (Hudson, 1989).

3. In some states where the statute does not specifically allow family members to make health care decisions for an incompetent family member, decisions about withholding life support are confused and run the risk of legal liability.

4. Physicians are never sure that the living will represents the continued choice of the patient; and also say that the living will does not cover the "exhaustive mix of conditions that interact on a critically ill patient" (Hudson, 1989)

5. There is confusion about the definition and interpretation of extraordinary/ordinary care. This wording refers to the language in some living wills that specifies that "no extraordinary means will be used to prolong my life should I become terminally or incurably ill." The

definition of extraordinary is subjective at best, and is confusing in some instances when applied in a medical treatment setting.

Health Care Power of Attorney

Some states have provided for a health care power of attorney (HCPA) statute, also called a durable power of attorney or a health care proxy in some states, which authorizes a person designated by the patient to make medical decisions for the patient, in the event of the patient's inability to make that decision for themselves. For purposes of this section, we will call it a health care power of attorney. The HCPA may also allow for the person holding the durable power of attorney to authorize the withdrawal or withholding of life support, although that right is not automatically granted to the designated person.

As one example of a health care power of attorney for health care statute, Ohio has just adopted a durable power of attorney for health care statute, which restricts who may be appointed as the decision-maker or "agent," restricts who may serve as a witness, and most significantly, restricts what decisions can be made by the agent" (Carlson, 1990).

As spelled out in Ohio law and described by Carlson (1990), the durable power of attorney statute requires that:

1. the document must specifically authorize the agent to make decisions when the patient has lost capacity;
2. it must be signed and dated by the maker;
3. any competent adult may be the agent except the following: the treating physician, the physician's agent or employee, or any employee or agent of the health-care facility;
4. the DPA/HC must either be witnessed or be notarized. If witnessed, there must be two eligible witnesses who personally know the maker. Those ineligible to be witnesses are: any person who is related to the patient by blood, marriage or adoption; any person who is entitled to benefit in any way from the death of the principal; any person designated as the agent in the document; and any physician or any employee or agent of a physician or of a health care facility;
5. the DPA/HC is valid for only up to seven years; however, if the maker is incompetent when it would expire, the DPA/HC continues.

It is important to note that the DPA/HC in Ohio is not a living will and it is not a set of treatment orders. Rather it is the election of an agent to make those decisions when they become necessary. However, the durable power of attorney statutes may differ in other states. In North Carolina, as in some other states with durable power of attorney statutes, the statute contains a clause authorizing the proxy (agent) to consent to medical treatment, but does not specifically mention refusal to consent or authority to instruct cessation of life-sustaining treatment. As a result of the Cruzan decision (which will be explicated later in this chapter), clarifying work in state legislatures is beginning on this topic in many states.

In addition to the living will and durable power of attorney statutes, some states have adopted very specific laws affecting the withdrawal of hydration and nutrition. As an example, Connecticut has adopted a Removal of Life-Support Systems Act. In Florida, the state constitution was amended to recognize a right to privacy in medical treatment decisions (Blum, 1990).

Patient Self-Determination Act

On November 5, 1990, President George Bush signed into law the Omnibus Budget Reconciliation Act of 1990. Sections 4206 and 4751, referred to as the "Patient Self-Determination Act" require providers of services under the Medicare and Medicaid programs to inform patients of their right to appoint a proxy and draw up written instructions for the desired limits to medical care to be activated if they become incapacitated. Hospitals and other health care providers were required to set up systems by December 1, 1991 to comply with the law. Senator John Danforth called the bill "the Miranda law for patients" (Hudson, 1991). The law was also designed to require those states without any advance directive statute to enact such legislation, as shown in Table 10.1.

Under the provisions of the law, any health care provider receiving Medicare or Medicaid dollars is required to ask admitted patients whether they have advance directives—either a living will or a health care power of attorney. If the patient does, the health care provider must document that fact in the patient's medical chart. The law required that the agency maintain written policies:

1. to provide written information to each individual concerning (a) his or her rights under state law (whether statutory or as recognized

by the courts) to make decisions concerning medical care, including the right to accept or refuse medical or surgical treatment and the right to formulate advance directives; and (b) the written policies of the provider or organization as to the implementation of such rights;

2. to document in the individual's medical record whether or not the individual has executed an advance directive;

3. not to condition the provision of care or otherwise discriminate against an individual based on whether or not the individual has executed an advance directive;

4. to ensure compliance with the requirements of state law respecting advance directives at facilities of the provider or organization; and

5. to provide (individually or with others) for education of staff and the community on issues concerning advance directives.

An observational cohort study was conducted for two years before and for two years after the enactment of the PSDA to assess the effectiveness of written advance directives in the care of seriously ill, hospitalized patients. The study, called the Study to Understand Prognoses and Preferences for Outcomes and Risks of Treatments (SUPPORT) focused on the impact of advance directives on how decisions were made about resuscitation (Teno et al., 1997). The SUPPORT study, widely known as the most significant study of seriously ill patients and their end of life care preferences, was funded by the Robert Wood Johnson Foundation and conducted at five teaching hospitals in the United States. The goal of the study was to improve end of life decision making and reduce the frequency of painful, prolonged patterns of dying (Greipp, 1996).

Hospitals in the study were required to provide PSDA mandated patient education about advance directives at hospital admission and documentation of patient wishes in the medical record. The additional intervention, provided by the SUPPORT study, included a nurse to facilitate communication among patients, family members, surrogates and physicians about preferences for treatment, and when appropriate, the completion of advance directives (Teno et al., 1997). Sixty-two percent of patients in the study were familiar with a living will, and 21% had an advance directive. Just 6% of these advance directives were mentioned in the medical records, which increased to 35% after the SUPPORT study interventions. Forty-three percent of patients with advance directives reported that they had discussed their wishes with a physician, compared to 30% of patients without advance directives. Twelve percent of patients with advance directives talked with a physician while completing their advance directives, and only 42% reported *ever* having discussed their wishes with their physician. By the second week of the study of these hospitalized patients, only one in four physicians was aware of the patient's advance directives (Teno et al., 1997).

Researchers concluded that advance directives, placed in the medical records of seriously ill patients, often did not guide medical decision making beyond the naming of a health care agent or proxy or documenting general preferences. The presence of advance directives did not, by themselves, enhance the physician–patient relationship or decision making about resuscitation. The SUPPORT study substantially improved documentation of existing advance directives, but did not ensure that the wishes in the advance directive were followed.

Do Not Resuscitate

The do-not-resuscitate (DNR) treatment decision has been the subject of intense interest in the last several years, focused especially on the terminally ill patient. The President's Commission for the Study of Ethical Problems in Medicine and Biomedical and Behavioral Research, as discussed by Enck, Longa, Warren, and McCann (1988), raises three critical points regarding DNR:

1. resuscitation is a very painful and intrusive procedure;
2. efforts to resuscitate a dying patient are only successful in approximately one-in-three attempts, and of those patients who survive, only one third are eventually discharged;
3. the success of resuscitation efforts is generally difficult to assess without the availability of a full range of resuscitation procedures.

The Commission made three chief recommendations to hospitals for the development of DNR policies: (1) Hospitals should develop explicit policies; "on the practice of writing and implementing DNR orders," (2) Hospital policies should recognize the need for balanced protection of patients, and respect the right of a competent patient to make an informed choice, and (3) Hospital policies should provide a means for appropriate resolution of conflicts, and also mandate internal review (President's, 1983). Since 1988, all hospitals are required to have formal DNR procedures for accreditation (Emanuel, 1989).

In 1988, the Emergency Medical Services Committee of the American College of Emergency Physicians adopted a position statement for the use of do-not-resuscitate orders in the prehospital setting. The development of such a policy was necessitated by the increasing numbers of terminally ill patients who are provided care in the outpatient or home setting, and whose wishes for resuscitation are unclear, especially to the emergency medical personnel. The American College of Emergency Physicians (ACEP) provided guidelines for appropriate EMS authorities for prehospital care providers to withhold CPR in patients who are known to be terminally ill. In their recommendations, the ACEP guidelines state that:

1. medical treatments limited by a "do not resuscitate" order should be clearly defined, and in the event of cardiopulmonary arrest, cardiac resuscitation would not be initiated. This would not imply that other medical therapies, such as IV fluids in the dehydrated patient, should be withheld in patients in whom they are medically indicated.
2. A legally valid, widely recognized form should be available for presentation to prehospital personnel when they are called to the scene of a "do not resuscitate" patient.
3. There should be an option not to execute a "do not resuscitate" order by the responding personnel if:
   a. The patient is able to express a wish to be resuscitated prior to cardiopulmonary arrest;
   b. Family members or the patient's designee expresses a wish to initiate resuscitation;
   c. The patient's responsible physician requests that resuscitation efforts be undertaken; or
   d. The prehospital personnel have any doubts about carrying out the "do not resuscitate" order.

The position statement has encouraged some states to develop do-not-resuscitate protocols for emergency medical personnel for use in the prehospital setting. Using a multi-disciplinary group of physicians, ethicists, attorneys, and representatives from hospitals, nursing homes, hospices, and home health agencies, a uniform method for alerting EMS personnel of the presence of a DNR order can be developed. Non-hospital DNR or EMS-DNR statutes have been enacted in 33 states, including AK, AZ, AR, CA, CO, CT, FL, GA, HI, ID, IL, KS, KY, MD, MI, MT, NV, NH, NM, NY, OH, OK, PA, RI, SC, TN, TX, UT, VA, WA, WV, WI, WY. A few other states, such as Oregon, have developed EMS-DNR protocols without special legislation (Sabatino, 1999).

Physician Assisted Suicide

Physician assisted suicide has become a lightening rod of regulatory issues in the United States, where concerns about patient self-determination mix with the legal, moral and ethical obligations of physicians and other health care providers.

As described by the State of Oregon Health Division, the Oregon Death with Dignity Act, a citizens' initiative, was first passed by Oregon voters in November 1994 by a margin of 51% in favor and 49% opposed. Immediate implementation of the Act was delayed by a legal injunction. After multiple legal proceedings, including a petition that was denied by the United States Supreme Court, the Ninth Circuit Court of Appeals lifted the injunction on October 27, 1997 and physician-assisted suicide then became a legal option for terminally ill patients in Oregon. In November 1997, Measure 51 (authorized by Oregon House Bill 2954) was placed on the general election ballot and asked Oregon voters to repeal the Death with Dignity Act. Voters chose to retain the Act by a margin of 60% to 40%.

The Death with Dignity Act allows terminally ill Oregon residents to obtain from their physicians and use prescriptions for self-administered, lethal medications. The Act states that ending one's life in accordance with the law does not constitute suicide. However, we have used the term "physician-assisted suicide" rather than "Death with Dignity" to describe the provisions of this law because physician-assisted suicide is the term used by the public, and by the medical literature, to describe ending life through the voluntary self-administration of lethal medications, expressly prescribed by a physician for that purpose. The Death with Dignity Act legalizes physician-assisted suicide, but specifically prohibits euthanasia, where a physician or other person directly administers a medication to end another's life.[1]

In 2000, a total of 39 prescriptions for lethal doses of medication were written, compared with 24 in 1998 and 33 in 1999. Twenty-six of the third-year prescription recipients died after ingesting the medication; eight died from their underlying disease; five were alive on December 31, 2000. In addition, one 1999 prescription recipient died in 2000 after ingesting

---

[1]Oregon Health Division, 2000 Annual Report.

the medication. In total, 27 patients ingested legally prescribed lethal medication in 2000 (26 patients who received prescriptions in 2000; 1 patient who received a prescription in 1999). During 1998 and 1999, 16 and 27 patients, respectively, died after ingesting the medications.[2]

The number of terminally ill patients using lethal medication in 2000 remains small, and is unchanged from 1999. Patients using PAS are better educated, but otherwise demographically comparable to other Oregonians dying of similar diseases. Physicians reported that patient concern about becoming a burden has increased during the last three years, though all patients expressed multiple concerns in the third year.[3]

In 2000, Maine had a ballot referendum on physician assisted suicide that was not passed by the voters. In a press release from the American Medical Association on November 8, 2000, the AMA states "The American Medical Association (AMA) is pleased that Maine voters have endorsed physicians' fundamental obligation 'to do no harm' by defeating a flawed ballot initiative that would have turned healers away from their primary purpose."

The Maine Medical Association and the Maine Citizens Against the Dangers of Physician-Assisted Suicide are to be commended for their work in upholding the notion that terminally-ill patients should not be abandoned.

The work of these concerned organizations to oppose the legalization of physician-assisted suicide certainly has prevented the introduction of deep ambiguity into the very definition of medical care.

Other states have taken actions to pass state laws making physician assisted suicide a crime. In 2001, there are challenges to the Oregon physician assisted suicide law by the U.S. Attorney General and by the Drug Enforcement Administration (DEA). One concern of the controversy over physician assisted suicide is that it may promote a chilling effect for physicians who prescribe narcotics for pain management, and the end result will be uncontrolled pain near the end of life.

Hospices and the Regulatory Process

In 2002, there were over 3,200 hospice locations throughout the United States (National Hospice and Palliative Care Organization, 2001). As pro-

---

[2]Oregon Health Division, 2000 Annual Report.
[3]OHD, 2000 Annual Report.

viders of health care to terminally ill persons and their families, hospices are confronted on a daily basis with the issues raised in this chapter. In 1982, Congress created the Medicare Hospice Benefit, which is reimbursed under Medicare Part A. As of January 2000, the Centers for Medicare and Medicaid Services (formerly the Health Care Financing Administration) announced that 2,273 hospices were Medicare certified.

Since the passage of the Balanced Budget Act of 1997, the benefit includes two initial 90-day benefit periods, followed by an unlimited number of 60-day periods. A physician must certify that the patient is terminally ill, and has six months or less to live if the disease runs its normal course. The benefit is separated into four levels of care—routine home care, general inpatient care, inpatient respite care, and continuous care. The Medicare and Medicaid Hospice Benefits are designed to pay a "prospective" daily rate for each day of care provided, no matter what the intensity of services.

Accreditation for hospice programs is provided by the Joint Commission on the Accreditation of Healthcare Organizations (JCAHO), Community Health Accreditation Program (CHAP), and the Accreditation Commission for Health Care (ACHC). JCAHO and CHAP have both sought deeming authority from the Centers for Medicare and Medicaid Services (CMS) to allow accreditation to take the place of the state survey process for Medicare certification for hospice. Forty four states have licensure laws for hospice programs, which regulate the use of the name, hospice, and specify the minimum standards that each hospice must meet. In some states, Medicare certification is often viewed by hospices in a state as a substitute for state licensure, and is effective for those programs who are Medicare certified.

As a part of the licensure process, some states have also developed rules for hospice inpatient units and hospice residences. Hospice inpatient units provide acute and subacute care for hospice patients who need a short term inpatient stay. The unit may be located at a hospital or nursing home, or could be a freestanding hospice inpatient unit not connected with another provider. Inpatient units receive reimbursement under the Medicare or Medicaid Hospice Benefit, and most private insurers at the inpatient level of care.

Hospice residences are designed for those patients without adequate caregivers, with frail caregivers, or for those patients who need supervised residential care. The hospice community believes that the need for hospice residences will increase dramatically as the population ages, as more elderly widows and widowers living alone need hospice care, and as families are living greater distances from each other and cannot provide care for elderly parents directly. The hospice residence is an important option for those patients. Currently there is no reimbursement for the room and board portion of hospice residential care.

A Certificate of Need (CON) law, which regulates the number of hospices that may provide care in a service area, is also in place for some states with licensing laws. In states where CON exists, a Certificate of Need application must be filed and approved before a hospice can begin providing care. The approval process considers how many hospice patients are already being served in the area, and whether the area needs another hospice program. Certificate of Need laws are in a constant state of flux by state legislators, as they consider how much regulation should be provided to hospice programs and other providers of health care. Some states have now abandoned their Certificate of Need laws for hospices and home health care agencies, and consequently, the number of hospice programs in a given area is increasing, resulting in competition for patients.

The hospice movement has matured since its beginnings in the 1970s and will continue to provide leadership for hospice and palliative care of terminally ill patients and their families. Hospice programs and their administrators will be challenged by the regulations which affect the care of the chronically and terminally ill, as well as those that affect hospice specifically.

The Future of Regulatory Issues

Regulatory and legal issues concerning death and dying will continue to increase in complexity, as health care technology increases in intensity and offers further challenges to decision makers. The Quinlan and Cruzan rulings are reflections of the legal impact on patient care and ethical decision making. As technology advances, new regulations will be drawn and new ethical decisions will need to be made. The area of regulation is fluid and will change as new situations present themselves. It can be hoped that the foundation has been laid for future decision making with the cases and issues presented in this chapter.

Discussion Questions

1. Why were the cases of Karen Ann Quinlan and Nancy Cruzan so important in raising public awareness of patient rights and advance care planning?

2. Supporters of physician-assisted suicide have used what philosophical argument?
3. What are the two common types of advance directives and how has their use evolved in the states?

References

American Bar Association. (2001). Olmstead: Catalyst to expand services for elderly. Commission on Legal Problems of the Elderly, Advocacy Alert. <http://www.abanet. org/elderly/olmstead.html>. 16 November 2001.

American Medical Association. (2000). Press release for Maine physician assisted referendum vote. <http://www.ama-assn.org/ama/pub/article/2403-3399.html> November 8, 2000.

Blum, J. D. (1990, May/June). The legal dilemma of stopping artificial feeding. *The American Journal of Hospice & Palliative Care, 7,* 42–48.

Byock, I. (1989). DNR orders and living wills. *Annals of Emergency Medicine, 18,* 911–912.

Carlson, R. A. (1990). Ohio's new law: What the durable power statute can do . . . and what it can't. *OHIO Medicine,* September/October, 435–440.

Chatzky, J. S. (2000). The last word—Making your final health-care wishes clear and comprehensive. 15 August 2000. <http://www.money.com/money/depts/investing/ moneytalk/archive/000 815c.html> 16 November 2001.

Covinsky, K. E., Fuller, J. D., Yaffe, K., Johnston, C. B., Hamel, M. B., Lynn, J., Teno, J. M., & Phillips, R. S. (2000). Communication and decision-making in seriously ill patients: Findings of the SUPPORT project. The Study to Understand Prognoses and Preferences for Outcomes and Risks of Treatments. *Journal of the American Geriatric Society, 48*(5 Suppl), S187–193.

Emanuel, E. J. (1988). A review of the ethical and legal aspects of terminating medical care. *The American Journal of Medicine, 84,* 291–301.

Emanuel, L. L. (1989). Does the DNR order need life-sustaining intervention? Time for comprehensive advance directives. *The American Journal of Medicine, 86,* 87–90.

Enck, R. E., Longa, D. R., Warren, Matthew, & McCann, B. A. (1988, November/ December). DNR policies in healthcare organizations with emphasis on hospice. *The American Journal of Hospice Care, 5,* 39–42.

Greipp, M. E. (1996). SUPPORT study results—Implications for hospice care. *American Journal of Hospice and Palliative Care, 13*(3), 38–39, 41–45.

Henderson, M. (1990). Beyond the living will. *The Gerontologist, 30,* 480–485.

Hudson, T. (1991, February 5). Hospitals work to provide advance directives information. *Hospitals,* 26–32.

Living will: How to write one. Mediscope. (2001). <http://www.mediscope.org/livingwill.htm> 16 November 2001.

Loewy, E. H. (1991). Weakening the bonds of friendship: An unfortunate outcome of the Cruzan decisions. *Journal of the American Geriatrics Society, 39,* 98–100.

Meagher, T. F. (1995). Hospice care in the long term facility. *Director, 3*(4), 149–150, 158.

Musgrave, C. F. (1987). The ethical and legal implications of hospice care. *Cancer Nursing, 10,* 183–189.

National Hospice and Palliative Care Organization. (2001). *NHPCO Facts and Figures.* November 8, 2001. <http://www.nhpco.org/public/articles/FactsFigures110801.pdf> 16 November 2001.

National Hospice and Palliative Care Organization. (2003, January). *NHPCO Facts and Figures.*

Oregon Department of Human Services, Oregon Health Division. (2001). <http://www.ohd.hr.state.or.us/chs/pas/pas.htm> November 16, 2001.

Pearlman, R. A. (1991). Clinical fallout from the Supreme Court decision on Nancy Cruzan: Chernobyl or Three Mile Island? *Journal of the American Geriatrics Society, 39,* 92–97.

Perkins, H. S. (2000). Time to move advance care planning beyond advance directives. *Chest, 117*(5), 228–231.

Rye, P. D., Wallston, K. A., Wallston, B. S., & Smith, R. A. (1985). The desire to control terminal health care and attitudes toward living wills. *American Journal of Preventive Medicine, 1*(3), 56–60.

Sabatino, C. P. 10 legal myths about advance medical directives. American Bar Association. <www.abanet.org/elderly/myths.html> 16 November 2001.

Schaffner, K. F. (1988). Philosophical, ethical and legal aspects of resuscitation medicine. II. Recognizing the tragic choice: Food, water, and the right to assisted suicide. *Critical Care Medicine, 16,* 1063–1068.

Sabatino, Charles P. JD, End-of-Life Care Legislative Directions 1999, Commission on Legal Problems of the Elderly, American Bar Association.

Siner, D. A. (1989). Advance directives in emergency medicine: Medical, legal and ethical implications. *Annals of Emergency Medicine, 18,* 1364–1369.

Teno, J. M., Licks, S., Lynn, J., Wenger, N., Connors, A. F., Phillips, R. S., O'Connor, M. A., Murphy, D. P., Fulkerson, W. J., Desbiens, N., & Knaus, W. A. (1997). Do advance directives provide instructions that direct care? SUPPORT Investigators. Study to Understand Prognoses and Preferences for Outcomes and Risks of Treatment. *Journal of the American Geriatric Society, 45*(4), 508–512.

Teno, J., Lynn, J., Wenger, N., Phillips, R. S., Murphy, D. P., Connors, A. F., Desbiens, N., Fulkerson, W., Bellamy, P., & Knaus, W. A. (1997). Advance directives for seriously ill hospitalized patients: Effectiveness with the patient self-determination act and the SUPPORT intervention. SUPPORT Investigators. Study to Understand Prognoses and Preferences for Outcomes and Risks of Treatment. *Journal of the American Geriatric Society, 45*(4), 500–507.

Tonelli, M. R. (1996). Pulling the plug on living wills, a critical analysis of advance directives. *Chest, 110,* 816–822.

U.S. Living Will Registry. (2000). U.S. living will registry helps hospitals educate public about advance directives. 11 December 2000. <http://www.uslivingwillregistry.com/pr_hospital.shtm> 16 November 2001.

Part Three

The Challenges of Grief and Bereavement

I Don't Know How to Grieve

Colleen Corcoran

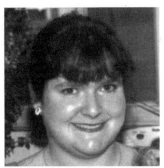

Colleen Corcoran is a research nurse prac-
titioner who has been involved in AIDS research for
the past several years. She has coauthored several
articles and has had publications in the Annals of
Internal Medicine, *the* Journal of the American
Medical Association, *and the* New England Journal of Medicine.

I don't know how to grieve. I am uncertain if I should gnash my teeth, pull my hair, hang dark cloth over the mirrors, wail, or throw myself on your funeral pyre. Perhaps I should quietly turn my suffering inward, as stoics are wont to do, and let my heart silently explode into a thousand unrecognizable pieces. I could reach for enlightenment and view your death as a Zen koan, as if I am the ready student and your death my new master. Or maybe I should follow in the footsteps of tragic heroes and drown my Ophelia self in a pool of tears or speak to skulls that cannot speak back. But I'm not a martyr nor a mystic nor a hero; I am none of those things. If you were my husband, I would be a widow, and perhaps I would find solace within that title and instinctively know how to mourn. But you were my brother, and there isn't a name for what I am, and I feel as lost as a small child in a crowd.

I thought part of grieving was to be angry at God, to shake one's fist in the air and demand an explanation for such suffering. Even though God and I parted company many years ago, it would be so tempting to turn to the breast of religion for solace, and root for comfort and sacred platitudes that assure me you truly are at peace. But I'm not angry at God, not at all. I refuse to be a foxhole convert, a fair-weather agnostic, and I will stand alone on this pedestal of grief and bite my tongue to stop from asking why, as if Jesus or Buddha or Mohammed or even Shiva could answer me back with an explanation that will heal my fractured soul. I think I know what truth exists in the darkest corner of the convert's heart, that no matter what God we choose from the catalogs of religion, there are no answers beyond what we make up to pacify ourselves. No deity can make sense of your death any better than they can justify all the endless waves of human suffering since the beginning of history. It is up to me to mourn you into purpose, to burn you into my heart and mind, so that your death can be reflected in some part of my life, and it is up to me to find out how to answer the "why" of my own sadness and loss.

To my profound horror, I discovered that life really does go on. The morning after you died, the sun came up, the day started like any other, and thoughtless people rose from their beds and went to work. Casseroles and hams and flowers and condolences arrived endlessly at our doorstep, and friends placed their sacrifices in our grieving hands and turned around and went back to their lives, as if they knew that the world would continue to spin, and other people's brothers would die, and death meant nothing to the sun and moon. But it mattered to me. Out of respect for you, I wanted the world to stop on its axis. I wanted the cessation of noise and light and children's play and the drudgery that defines our most basic of days. I waited for the stars to fall out of their cold, still place in the sky and the earth to be knocked out of its orbit, out of respect for the death of one of its children. But the irreverent sky continued to introduce day and night repeatedly, even after we put you in the ground, and I began to acknowledge the universe's profound indifference. If life itself can't create space to mourn you, how can I?

I have been running blindly since your death, only occasionally lifting up my black veil to look around when I run into walls in this maze of pain. My scientific mind is desperate to find an escape, and I want to plug this grief into a formula to get a solution, an end, an exit. I want to be able to calculate the number of tears I have to shed before this ache in my heart disappears, or how many support groups or therapists I have to embrace before I can close my eyes at night and not picture you laying in the mahogany casket I picked out. I reach desperately for a promise, a contract, money-back guarantee, pass go and collect $200, something or someone who will assure me that I am entitled to peace and happiness and blissful amnesia, if I only finish grieving. Those who have walked where I am walking now shake their heads at my entitlement and tell me that the grief never really ceases, but is a tide that ebbs and flows and sculpts contours on the soul, so that we are never the same person again.

I am afraid of the new person I seem destined to be molded into, this woman without a brother. I am afraid the grief will eat away at some fundamental part of my core self, and I will be less than I was before. Perhaps this is the way it is supposed to be: We mourn by letting small parts of ourselves die. Perhaps grief is the language of the dead, and my sorrow and loss and the small corners of my soul that are in tatters are the only sacrifices I can make at your alter, the only way I can tell you that I miss you deeply.

If only I knew how to grieve.

Eleven

The Bereavement Process: Loss, Grief, and Resolution*

Joseph T. Mullan, Marilyn M. Skaff, and Leonard I. Pearlin

Joseph T. Mullan was trained in the Program on Human Development at the University of Chicago, where he was awarded his PhD in 1981. His research focuses on how people marshal their psychological and social resources when facing difficult life circumstances, such as caregiving, illness, and death. He is currently an adjunct assistant professor in the Department of Social and Behavioral Sciences at the University of California, San Francisco. He has collaborated with Leonard I. Pearlin on two large multi-year longitudinal studies of informal caregivers to people with chronic, debilitating ill- 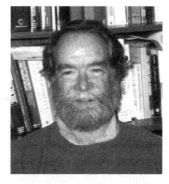 *nesses, those with a progressive dementia, such as Alzheimer's disease, and those with HIV symptoms or AIDS.*

Marilyn M. Skaff received her PhD in human development and aging in 1990 from the University of California, San Francisco. During her doctoral studies, she worked on the Alzheimer's caregiver study with Drs. Pearlin and Mullan, and her dissertation was based on data from that study. She is currently an assistant adjunct professor with the Department of Family and Community Medicine at the University of California, San Francisco, where her work fo-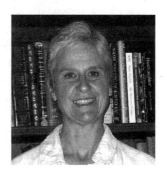

*Support for this work was provided in part by grants from the National Institute on Aging no. AG12910 and the National Institute of Mental Health nos. MH42122 and MH23653.

*cuses on sense of control and its effects on health
across diverse ethnic groups.*

*Leonard I. Pearlin took his PhD in Sociology in
1956 from Columbia University. He is currently
graduate professor of sociology at the University of
Maryland, College Park, where he runs the stress
and health project. Prior to that, he was professor of
medical sociology at the University of California,
San Francisco, and a research scientist at the National Institutes of Mental Health. His writings and
research have mostly centered on the causes and consequences of chronic stress.*

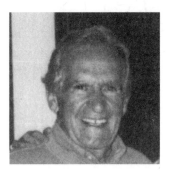

Bereavement is a complex psychosocial process, its complexity stemming
in part from the fact that the death of an individual reverberates throughout
a survivor's life at many different levels. Moreover, a single death can
trigger emotional and material repercussions throughout the reaches of
the deceased person's social network. Because the life-narratives of those
constituting the network had been intertwined, the death of one may have
far-reaching effects on the lives of others (Walsh & McGoldrick, 1991).
Death is a biological event, but it is no less a psychosocial event: It can
initiate or hasten a process entailing loss, grief, and resolution and their
interrelationships, a process that often persists among survivors long after
the death has occurred. This chapter is aimed at describing and explicating
some of this process and its components.

Many of the views and observations presented here are based on two
research projects the authors have conducted. One is a study of spouses
and adult children caring for relatives with Alzheimer's disease. Because
this is characteristically a disease of older people, the death of the impaired
person is commonly experienced by caregivers. Although the death sometimes follows a brief period of caregiving, in most instances, the caregiving
has gone on for many years. The second study is of friends, lovers, and
family members caring for people with AIDS. Most of these caregivers are
young, and some of them share the same life-style (and similar health
problems) as those for whom they are caring. For these people, survivorship
may include not only the loss of one special person, but also a grim preview
of their own life-course and its end. We have had the opportunity to follow
the survivors in both of these studies from the time they were active
caregivers to more than 3 years following the death of the care recipients
(Aneshensel, Pearlin, Mullan, Zarit, & Whitlatch, 1995; Mullan, 1998).

Although there are some striking differences between these two groups of caregivers—differences to which we return later—there are some important similarities. Most notably, in each group, the death of the loved one approaches gradually and is thus foreseen in advance of the death. In each group, too, caregivers may witness a profound physical and/or mental transformation taking place prior to death. The foreseeable nature of the deaths, and the transformations that may precede death, both contribute in these groups to the initiation of the bereavement process before the death occurs. Together, these two studies obviously embrace only a very small sample, either of the circumstances under which people die, or of circumstances that must be confronted by survivors; consequently, no claims can be made for the generalizability of our findings or speculations. Nevertheless, these two groups of caregivers enable us to observe with unusual clarity not only the acute phases of bereavement but also its early beginnings and later stages.

As we see it, there are three closely interrelated components making up the bereavement process: loss, grief, and resolution. We regard all three of these components as being subsumed by the overarching construct of bereavement. *Loss* refers to the separation from a part of one's life to which one was emotionally attached. *Grief* refers to the complex emotional, cognitive, and perceptual reactions that accompany loss. It may assume a variety of trajectories and expressions whose character may be shaped by the nature and intensity of the losses that are experienced. *Resolution* is the final component in surviving the death of a loved one. We use this term to refer not to an end point of grief, but to the process whereby individuals manage the circumstances of their lives, as time goes on. This process is conditioned by the nature of the losses they have experienced, the psychological, social, and economic resources they can call upon to deal with grief, and their ability to restructure their lives.

Although loss, grief, and resolution are conceptually discrete, they are not necessarily temporally discrete. Each is a process that may emerge slowly and gradually and, perhaps, may never completely displace the process that preceded it. Particularly, among those witnessing death after a lengthy physical or cognitive decline, for example, elements of loss may begin to surface long before death, but continue to be freshly confronted after the time that death has occurred and grief is actively underway. Thus, in addition to those losses that might be experienced prior to or immediately after death, others may periodically come into focus following a considerable time interval. Similarly, grief may be coextensive with loss, including loss that occurs before death, and it may also overlap with the process of resolution. People may have profoundly restructured their lives since caregiving and death, and may still feel flashes of pain (Wortman & Silver, 1990). Indeed, we assume that episodes of grief may pepper the entirety of a survivor's life. This is particularly likely to be the case among those who stood in close relationship to the deceased person; that is, partners, children, and parents.

Loss, grief, and resolution, then, may begin in advance of death and continue on afterward. Moreover, they may overlap in time, thus having no clear or discrete experiential boundaries. For simplicity, however, our discussions of each will be separate.

Death, of course, is the key juncture in the bereavement process, surrounded by loss, grief, and resolution. These three constructs, however, are themselves rather global, each containing multiple dimensions around which there is considerable variability. Much of this chapter is aimed at identifying the dimensions of the constructs and their interconnections. In this way, we believe, we can illuminate the process underlying the survival of the death of a loved one.

Loss

We usually think of loss as entailing the involuntary separation of ourselves from something that had been a valued part of our lives. As we suggested earlier, death can accelerate loss, but loss may have begun well before the death. We can assume that loss is most severe when it involves the death of a person who was an integral part of the survivors' lives. That is, when attachment to and identification with the deceased person were strong, when there was a functional and emotional intertwining of lives, and when the relationship was of long duration and spanned a broad range of shared experience and history, death will leave the survivor feeling profoundly bereft. Each death brings with it many losses. Especially in the case of caregivers, the actual death may be only a single, albeit powerful, marker in the process of loss that precedes death. We discuss four general classes of losses: losses associated with the relationship, life-style, biography, and the self.

Relationship Losses

Let us first consider losses related directly to the dyadic relationship that the survivor had with the deceased. A central loss obviously is the loss of intimacy, the end of expressive and affectional support and exchange formerly provided by the impaired person. In the case of spouses and lovers, the loss of emotional and sexual intimacy may occur insidiously as the disease progresses, but leave an emotional and physical gap (Parkes, 1987). To the extent that the transformed or deceased person was a source of esteem and self-validation, death may leave the life of the survivor in an expressive vacuum.

Loss of the companionship that was habitually shared with the relative or friend is also likely to be strongly felt. This may involve missing the daily conversation previously shared with a friend or partner, or the mutual activities engaged in with someone. The collapse of deeply ingrained daily routines can leave caregivers with large empty spaces in their lives.

Another aspect of the survivor–deceased relationship, around which loss is experienced, concerns instrumental support. Like affection and companionship, this involves something that had been built into everyday life and the loss of which is capable of imposing considerable hardship. In long-standing relationships, death can destroy an intricate division of labor that was established. With the decline of the patient's vitality, or the occurrence of death, the caregiving partner is frequently left without the skills, time, or energy to compensate for the instrumental activities that the deceased person had brought to the relationship.

Still looking at the dyadic relationship, there is a somewhat different kind of loss that can occur: the loss of mattering. Mattering refers to the gratification one feels as a result of being needed, being important to another person, and being able to do something for that person (Rosenberg & McCullough, 1981). It is the other side of social support. One of the consequences of caregiving is the fulfilling experience of making a differ-ence in another's life. To the extent that caregiving had become a central element in the lives of caregivers, the death of the patient may deprive the survivor of a role from which they were able to extract a sense of purpose (Wortman & Silver, 1990). In no longer having a person to whom they matter, survivors can be left feeling that they have been stripped of some meaning and mission from their own lives.

Finally, there is the loss of persona, something that is especially apparent in the experiences of Alzheimer's caregivers. Many caregivers are destined to observe dramatic and disheartening mental and physical transformations in those for whom they are caring. The progressive cognitive and functional deterioration in the person who is ill can leave caregivers feeling that the quintessential loved one no longer exists. Biological life goes on, but the person with whom attachments were forged in past times has largely disappeared. With the transformation of the impaired person, many of the elements of the caregiver's relationship with that person must also undergo a transformation and disappearance. Our respondents, of course, are keenly sensitive to this loss of persona and the accompanying loss of relationship. As one widow put it:

> He couldn't speak anymore. Half the time I don't know if he even knew me. I think he knew I belonged to him, but he'd lost the relationship along the way. . . . The person that you found unique was gone. . . . He was gone 2 years before he finally passed away. As I say, his mind went, he was incontinent, he was totally helpless. Everything that he had been—a witty, intelligent person— and there was nothing left, just a shell.

These caregivers are certainly not representative of the entire population of people that experience the death of a loved one. But they do reveal a great deal about a type of loss experienced in relationships in which one of the parties is destructively altered by a disease.

Losses of Life-Style

The transformation of a loved one, and the disappearance of affectionate exchange, emotional and instrumental support, and mattering have in common the fact that they each involve losses that are rooted in the structure of the dyadic relationship between the caregiver and the impaired or deceased person. Other losses are broader in scope and involve activities, roles, and relationships other than those centering on the dyadic relationship. Collectively, they may be thought of as losses of previously established life-style. One of these entails the survivor's loss of status in the community. In instances in which the survivor's status was dependent on the occupation or activities of the deceased individual, the survivor may experience a fall from status after the death. The signs that a loss of status has occurred may be diverse: The survivor no longer receives invitations from those who earlier extended them to the pair, or subtle signs of homage are no longer accorded. In general, if the friends and associates affiliated with the deceased were of higher status than those primarily allied with the survivor, then the survivor may experience a loss of status.

Of course, an attenuation of social ties can occur for reasons other than the loss of status conferral. A "couple identity," and the social network in which it is embedded, often has a structuring effect on social life. Survivors may experience a gradual loss of contact with former social ties made up of other couples. Such constriction frequently occurs before death, among caregivers, who report a loss of contact with other people as the demands of care progress. Caregivers themselves may have little time or energy for social contacts. Friends may no longer feel comfortable being around the impaired person, or the behavior or physical condition of the patient may preclude involvement in social activities. In the case of Alzheimer's caregivers whose partners are placed in a care facility, the caregiver may experience the "social widowhood" of a person without a partner, yet still feel the ties of marriage. Even friends and adult children may find that contact with the larger social network is diminished. This is particularly likely to be the case when the impaired or deceased person was the one who actively maintained social ties and rituals, usually referred to as the "kinkeeper" in traditional family studies (Troll & Bengtson, 1992).

Related to status and affiliative losses that the survivor may experience is a loss of material resources. If death results in diminished finances or reduced income, the survivor might find that the material footing on which he/she earlier stood is no longer there. We know from previous studies that, when the loss of a loved one is accompanied by the loss of income, the impact of the death is more severe than in instances in which these resources are left intact (Pearlin & Lieberman, 1979; Umberson, Wortman, & Kessler, 1992).

Loss of Biography

Thus far, we have discussed losses involving the decline or disappearance of elements of the dyadic relationship, as well as broader losses involving status, resources, and network. A third genre of loss entails the loss of biography. Concerning loss of the personal past, there is some indication from our studies that the disruption of certain relationships by death can leave survivors feeling cut off from their own biography. Shared memories may be lost. When crucial people are lost, so too is the recounting of that portion of the survivor's life. No one is left to fill in the blank spots. Parents, of course, are the chroniclers of their children's distant past, and the death of the last parent may leave a surviving adult forever separated from that part of their own childhood that was known only to their parents.

As distinct from personal history, the death may similarly entail the loss of group history. This history is more than a genealogy: It is a journal of past relationships that helps make sense out of the present. As people from a group die, especially the oldest generation, skeletons (or genies) are unlikely to be let out of the closet, and the hidden flaws and follies of members of the group will probably forever remain hidden. For adult children, the opportunity may be lost to learn more about their parents as people and about that small subculture that was unique to the family.

Concerning a loss of future, we find that debility and death often disrupt the visions of the future that survivors had shared with their loved ones. A variety of plans and expectations may be shattered: for travel, for love and companionship, for the pursuit of deferred goals and interests, for retirement, and, in general, for the enjoyment of the hard-earned fruits of years of labor and waiting. For parents, the death of a child is a painful affront to life-course expectations, closing off the possibility of observing how another future is taking shape. The loss of a cherished future, often nurtured by long-standing dreams and hopes, can understandably be a bitter pill.

Loss of Self

Finally, we come to a loss of self or of identity, often noted in the literature (Lopata, 1975; Marris, 1974; Moss & Moss, 1989; Parkes, 1987; Stroebe & Stroebe, 1987). To a great extent, the loss of self is inseparable from the losses we have discussed above. Thus, the loss of relationship, of community standing, and of the continuity of one's own life course are all likely to have an impact on one's understanding of oneself. To the extent that what has been lost was central to the organization of the thoughts, activities, and emotions of the caregiver, the self that survives death will not be the same as the self who had existed before death and disability. This altered self leads people to grieve not only for their departed loved ones, but also for their departed selves (Marris, 1974).

The self, in many instances, is not merely changed from its previous composition, but is diminished. People can feel that they have become lesser beings. This is a result of two conditions. One exists when the deceased or disabled person was a major source of positive feedback to the survivor, reaffirming and reinforcing the elements of self that the survivor prized. In the absence of this feedback, these prized elements may wither and recede. Second, caregiving can expand to the point that it drives out other activities and roles in a life. We refer to this phenomenon as *role engulfment*, a situation that may leave a person with limited sources of feedback about themselves, other than those tied directly to the incapacitated or deceased person (Skaff & Pearlin, 1992). Consequently, survivors may begin to feel that they have lost their former identity or self.

What we wish to emphasize in this discussion is that loss is not an undifferentiated experience. On the contrary, it is possible to identify a wide array of losses: the loss of affective exchange, of instrumental and emotional support, of mattering to another person, of companionship and the activities it entailed, of network and social affiliation and status and economic resources, of life-course continuity, and of self and identity. Among people who have experienced the death of a person with whom they had stood in a close relationship, therefore, there is likely to be considerable variation in the substance and intensity of the losses that they encounter. Moreover, we should not assume that loss is synonymous with death, for some losses may begin to emerge prior to death.

Much of our discussion that follows assumes that both grief and resolution are somewhat dependent on the nature of the losses that are experienced. The recognition and assessment of the multiple dimensions of loss, therefore, is an essential step toward understanding the process that influences how survivors ultimately fare after the death of a closely related person. If we are able to identify the dimensions of loss and their scope, we submit, some of the mystery surrounding survivors' adjustments to death will be dissipated.

Grief

We define *grief* as the complicated set of emotional and cognitive responses that accompany loss. As we have explained, loss is not a uniform experience; as a result, grief varies in form, intensity, and duration. No consensus exists in the literature on the variety of emotions that grief includes. However, clearly the principal emotion associated with grief is depression. It may be a low-grade dysphoria in people who continue to function in their usual social roles, but who live their lives in an emotional valley. Or it may be more severe, immobilizing the survivor psychologically.

Beyond the emotional components of grief, there are also more ideational or cognitive components of grief, which we shall emphasize here. We label them cognitive, but not to imply that they lack any emotional aura—far from it. They involve thoughts and echoes from the past, changing images of the deceased, and efforts to maintain ties and to separate oneself from the deceased. These manifestations of grief are likely to come and go, as the survivor alternately forgets and then realizes with a jolt that a loved one has died. We shall outline several of these manifestations of grief. Not everyone experiences all of them, nor with the same intensity, but probably some are experienced by most people following the death of someone close.

Often, thoughts and memories of the deceased person occupy the bereaved. These memories and images may come unbidden; they may intrude into consciousness even when the survivor is making a concerted effort to concentrate on something else. People often talk of finding themselves thinking about the person or remembering things they had not thought about in years. For some, these thoughts and memories may persist and constitute a stable backdrop to ordinary consciousness, as though reviewing the deceased person's actions, mannerisms, and moods helps to consolidate images in a form in which they can comfortably endure in memory. Perhaps this process is a way of holding onto the person, or an idealized composite of him or her, even while confronting the reality of the loss.

Perceptual illusions can also occur—seeing, hearing, or sensing things that are not there—sometimes causing people to worry about the state of their own mental health. But these fleeting moments are often understood for what they are, a misinterpretation of a sound or sight. At times, these illusions may be part of the normal perceptual process that one employs to fill in the blanks in the world, sustaining the habits and perceiving the continuity that had been there until the death. Or, as attachment theorists suggest, perhaps these perceptual illusions are understandable as part of a normal search in which the survivor is trying to find the deceased by picking up some sign of him or her (Parkes, 1987). These illusions may signal an underlying tension between the need to recognize the reality of death and a desire to hold onto the past, a tension sustained by the longing for the deceased person, which accompanies bereavement. This wish to be reunited with the deceased is often spoken of as an intense yearning that comes suddenly and initially causes pain, for it inevitably is accompanied by the aching knowledge that the wish will be unfulfilled.

Particularly in the acute phase of grief, people often report a kind of dissociation from the normal flow of events in the world and from their characteristic sense of connectedness to it. As they struggle between grasping a new reality and clinging to an old bond, they may feel numb, that their sense of time is disrupted, and that they are watching things from a distance. This unsettling mix of feelings and dissociations seems to be the internal counterpart of the external discontinuity brought on by death.

These common grief reactions seem understandable enough as people grapple with the tension between facing and accepting the reality of death and trying to preserve some continuity in their world. At times, this "conservative impulse" to hold onto the past, as Marris (1974, p. 5) calls it, may involve brushing the reality of death aside. In any case, the intellectual recognition of death is accompanied by a deeper emotional sense of the loss.

As loss takes place within the context of a relationship, grief will inevitably be affected by the history of the relationship. This history includes not only the closeness between the survivor and the deceased and the amount of conflict they experienced, but also any "unfinished business" left by the death (Lopata, 1975). After the burdens of providing care, not surprisingly, some of the bereaved caregivers whom we have studied feel regrets and guilt about how they acted toward the deceased person. They feel a sense of having broken a standard, of having treated a dependent person less kindly than they should have. If anything, it is surprising that more caregivers do not feel these regrets, for the caregiver role is a setting in which guilt may easily arise: It is a difficult and enduring set of demands that often cannot be met; patient behavior may seem bewildering, especially as cognitive and emotional difficulties occur; and even if the past relationship was generally positive, the demands of the role can give rise to frustration and anger, and the guilty wish for relief.

Fundamental to the distinction we make between loss and grief is the difference between the objective loss of an important element in life and the recognition and realization of the loss. Although the loss and the realization of loss may coincide at death, this neat simultaneity rarely exists, in our experience. That is, as we discussed earlier, caregivers facing the transformation of a cognitively impaired relative often develop a strong sense of having lost the person and important elements in their relationship, such as companionship, expressive support, and intimacy, well before their relative's biological death. Conversely, survivors may not recognize immediately all that has been lost with the death of their impaired relative. It may take some time for them to realize just how much they depended on the person's presence to structure their days, and more than this, how much they depended on the person's needs to provide meaning and purpose to their lives.

We mention this disjunction, between objective loss and sense of loss, because both may affect the form and duration of grief, before and after death occurs. For example, when a person becomes progressively impaired, a caregiver must begin to make adjustments in her life to compensate for his impairments. These adjustments may begin to take their toll on her energy and well-being before she has recognized exactly what has happened. Because many dementing illnesses, in particular, are insidious in their onset and progress rather slowly, caregivers may not immediately recognize declines in functioning and the consequent losses with which they are dealing.

If recognition is the first step in the development of a sense of loss, realization is the second. It is the subtle process whereby people move from the simple ability to recognize a deficit to the deeper realization that something is irrecoverably missing from their lives. At the simplest level, the first psychological task is to recognize the losses one is facing. Immediately after the death, this basic understanding may come and go; as survivors engage in familiar plans and activities, they may temporarily forget that the person is no longer alive. But typical patterns of thoughts, feelings, and behavior elicited by familiar circumstances no longer fit the new situation. This lack of a fit is one sign that change is needed, and it engenders in survivors a sense that things are out of kilter. The common patterns of responding assume that the world has remained constant and continuous, that one's typical ways of reacting to things will be appropriate. Death is a breach in this continuity, which throws into question the meanings sustained by these experiences.

For many caregivers, the immediate impact of death is dramatic. However much they may have realized the losses they were experiencing, and may even have grieved to some extent for them, death is immediately related to intense grief. Our impression is that intense grief is associated with the realization of some losses more than others: Losses involving the relationship with the deceased appear to affect grief more immediately than those involving the less personal aspects of the deceased, such as social status or network relationships.

Over time, these intense feelings, particularly depression, illusory experiences, and the sense of unreality, diminish. Many survivors, however, continue to review images and memories of the person, but these images are less and less associated with pain. Initially, the review of their relationship with the deceased may increase their sense of loss, for this is the time in which they uncover the many things they have lost with the illness and death. The bouts of grief noted by others (Bowlby, 1980) may be related to these successive discoveries. But as this grief process continues, what remains, particularly for those whose sense of self has not been undermined by the losses encountered, may contain many positive elements. Survivors may recognize their accomplishments as caregivers; they may take satisfaction in having performed a difficult job in a loving way; and they may realize their own strengths in relationships, as friend, lover, partner, or companion. And these realizations may represent the first steps in the process of resolution, to which we now turn our attention.

Resolution

For most caregivers, much of the work of resolution follows the initial grief associated with the losses experienced. We refer to the *work* of resolution, because people actively participate in finding a way to come to grips with their losses and the grief and emotions associated with those losses. *Resolution* is meant to convey, with a neutral term, a complex process that involves a restructuring, however subtle, of the social world and the sense of self. This restructuring may involve resuming old activities, assuming new activities and roles, and developing a changed perception of the world and of the self.

What hastens someone's movement through bereavement? There is no simple answer to this question, because adaptive behaviors can be enormously varied (Stroebe & Schut, 2001). Further, just what comprises resolution is not clear (Silverman & Nickman, 1996); some symptoms of grief can recur for many years (Wortman & Silver, 2001). Thus, resolution does not necessarily mean returning to a previous level of functioning (Wortman & Silver, 1990), or dissolving the connection to the deceased (Klass, Silverman, & Nickman, 1996). For some, it may mean an opportunity for positive growth, a new life-style, or a sense of mastery and competence (Skaff, Pearlin, & Mullan, 1996). But, despite these kinds of unanswered questions and unresolved issues, some focus to the matter of resolution can be achieved. Our discussion of resolution parallels in some way the emerging view that bereavement encompasses two complementary tasks, restructuring life activities and managing the cognitive–emotional consequences of loss and grief (Archer, 2001; Bonanno & Kaltman, 1999; Stroebe & Schut, 1999).

We begin by noting that the course of resolution probably depends, at least to some extent, on the nature of the losses one has experienced. More specifically, it depends on whether losses are reversible or substitutable. Reversible losses can be turned around or retrieved. We do not mean to trivialize profound losses. However, although the death of a person is irreversible, the associated losses may be at least partially reversible (Marris, 1974). Referring to our catalogue of losses, let us suppose, for example, that the survivor has suffered a loss of status or of financial resources following the death. These kinds of losses may not be reversed, but they are not intrinsically permanent. Similarly, any constriction in the range of the survivor's social network is also potentially reversible. One begins to make new friends, reactivate old friendships, become engaged in leisure-time pursuits, or join clubs and organizations. Essentially, then, some losses can be reversed through social reintegration and, we believe, the more quickly and completely such reversals occur, the faster will be the psychological resolution of bereavement.

Of course, these assertions are difficult to substantiate empirically. It is simple enough to determine whether decreases in the duration of psychological distress are correlated with the reversal of social losses. What is not clear is whether reintegration frees one from distress, if relief from distress enables one to seek reintegration, or if their influence is mutual. To discern the directions of effect, longitudinal observations are needed.

Some losses that are not reversible are substitutable, "alternative rewards," as Moos and Schaefer (1986) have written. For example, the affection and support that the deceased once provided may be supplied by others. Indeed, survivors may bond to others with the hope that the love and understanding they had before will be provided by new relationships. In addition, one of the forces that drives intimacy and caregiving is the desire to matter to another person, to be important to that person's welfare. Resolution may involve not only finding others from whom one can receive support and affection, but also others to whom one can again matter by giving support and affection. Finding replacements for those roles that have been lost is another part of the resolution process that may involve substitution of new roles (Stroebe & Stroebe, 1987). This, of course, can be more difficult for older people who may have fewer opportunities for engaging in new roles. Among informal AIDS caregivers, it is not unusual for the survivor to assume caregiving activities with another person. Although these activities may be directed by personal attachment and a sense of mission, these survivors may also be able to retrieve a sense of mattering through such relationships.

Resolution, then, can be partially charted by the survivor's efforts to reverse losses or, when they are irreversible, to find substitutes or compensations for what cannot be retrieved. We believe that resolution can also be discerned on a different and more subtle level, as survivors restructure their cognitive–emotional lives in the aftermath of loss and grief. The past is constantly being reworked, as individuals revisit images and memories of the people they have lost. We believe that, in this review process, people often find a way to consolidate images of the deceased person so that they can be stored comfortably in memory. This is probably an important issue, because, if the images remain entirely and deeply painful, a part of the past may remain inaccessible, as survivors confront the challenges of their lives.

This internal restructuring takes some time, and bereavement adaptation at 1 year is different from bereavement adaptation at 3 years. Immediately after a death, many survivors experience pain and depression. Memories are often only painful reminders of what has been lost. Although there may be times of comfort when the deceased person is recalled, as often, the thoughts are loaded with depressive affect and the person feels out of sync, dissociated from day-to-day life.

Gradually, however, more of the memories and images of the deceased can be experienced apart from sadness; indeed, many report that their memories can also bring comfort. Thus, at this point in bereavement, people may be consolidating images and memories of the deceased, even as they restructure their lives.

Earlier, we discussed the multiple aspects of loss of self or identity that may occur, both preceding and following the death of someone close. But resolution in relation to the self may involve not only loss, but also transformation, with the potential for positive growth and enrichment of self (Moss & Moss, 1989; Wortman & Silver, 1990). For widows and widowers, the resolution process may involve establishing a new identity as a single person (Lopata, 1996). Although this may be painful and slow, it carries the potential for a new and more positive sense of self (Lopata, 1996; Parkes, 1987). As one widow put it, "I'm more self-reliant. Doing my own thinking, not looking to see if he approves of what I'm doing." Some of the tasks include finding new roles to replace those lost, establishing a new social life as a single person, and revising one's view of oneself in terms of future hopes and plans.

Adult children may experience rather paradoxical feelings at the death of a parent. On the one hand, they keenly feel the losses that we have described; on the other hand, however, they often feel a sense of personal growth or enrichment (Moss & Moss, 1989). Thus, although they may lose a lifelong source of positive feedback about the self that had been provided by the parent, they frequently gain a new sense of "coming into one's own" (Kowalski, 1986). The death of a parent may also remind them of their own mortality and the time left to accomplish their own goals. Adult children who lived with the parent before death, and who may have forfeited significant portions of their own lives, may find the restructuring of their own separate identities to be particularly difficult and rewarding.

For spouses and adult children who cared for their relative for an extended period of time, the death of that relative is even more likely to have both positive and negative effects on the sense of self. The loss of self, which some of our Alzheimer's caregivers experienced prior to the death of their relative, may be lifted as they are relieved from the role that had so engulfed them. The resolution of a former sense of self, or rebuilding a new sense of self, will, we believe, depend upon how well the caregivers are able to find new sources of self-evaluation by establishing new roles or by re-engaging in old ones.

For anyone who experiences the illness and death of someone close to them, there is the potential for that experience to lead to a new sense of self-confidence, competence, and mastery (Calhoun & Tedeschi, 1989–1990; Schaefer & Moos, 2001). Being relieved of the burden of caregiving, but also knowing that one was able to deal with a very difficult situation, appears to have a positive effect on sense of self. Analyses of data on our Alzheimer's caregivers reveal an increase in a sense of mastery among those recently bereaved (Mullan, 1992; Skaff et al., 1996).

We are only at the beginning of our quest to understand resolution. Yet we are confident that it represents more than the simple wearing away of grief with time. As important as time may be as a healer, resolution depends on the active efforts and cognitive realignments of the survivors. It also depends on the situational contexts in which loss and bereavement occur.

Bereavement and the Historical Moment

To this point, we have been emphasizing the similarities between the two groups of bereaved caregivers, suggesting implicitly that the differences found between them reflect the particular losses they experience. However, emphasizing some striking contrasts between the Alzheimer's and AIDS caregivers is important—contrasts that can lead to an altered course of bereavement, with qualitatively different losses, changed grief responses, and a recasting of the work of resolution. Among the many differences between the two groups of caregivers, we note what seem the most salient: AIDS has a compressed time frame, and the stigma associated with AIDS and its victims may extend to the caregivers. Two other contrasts between AIDS and Alzheimer's caregivers seem most clearly to affect the course of bereavement: first, the untimeliness of AIDS, affecting younger people who are not expected in our culture to be ill; and second, the extraordinary number of deaths confronted by AIDS caregivers at the time of our study, in the early 1990s.

The reality of the AIDS epidemic was that young adults often became the primary caregivers to their young friends and partners. For these young adults, caregiving is an "off-time" activity, not compatible with the culture's expectation of the typical developmental tasks of that life stage, when people are typically establishing their identities, their occupational directions, and their social bonds, especially intimate ones. We do not expect young people to be held down by inflexible obligations, such as caregiving, nor to regularly confront illness and death.

To measure such complicated processes is, of course, difficult—for example, the developmental losses incurred as people are preoccupied with the illness and death of someone close to them. Among the AIDS caregivers, however, we certainly see evidence consistent with the notion that caregiving seems most difficult and stressful for those off-time: the younger men and women caregivers are more overloaded, frustrated, and depressed, compared with their older counterparts (Mullan, 1998).

We expected that the higher levels of caregiving distress would mean more distress for the younger caregivers following the death of the care recipient, but, in fact, we could discern no clear differences in grief between the older and younger survivors. One hypothesis is that younger caregivers do have a somewhat more difficult time managing the death, but that this is offset by the depth and breadth of the losses experienced by the older caregivers, whose lives are more interconnected with those who have died. Older caregivers have simply had more time to become involved in social networks that were being decimated by AIDS.

Obviously, entire communities were being affected. By contrast, Alzheimer's caregivers sometimes construct a community of other caregivers, but it is a voluntary community, and, often enough, one to which they are only intermittently connected. By contrast, in the early 1990s, AIDS caregivers were involuntarily engulfed by illness and death. They soon realized that their entire community was under siege, and that they faced a world of loss.

These losses were extensive, even among people caring for family members, often thought to be removed from the large-scale community losses. The figures are staggering. In our sample, about 90% of the nonfamily caregivers reported a close death from AIDS, at the initial interview. One half of the traditional family caregivers reported a close AIDS death. Over the next year, 50% of the caregivers had suffered the loss of the person for whom they had been caring. In addition, about 50% of nonfamily and 25% of family caregivers reported additional close deaths from AIDS over that year.

Such losses challenge our theories of bereavement, which are based on adaptation to individual deaths (Nord, 1997; Schwartzberg, 1992). Indeed, we had expected to find increased grief and depression as the number of close deaths increased, but we did not. Early in the epidemic, Martin (1988) had detected a strong relationship between multiple deaths and well-being. However, later studies have not found such clear effects (Kemeny et al., 1994; Neugebauer et al., 1992; Siegel, Karus, & Raveis, 1997).

We are baffled by how the caregivers managed to survive psychologically in the midst of such dramatic and continuous losses. And yet, as we examine our AIDS caregivers' responses to the death of the care recipients, they seem almost indistinguishable from those of the Alzheimer's caregivers: The death leads immediately to the typical levels of depressive feelings and the patterns of grief that we have described, then we see a decline over time, as people re-engage in a variety of ways with their lives. But if each death involves such a process, why do we not see a clear effect of the multiple losses that AIDS caregivers experienced?

One historical explanation has been offered: that the meaning of death has been changed by the epidemic. Early on, the numbers of deaths were shocking, because they violated life-course expectations and occurred in communities that were unprepared for them. By the time that we talked with our caregivers in the mid-1990s, the deaths had become part of the expectations that people brought to their lives, having been surrounded by illness and death (Neugebauer et al., 1992).

If we have yet to understand fully the complicated set of losses and subsequent grief reactions that follow one death, not surprisingly we cannot explain clearly the impact of an enormous number of deaths. Traditional models of bereavement lack a language for discussing such widespread loss. Perhaps our focus on typical patterns of grief is misplaced, and we should be asking about symptoms of trauma instead. However, our respondents have suggested another avenue to explore: Many reported that they have felt numb and emotionally shut down in the face of such devastation (see also Nord, 1997). This muted emotional response may indicate that they are selectively responding to losses, with strong feelings evoked only by deaths that symbolize their most precious losses. In effect, there may exist an economy of grief, limiting a person's response, at least for periods of time. In any case, clearly we know relatively little about one of the major ways that AIDS has affected millions of people. Thus, a major consequence of the AIDS epidemic has gone mostly unstudied and not understood.

Discussion

Dying and death are unique experiences for survivors. In a multitude of ways, the surrounding conditions may combine to make each person's confrontation with the death of a loved one different from that of others. Yet, certain threads seem to cut across the unique aspects of survivorship. Together, these threads enable us to describe not only how individuals and groups may differ in their survivorship, but also how, at some level, they may be seen as sharing an experience.

These things are loss, grief, and resolution—constructs very familiar to students of death and dying. What we have sought in this chapter is, first, to give some elaboration to these constructs. Although they are familiar, their substance and dimensions are not yet satisfactorily specified. Second, we have attempted to identify some of the linkages among the three constructs. This attempt is guided by the assumption that adaptation to the death of a loved one is best understood within the framework of a process encompassing loss, grief, and resolution. We do not assume that these are three discrete stages of bereavement. But we do believe that they constitute the foundations for describing the experiential trajectories of survivors and for identifying the conditions that help to explain variations in these trajectories.

Our perspectives on bereavement, and the processes that we believe give it meaning and direction, are colored by the two groups of former caregivers we are studying. The striking differences between these groups help to highlight their common experiences.

On average, the Alzheimer's group will have been active caregivers for a longer time than the AIDS groups. Yet, in each case, circumstances have forced a recasting of reciprocal relationships into relationships mostly based on one person giving and the other receiving. This recasting itself may produce a swirl of emotions and conflicts that must be dealt with along the entire course of the survival process.

Although, among the children of parents with Alzheimer's disease, there is some fear that the disease may be inherited, it is the AIDS caregivers, particularly close friends and lovers, who may read into death a scenario of their own fates. To some extent, then, resolution depends on members of both groups reconciling themselves to losses created by illness and death, and also to threats they may feel to their own lives. This task is greater among AIDS caregivers. These caregivers, too, often experience multiple deaths. When the caregiver and person with AIDS are part of a larger community with which they closely identify themselves, as is often the case, then the death of one individual can also be interpreted as a gradual chipping away of the collectivity. In a real sense, there is the loss of community by attrition, and, although the survivor might eventually recover from the death of a loved one, he may never recover from the loss of community.

In thinking about surviving the death of a loved one, as a process, loss and its many dimensions seem to us to be the key to much of what follows. The sheer range of losses that are experienced, and the intensity of the losses, would be major factors regulating the cognitive substance, emotional sensitivity, and length of active grieving. As we have discussed, we similarly regard resolution as closely dependent on loss. Although we can offer no empirical evidence to support this assumption, it seems reasonable to suppose that, to a substantial extent, resolution occurs as people are able to reverse losses that are reversible and to find substitutes for those that are not.

We have emphasized some of the compensatory processes of resolution, because they follow from the recognition that loss is multifaceted, varying both in the kinds and intensity of the losses experienced, as well as the variety of effects the losses can have on individuals. We have learned that some appear to experience little in the way of traditional grief reactions (Wortman & Silver, 2001); that people experience positive emotional states, even as they grieve (Folkman, 1997); and that part of the bereavement process for many people is the ability to remain connected to positive images of the deceased person, incorporating them into a living memory accessible over time (Klass et al., 1996).

As we have seen, bereavement adaptation involves more than managing loss, grief, and depression. It often involves a restructuring of major life domains: one's time, social relationships, occupational life, financial situation, and plans for the future. Each of these domains, and more, can be affected by a death. The bereaved may gradually restructure components of the self, as they adjust to the new reality of life without the deceased person. We have little understanding of how the images of the deceased person come to be incorporated into the self concept that people form in the aftermath of the death. But certainly the bereaved person remains connected to the person who died (Klass et al., 1996).

A major perspective we hope to convey with this chapter is that survivorship and the process it entails are highly complex and variable. Although there is much that we do not know, we are learning to raise the kinds of questions that will guide future research into bereavement.

Discussion Questions

1. How can a personal experience like bereavement be affected by historical processes?
2. Provide a critique of the term 'resolution.' What other terms might be used instead? Should it be avoided in discussions of bereavement?
3. Imagine developing a set of bereavement services consistent with the model of bereavement outlined in the chapter. What assessments need to be conducted? What kinds of services would need to be available?
4. Consider bereavement among people who have not been caregivers. In what ways does studying caregivers limit our perspective on the processes of loss, grief, and resolution?

References

Aneshensel, C. S., Pearlin, L. I., Mullan, J. T., Zarit, S. H., & Whitlatch, C. J. (1995). *Profiles in caregiving: The unexpected career.* San Diego, CA: Academic Press.

Archer, J. (2001). Broad and narrow perspectives in grief theory: Comment on Bonanno and Kaltman (1999). *Psychological Bulletin, 127*(4), 554–560.

Bonanno, G. A., & Kaltman, S. (1999). Toward an integrative perspective on bereavement. *Psychological Bulletin, 125*(6), 760–776.

Bowlby, J. (1980). *Loss* (Vol. 3). New York: Basic Books.

Calhoun, L. G., & Tedeschi, R. G. (1989–1990). Positive aspects of critical life problems: Recollections of grief. *Omega: Journal of Death & Dying, 20*(4), 265–272.

Folkman, S. (1997). Positive psychological states and coping with severe stress. *Social Science & Medicine, 45*(8), 1207–1221.

Kemeny, M. E., Weiner, H., Taylor, S. E., Schneider, S., Visscher, B. R., & Fahey, J. L. (1994). Repeated bereavement, depressed mood, and immune parameters in hiv seropositive and seronegative gay men. *Health Psychology, 13*(1), 14–24.

Klass, D., Silverman, P. R., & Nickman, S. L. (Eds.). (1996). *Continuing bonds: New understandings of grief.* Philadelphia: Taylor & Francis.

Kowalski, N. C. (1986). Anticipating the death of an elderly parent. In T. A. Rando (Ed.), *Loss and anticipatory grief* (pp. 187–199). Lexington, MA: D. C. Heath.

Lopata, H. Z. (1975). Grief work and identity reconstruction. *Journal of Geriatric Psychiatry, 8*(1), 41–55.

Lopata, H. Z. (1996). *Current widowhood: Myths & realities.* Thousand Oaks, CA: Sage Publications.

Marris, P. (1974). *Loss and change.* New York: Pantheon.

Martin, J. L. (1988). Psychological consequences of AIDS-related bereavement among gay men. *Journal of Consulting and Clinical Psychology, 56*(6), 856–862.

Moos, R. H., & Schaefer, J. A. (1986). Life transitions and crises: A conceptual overview. In R. H. Moos (Ed.), *Coping with life crises: An integrated approach* (pp. 3–28). New York: Plenum.

Moss, M. S., & Moss, S. Z. (1989). The death of a parent. In R. A. Kalish (Ed.), *Midlife loss: Coping strategies* (pp. 89–114). Newbury Park, CA: Sage.

Mullan, J. T. (1992). The bereaved caregiver: A prospective study of changes in well-being. *Gerontologist, 32*(5), 673–683.

Mullan, J. T. (1998). Aging and informal caregiving to people with HIV/AIDS. *Research on Aging, 20*(6), 712–738.

Neugebauer, R., Rabkin, J. G., Williams, J. B. W., Remien, R. H., Goetz, R., & Gorman, J. M. (1992). Bereavement reactions among homosexual men experiencing multiple losses in the AIDS epidemic. *American Journal of Psychiatry, 149*(10), 1374–1379.

Nord, D. (1997). *Multiple AIDS-related loss: A handbook for understanding and surviving a perpetual fall.* Washington, DC: Taylor & Francis.

Parkes, C. M. (1987). *Bereavement: Studies of grief in adult life.* Madison, CT: International Universities Press.

Pearlin, L. I., & Lieberman, M. A. (1979). Social sources of emotional distress. In Roberta G. Simmons (Ed.), *Research in community and mental health: An annual compilation of research* (Vol. 1., pp. 217–248).

Rosenberg, M., & McCullough, B. C. (1981). Mattering: Inferred significance and mental health among adolescents. *Research in community and mental health: A research annual* (Vol. 2, pp. 163–182).

Schaefer, J. A., & Moos, R. H. (2001). Bereavement experiences and personal growth. In M. S. Stroebe, R. O. Hansson, W. Stroebe, & H. Schut (Eds.), *Handbook of bereavement research: Consequences, coping, and care* (pp. 145–167). Washington, DC: American Psychological Association.

Schwartzberg, S. S. (1992). AIDS-related bereavement among gay men: The inadequacy of current theories of grief. *Psychotherapy, 29*(3), 422–429.

Siegel, K., Karus, D., & Raveis, V. H. (1997). Correlates of change in depressive symptomatology among gay men with AIDS. *Health Psychology, 16*(3), 230–238.

Silverman, P. R., & Nickman, S. L. (1996). Concluding thoughts. In D. Klass, P. R. Silverman, & S. L. Nickman (Eds.), *Continuing bonds: New understandings of grief* (pp. 73–86). Philadelphia: Taylor & Francis.

Skaff, M. M., & Pearlin, L. I. (1992). Caregiving: Role engulfment and the loss of self. *Gerontologist, 32*(5), 656–664.

Skaff, M. M., Pearlin, L. I., & Mullan, J. T. (1996). Transitions in the caregiving career: Effects on sense of mastery. *Psychology & Aging, 11*(2), 247–257.

Stroebe, M., & Schut, H. (1999). The dual process model of coping with bereavement: Rationale and description. *Death Studies, 23*(3), 197–224.

Stroebe, M. S., & Schut, H. (2001). Models of coping with bereavement: A review. In M. S. Stroebe, R. O. Hansson, W. Stroebe, & H. Schut (Eds.), *Handbook of bereavement research: Consequences, coping, and care* (pp. 375–403). Washington, DC: American Psychological Association.

Stroebe, W., & Stroebe, M. S. (1987). *Bereavement and health: The psychological and physical consequences of partner loss.* Cambridge, England: Cambridge University Press.

Troll, L. E., & Bengtson, V. L. (1992). The oldest-old in families: An intergenerational perspective. *Generations, 16*(3), 39–44.

Umberson, D., Wortman, C. B., & Kessler, R. C. (1992). Widowhood and depression: Explaining long-term gender differences in vulnerability. *Journal of Health and Social Behavior, 33*(1), 10–24.

Walsh, F., & McGoldrick, M. (1991). Loss and the family: A systemic perspective. In F. Walsh & M. McGoldrick (Eds.), *Living beyond loss: Death in the family* (pp. 1–29). New York: W. W. Norton.

Wortman, C. B., & Silver, R. C. (1990). Successful mastery of bereavement and widowhood: A life course perspective. In P. B. Baltes & M. M. Baltes (Eds.), *Successful aging: Perspectives from the behavioral sciences* (pp. 225–264). Cambridge, MA: Cambridge University Press.

Wortman, C. B., & Silver, R. C. (2001). The myths of coping with loss revisited. In M. S. Stroebe & R. O. Hansson (Eds.), *Handbook of bereavement research: Consequences, coping, and care* (pp. 405–429). Washington, DC: American Psychological Association.

Twelve

Social Support and Mutual Help for the Bereaved

Phyllis R. Silverman

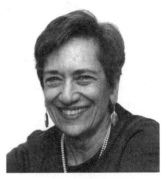

Phyllis R. Silverman, PhD, Lic. SW, is professor emerita at the MGH Institute of Health Professions, an associate in social welfare in the Department of Psychiatry at Massachusetts General Hospital and Harvard Medical School, and scholar-in-residence at the Women's Studies Research Center at Brandeis University. She developed the concept of the widow-to-widow program and directed the research project that demonstrated its effectiveness. She is the recipient of the 1991 presidential medal from Brooklyn College, City University of New York, for her out- standing contributions to the fields of bereavement and social welfare. The National Center for Death Education recognized her as a pio- neer in the field of thanatology with its 1994 award. In addition to her social work de- gree from Smith College School for Social Work, she holds an ScM in hygiene from Harvard School of Public Health and a PhD from the Florence Heller School for Ad- vanced Studies in Social Welfare at Brandeis University. She has published extensively in professional journals and has written several books on widowhood and mutual help groups. Her most recent book, Never Too Young to Know: Death in Children's Lives, *was published in 2000.*

The Nature of Social Support

Murphy observed, in studying development in children, that most prac- titioners and researchers focus primarily on the achievement of autonomy as the goal of development. Competent children, she observed, not only know when they need help, but know how to solicit such help, be it for approval and love or for concrete assistance (Murphy, 1974). Murphy's observation points to the fact that we are social creatures, and the need for others is essential to human life. To deal with the various vicissitudes and stresses of living, we must acknowledge the importance of relationships and the interdependencies among people that make a viable life possible. This is true not only in the young, but throughout the life cycle. The literature on the new psychology of women has made these truths even clearer (Gilligan, 1982; Miller, 1986; Brown & Gilligan, 1992; Belenky, Clinchy, Goldberger, & Tarule, 1996). These researchers are talking about the centrality to human life of connection and care between people; they are saying that only in relationships do we grow, develop, and adapt.

These observations from Murphy's research into the effect of stress, and from studies of the psychology of women, are in some ways joined, as we turn to research on social support (Belle, 1987; Barnett, Biener, & Baruch, 1987). This research, focusing primarily on periods of stress, documents the value of social support as a mediator of this stress (Garmezy, 1987). The availability of support, which means the availability of others, seems to be correlated with adaptive behavior. Adaptive behavior involves coping effectively with the stress, so that it is possible to carry on with life, compared to maladaptive behavior that can be dysfunctional, given the nature of the stress (Belle, 1989; Gottlieb, 1981; Folkman, 2001).

Cobb (1976), one of the earliest researchers to study the phenomenon, defined *social support* as information leading to the subject believing that he is cared for and loved, that he is esteemed and valued, and that he belongs to a network of communication and mutual obligation. Caplan (1976) defined support in terms of the functioning of a support system that is a continuing social aggregate that provides individuals with opportunities for feedback about themselves and for validation of their expectations about others, which may offset deficiencies in these communications within the larger community context. In such relations, Caplan continues, the individual is dealt with in a personalized way: People speak his or her language, guide him or her in what to do, offer feedback about what he or she is doing, and can provide extra supplies of money, materials, and skills. Eckenrode and Gore (1981), Folkman (2001), and Folkman and Moskowitz (2000b) noted that understanding the value of support is not possible without looking at the context in which it occurs and the responses of the recipients. They suggested looking at the social network in which the stress and available support are embedded. A focus on the social network brings to the fore those who are actors in the network, how they interact, and what help they provide (Gottlieb, 1981; Vachon, 1979).

Stylianos and Vachon (1993), in their review of the growing literature on social support, define support as a transactional process requiring a fit between the donor, the recipient, and the particular circumstances. Gottlieb (1990) reinforces this point by reminding us that support is a process, and that understanding the nature of support and its effectiveness is essential to understanding the interaction between those involved, how it gets expressed, and to what it leads.

For example, Belle (1982) found that depressed low-income women often had many people with whom they were in contact and from whom help might be expected. Nonetheless, these women often felt isolated and unsupported. Belle found that potential helpers in the network were more interested in taking than in giving, in spite of the clear need in others. Folkman (1997) and Folkman and Moskowitz (2000a) found that recipients of help who had a more positive approach to life, and an acceptance of their need for assistance, were better able to use the support offered after the death from AIDS of someone close to them. There is a need, then, to not only identify the actors in the situation, but their resources, attitudes towards help from others, and ability to respond to their own needs and the needs of others.

Another factor to consider, in both the provision and the receipt of support, is the gender of those involved. Differences may emerge between how men and women define their needs, and what they define as appropriate help, as well as the kind of help they themselves can provide. Barnett et al. (1987), Gilligan, Ward, and Taylor (1988), and Miller and Striver (1997) have suggested that we will learn more about care and connection from studying women's experience. Lyons (1989), in a study of how adolescent girls develop, points to the growing concern of these young women to learn to care for others and to respect the reality of others. These adolescents were not striving for individuation and separation, which are typically considered the primary developmental issues of adolescence. Instead, these girls aspire to be interdependent, that is, to be in relationship with others in a new way.

Using men's experience (Levinson, 1978) as the norm has led to a focus on individuation and autonomy as the goal of development. The consequence of this focus became clear in my studies of the widowed (Silverman, 1987). Widowers, for example, talk of needing to learn to reach out to others and take responsibility for their social life, which was usually a role their wives had played in their marriage. They have no trouble making decisions, particularly about work-related issues, and their sense of integrity and self remain intact. Widows report needing to learn to make decisions, to speak out for themselves, and to develop a new sense of self. They usually report knowing themselves in terms of their relationship to others, that is, as wife or mother (Silverman, 1987). Men seem to have difficulty reaching out for help of any kind: They seem to think they should be able to manage by themselves (Boerner & Silverman, 2002; Cook, 1988; Silverman, 1987). Some men found it easier to join a poker group, where they in fact got a good deal of support, but would not choose to come together to simply talk about feelings (Campbell & Silverman, 1996).

A study of widows and widowers caring for dependent children (Silverman & Worden, 1992) found that the vast majority of both men and women reached out to women for assistance and support. Women have been the providers of support in our society. They are accustomed to this role and accept themselves in this role. Women talk of needing to be needed. Widowers talked of learning to care as one of the lessons learned by the few who joined together with other widowed people. It was a new experience to be helpful by exchanging feelings with others and to have a male friend with whom they shared details of their daily lives (Silverman, 1987; Campbell & Silverman, 1996). When we talk, then, of support, we are talking about the fundamental nature of relationships and of care that is only possible in the context of these relationships and that makes for special bonds between people. We need to understand how this care is expressed in any given community and whether the community values the need for such care, not only in response to a given problem, but as part of the essence of the human condition.

In looking at stressful situations that lead to the need for support, we often consider them static, constant over time, and unrelated to the context in which those affected are acting (Silverman, 2000). A stress is rarely a single event or activity. For example, if we assume that a widowed person is simply reacting to the death of the spouse, we are overlooking a large part of the stress the widowed person is experiencing.

Stress, for the widowed, may come from the exhaustion, and perhaps relief, after having watched a spouse suffer a long illness, which the death ended; from young children who must grow up in a single-parent household and who make new demands on their sole parent; or from the fact that they are themselves old and not well and for the first time find themselves living alone. Stress also occurs for some families who have never faced death, and have no way of seeing it as an expected part of the life cycle. Stress may also emanate from others in the network, who cannot tolerate the pain associated with bereavement and that is so much a part of the reality of the newly widowed. These others may withdraw or pressure the widowed to be "over" their loss in a very short period of time (Silverman, 1981, 1986, 1999). Stress, then, emanates not only from the sadness and sense of loss, but from the changes in the social context in which the survivors must live the rest of their lives. With the passing of time, the bereaved's needs will change, as will their circumstances. These changes will not occur in a vacuum, but as a result of interaction among the actors at work in this system, some as helpers, some as beneficiaries, some as both. Help or support, then, cannot remain the same, but has to respond to the new conditions and new problems (Belenky, Bond, & Weinstock, 1997; Gottlieb, 1990; Silverman, 1966, 1986; Stylianos & Vachon, 1993).

This chapter focuses on the needs of the bereaved. Death of a loved one is something that all of us will experience. Although we may see many deaths as untimely and out of turn in the life cycle, death itself ultimately cannot be avoided. It is the price that we all pay for being alive, and we will all be bereaved, if we are involved in relationships. We are looking, then, at a universal stressor to which we all need to learn to respond. When we talk about the availability of social support in a community at the time of a death, we are talking about the very basic quality of life in that community.

This quality is related to how people understand bereavement. Do they see it as an illness that needs to be expunged like a germ, or as a legitimate human expression of pain and sadness that brings with it a need for change (Silverman, 2000)? Quality of life in a community is also related to what help is available and how people utilize it. If we agree that the help should be responsive to the need, these two considerations are really very much related (Belenky et al., 1997). The remainder of the chapter will focus on the needs of the bereaved and how they are met by the available helping networks in their communities, and the support these networks can provide, with particular emphasis on mutual help.

The Nature of the Bereavement Process

The understanding we have of bereavement is reflected in the vocabulary available for describing the widowed person's grief. We talk of a "time of healing," of "getting over it," and of "working it through." We say, "You will recover." The images associated with these phrases imply that grief is an illness from which one recovers with appropriate treatment. The expectation of such treatment is that it will, at the least, relieve the mourner's pain, and, at the most, remove it entirely. Implicit too is that grief ends, and that people will pick up their lives and carry on as before. The affective and psychological aspects of grief are emphasized in this approach, so that the crying, sadness, pining, feeling alone, and feeling cheated by the loss come into focus as the primary issues to be attended to. This approach can result in major deception of the bereaved, as they try to conform to the expectations of their social network. With the diminution of these feelings, they expect that their grief will be "resolved." When they are unable to achieve this goal, they can feel defective and stigmatized, as if something must be wrong with them. Their grief is long and pervades most aspects of their lives, which are irrevocably changed and cannot be reconstituted as before (Silverman, 1981, 2000; Lopata, 1988). The death of a spouse, or of any other person who was very much a part of the survivor's life, leads to major disruptions in the way the mourner's world is constructed, the way they see themselves in relationship to that world, and in the very habits of daily living (Silverman, 1986, 2000; Neimeyer, 1998, Klass; 1988; Shamgar-Handleman, 1986).

In reality, pain may be tempered by time, but time does not heal. The widowed do not recover; rather, they make an accommodation to their new situation. This involves dealing with the inner sense of loss, accepting the pain as part of living, and learning to remember the deceased with ease and satisfaction. Ultimately, finding a new sense of self requires finding a new place for one's self in the world as a formerly married, now single person. Help for the widowed must be responsive to their need to legitimate their feelings and to learn to live in a new way in the world (Silverman, 1966, 1969, 1976).

Helping Networks

As we look at the nature of help that is available in any community, we begin with the central unit of the family and move beyond that to the neighborhood, to the community, then to the professional helping system. The primary unit of social support is the family (Shapiro, 1994; Nadeau, 1999). Caplan (1976) identified how the family functions as a provider of care, of approbation, of material needs, and of feedback. The family anchors the individual in a social network and in the larger society. Gottlieb (1981) looks at the helping networks in any given community and considers the social distance between them. He considers the access to the system and whether or not people working in the system receive remuneration for this work. Gottlieb finds that the further away from the nuclear family unit the helping system is, the less personal are the services provided. The family maintains a system of mutual obligation to its members, who are connected by marriage, birth, or adoption. Providers of service in the professional community offer care and services because they have a societal mandate to do so, and there is a fee for this service. Payment for services is the primary obligation of the client or patient; the other obligation may be to comply with the advice of the professional (Hughes, 1971). There is no expectation of reciprocity. Help is more specialized, and division of labor is clear. In the family, in the neighborhood, and in friendship, help is offered as a matter of personal obligation, and there is a sense of mutuality and reciprocity. The helpers' expertise in this informal system comes from their knowledge of the recipient and from their experience and their own value system (Gottlieb, 1981; Belenky et al., 1997).

As we look at the impact of the death of a spouse, we return to the social impact of this loss. In their roles as husbands and wives, men and women find a way of framing and focusing their daily lives and of providing each other with appropriate support. This unit is irreparably disrupted when one of the spouses dies. This source of support is gone. The nature of this support can vary. The widowed individual can lose, for example, a companion with whom to share ideas, the primary financial provider in the family, or the primary nurturer of the family. Exactly what is lost depends on the way these individuals constructed their marriage, as well as the dictates of the community, which provides a major frame for defining the meaning of marriage (Silverman, 1986). The widowed individual has to turn for assistance to family members, friends, neighbors, and beyond.

The bereaved (and there is rarely a single mourner, even in the death of a spouse) need each other and their families to share their feelings about the deceased, to remember together, and to support each other as they acknowledge their pain and loss. They need friends to help with the concrete tasks of living and managing their family, from the time before the funeral to afterwards, as they try to establish a life-style appropriate to their new situation. They need the funeral director and the clergy to help with burial and mourning rituals. In the long run, religion can be very important in trying to find a way of living with the fact that people die.

When such a profound and complex disruption has occurred, however, no one kind of assistance is usually sufficient. Dakoff and Taylor (1990) have documented that different kinds of help are expected from different helpers in a helping network, and therefore the helpfulness of any given act is in part related to its source. For example, in that study, esteem and emotional support were valued from family members and not from physicians. When physicians provided specific information, they were seen as very helpful to people with cancer. What happens when these helpers are not able to respond to the bereaved in a way that is helpful? Often the mourner is referred to professionals for assistance (Osterweis, Solomon, & Greene, 1984). These professionals could be clergy, physicians, or mental health therapists. Clergy, unless they have a psychological orientation, may rely on prayer and concrete advice. Physicians usually prescribe medication to relieve what are designated as symptoms of grief. The mental health professional generally focuses on the psychological aspects of the process (Jacobs, 1999). Whatever the help may be, the message to the bereaved is that there is something wrong, and, with the correct professional help, he or she will get over the grief. This can further stigmatize an individual who already is feeling disoriented in the face of a disrupted sense of self (Silverman, 2000). On the other hand, this type of assistance may be very useful to people and should not be discounted outright.

There is still another dimension of support, which comes from anyone who has had a personal experience with widowhood. The widowed need to know that most widowed people have similar experiences, and they need to find role models for how they can build their lives anew. We talk a good deal about peer influence on adolescents, but we need to consider that this may be a need throughout the life cycle. At each new stage or phase, we seek others who have gone before us, to learn from them. If the widowed do not have people in their network who have been widowed, they may seek others outside this network. The growth of mutual help organizations has made us increasingly aware of this need for others who have had a similar experience. Hamburg and Adams (1967) pointed out that learning is made easier when the helper is one step ahead of the person in need and has experience with the problem. These organizations are based on the premise that, in times of stress, people need others, as role models and teachers, who have had a similar experience (Silverman, 1966, 1969, 1978, 1980, 1986; Gartner & Riessman, 1977; Lieberman et al., 1979; Powell, 1987).

Gottlieb (1981), looking at the continuum of help available in the community, talks about intentional communities. These are places that people establish or seek, to meet needs that cannot be met in their existing networks. Belenky et al. (1997) provide an excellent historical review and description of this process. These are in contrast to what is called the informal helping network, consisting of family and friends, or formal professional networks. Some researchers have talked about these intentional communities as natural helping efforts (Pancoast, Parker, & Froland, 1983). *Intentional* seems a more accurate term, because such initiatives are consciously designed and carried forward. They are not based on professional knowledge, which is used in the more formal system, but on experiential knowledge (Borkman, 1978), mutual reciprocity, and peer relationships. People join together as members of the organization, not as clients, and the members control the resources and determine what help the organization will provide and who will provide that help. These organizations have a formal structure resembling a club or other type of voluntary association (Silverman, 1978, 1982).

Mutual Help and the Bereaved

Historically, the bereaved have probably been helping each other since people have been living in communities and mourners needed solace. Habits of the past often fall into disuse. As society became more specialized, especially in the past century, we have witnessed the professionalization of services once performed by citizens for each other. People became self-conscious about their lack of credentials to help in times of stress and no longer recognized as legitimate the experience they may have amassed from living. Informally, people helped each other, and, sometimes, without much fanfare set up programs to help each other in churches and community centers (Silverman, Mackenzie, Pettipas, & Wilson, 1975). Not only did people in general not legitimize this type of help, but those responsible for planning community services did not recognize this mutual assistance as important or relevant.

Over the past three decades, this has been turning around, as more and more professionals have recognized the limitations of their efforts. This has been accompanied by a growing recognition of the fact that, in most communities, there are people who are known for their helping qualities. They were identified as natural helpers, and some professionals aligned themselves with them in helping programs (Pancoast et al., 1983; Belenky et al., 1997). The New Careers for the Poor Program, in New York (Pearl & Riessman, 1965), recognized that residents of a given community were more successful than the professionals in engaging disadvantaged families from that community, in helping programs. People with problems were not waiting for the professionals to help them. They never really abdicated this responsibility. Alcoholics Anonymous had already established their efficacy as a resource for alcoholics, with much greater success than any professional initiative. Katz (1970) had documented the early efforts of parents of retarded children and children with mental illness, who took the initiative in developing services for their children through mutual help organizations. Consciousness was growing, among professionals, of the positive impact of these efforts of people with common problems to develop intentional communities, through which they could help themselves and each other (Gartner & Riessman, 1977). This awareness was enhanced by the President's Commission on Mental Health (1978), which recommended that there be clearinghouses in every community to make information available about mutual help groups in that community. There are now a number of clearinghouses throughout North America and in many parts of Europe (White & Madera, 2002).

In the late 1960s, there were two parallel initiatives that led to lasting mutual help programs for the widowed and for bereaved parents, and that changed the nature of services available today for the bereaved in any given community. Compassionate Friends is an organization for bereaved parents, which was developed by the chaplain in an English hospital, in response to his growing awareness of the sense of aloneness and isolation experienced by parents whose children died in that hospital (Stephens, 1972). This program was imported to the United States in the 1970s (Klass, 1988, 2000). Although professionals are consultants to this organization, bereaved parents provide the leadership and are the primary helpers.

The Widow-to-Widow program was a demonstration–research project at Harvard Medical School (Silverman, 1966, 1986, 2000). It was based on the finding that the only people who seemed to be helpful to the newly widowed were other widowed people (Maddison & Walker, 1967). The goal of the original program was to develop an early intervention program for the newly widowed that might prevent their developing subsequent emotional problems. A target community was designated, and five widows reached out to every newly widowed woman under the age of 65 years, in that community. The program demonstrated the value of early outreach, that is, that an unsolicited call from another widow was appreciated by the newly widowed. The widowed helper was able to use her own experience in helping the newly bereaved acknowledge and deal with her grief and to find new direction in her life. This program became the model for grass roots efforts in many communities in the United States and abroad (Silverman, 1986). It also served as the model for the Widowed Persons Service (WPS) sponsored by the American Association of Retired Persons (1999). In England, it served as the model for the National Widows Service.

Vachon, Lyall, Rogers, Freedman-Letofsky, and Freeman (1980), in Canada, demonstrated the effectiveness of the Widow-to-Widow approach, in a replication of the original program. However, they had a control population of newly widowed women who were not invited to participate in the intervention. They identified a high-distress group, and a sample of these women were assigned to the intervention program. At 6, 12, and 24 months, the women in the intervention group reported better physical health, less anticipation of further difficulty in adjusting to their loss, less contact with old friends, and more investment in new relationships, than did control subjects. Lieberman and Videka-Sherman (1986) found that participation in mutual help groups had specific positive mental health effects, compared to a control group who did not have this experience.

Tracy and Toro (1989) compared natural or mutual help and professional helping processes. Different types of helpers were found to react differently to clients, but all clients felt helped by a sequence in which helpers provided some direction, in response to the client emotionally examining what was happening. Successful mutual help leaders were more likely to use self-disclosure as a helping technique The most important part of Tracy and Toro's findings is that each of these types of helpers seem to be training the client in a unique manner of behavior and responses. Other studies have looked at the value of mutual help groups, compared to, for example, brief psychotherapy (Marmar, Horowitz, Weiss, Wilner, & Katreider, 1988; Lund, 1989). They juxtapose these two helping modalities, as if they are mutually exclusive. They also look at the mutual help experience as if help that is provided is mainly in a group experience similar to what is offered in group therapy, with the main difference being in the preparation and experience of the leader. No differences were found in outcome, as far as who was leading the group (Lund, 1989). It may be that being in a group is a helpful experience to the newly bereaved, as Yalom, Vinogradov, Stone, and Maclennan (1988) observed. Lieberman (1993) pointed out that it is very difficult to generalize about the value of self-help groups for the bereaved, since they do not represent a homogeneous form of help and are responding at many different levels to the needs of their constituents. Studies need to recognize that mutual help involves more than a group experience and that the context in which the help is provided may also impact its success. In a mutual help organization, members are peers who make their own decisions about what happens and who can move from the role of recipient of help to that of helper (Silverman, 1976). Help is offered in many ways: through one-to-one outreach, telephone hotlines, social activities, newsletters, educational meetings, group discussions, legislation and advocacy activities, and through becoming leaders and helpers in turn.

In a professionally led support group, members are screened by the agency and are in the subordinate role of client. They have no ongoing relationship to the agency and are not responsible for the continuing life of this helping experience. Help is primarily through psychological or educational counseling, in group or in individual sessions (Lieberman & Borman, 1979; Silverman, 1976, 1980; Yalom et al., 1988). We need to keep in mind that the help offered in one setting should not compete with help in another setting. They are not mutually exclusive, since they are not the same type of help.

A mutual help setting has its own dynamic. Help is effective because people

1. find others, so that they feel less alone and less unique;
2. have their feelings legitimized;
3. get specific information about their problems and a sense that there is something they can do about them;
4. have role models who can provide alternative ways of solving problems and with whom they can identify;
5. can and do assume responsibility for the ongoing life of the organization; and
6. find the ability to help others.

As they move away from the death event, meaningful help also involves extended social activity. Their affiliations provide the opportunity to "re-people their lives" (Silverman, 1970).

The remainder of this chapter presents direct quotes from members of mutual help organizations about the help they received in this context. The focus is on finding others like themselves, getting new perspectives on their widowhood, and becoming helpers in turn (Silverman, 1988a, 1988b, 1988c).

The Value of Finding Other Widowed People

Most people are surprised at their reaction to first meeting another widowed person. They did not expect such responsiveness.

> The people really understood what I was going through. I could bare my soul and no one turned a deaf ear.

> When I said Sunday was so long, it was nice to have someone else agree with me.

Most of these widows and widowers were involved with family and friends, but meeting others "in the same boat" had a special meaning. Not only were there others to listen, to say "I felt the same way," but the others were there for as long as they were needed.

> Since we take time to listen to each other, I got it out of my system by telling it over and over again about his last days, the conversations we had, the finding him dead, the doctor coming, seeing his body go out of the house.

> I often wondered how I would have survived. The first year, all we did was share our feelings and emotions every step of the way.

Feelings were legitimized, and the widowed no longer felt so alone.

> I realized for the first time that I am not the only person who lost a spouse.

> I realized that the things I was experiencing and feeling were normal.

> It helped me get involved in new friendships. It kept me connected to others. My friends had disappeared and every other group I went to were couples.

People talked of developing a sense of optimism and hope, as a result of this sharing. They also found role models. Information they received was as helpful as being listened to.

> The lectures were helpful and the grief workshops were very good. Widowed people need perspective on what is happening to them.

Learning from Others Like Themselves

The widowed began to see alternatives to how they defined themselves and how they lived their lives.

> You have to let widowed people know that there are no quick fixes, no easy answers, that, through the hurts and upsets of a big adjustment, one evolved into something that surprises even yourself, that each of us is loaded with gifts and untapped talents.

Several widows reflected on how their participation helped them change.

> The most important thing a widow must learn is to like herself and believe in herself and her own abilities. She has to learn to choose her own priorities in life.

Some, especially the men, began talking about developing empathic qualities.

> I became much less selfish with my time for others. I became much more understanding of the problems of the newly widowed. It got me out with a lot more friends.

Women, in contrast, talked about new confidence they were developing, as well as their growing independence, and how the groups helped them achieve this.

> It (the organization) gave me permission to be a different person. It made me feel and understand that there is no written creed that says you have to be married to be happy. It became clear that I was going to have to make a new life for myself.

Helping Others

Both widows and widowers reported new ways of being connected to others through membership in these organizations. This was not simply because of the help they received, but because of the new opportunities for mutuality that they found, not only in their social lives, but in their ability to help others. These people had rediscovered Riessman's (1965) observation that helping others is a very effective way of helping oneself.

> Working with WPS has given me a purpose in life. It keeps me busy and allows me to give service to widowed persons, especially the newly bereaved. I need to be needed, and I am.

> I can understand the newly widowed, because I could not forget such a lost-soul feeling as I had. I am better because, in turn, I am helping someone else.

The men talked of helping themselves, through helping others, as a brand new experience.

> It's the secret—by helping others you help yourself. Other than my children, TLA [To Live Again], and the work I do with it, is the most important thing in my life. I feel I am really doing something worthwhile, and it makes me feel a sense of real accomplishment.

Most people mentioned that the feeling of being needed gave them purpose in life. In the role of helper, people found a valuable and meaningful way of being connected to others and to themselves: "In helping others, I help myself." This is the real meaning of mutual help—the exchange and mutuality that takes place between people as they cope with common problems.

Conclusions

The importance of connection to others, and being involved in caring relationships, cannot be underestimated, especially at times of stress in people's lives. Not only does care need to be offered, but people also need to accept it as appropriate. Providing this attention to people in need is not only the province of professionals mandated by society. It is beholden on each of us to be involved in helping and caring networks. These networks make the human condition viable and meaningful. Mutual help efforts are one such caring enterprise, and are particularly helpful when a death occurs.

Discussion Questions

1. How does bringing in the concepts of relationship, gender, and changing the goals of development from individuation to interdependency change the concept of support, and how it is applied?
2. How does it change the concept of help?
3. By eliminating the concept of recovery and getting over it from our paradigm of grief, how is this paradigm different?
4. Describe the components of mutual help and how a relationship with another widowed person facilitates coping with the death of a spouse.

References

American Association for Retired Persons. (1999). *Widowed persons service: Directory of services for the widowed in the United States and Canada*. Washington, DC: American Association for Retired Persons.

Barnett, R. C., Biener, L., & Baruch, G. K. (1987). *Gender & stress*. New York: Free Press.

Belenky, M., Clinchy, B., Goldberger, N., & Tarule, J. (1996). *Women's ways of knowing*. New York: Basic Books.

Belenky, M., Bond, L. A., & Weinstock, J. S. (1997). *A tradition that has no name: Nurturing the development of people, families, and communities*. New York: Basic Books.

Belle, D. (1982). *Lives in stress: Women and depression*. Beverly Hills, CA: Sage.

Belle, D. (1987). Gender differences in the social moderators of stress. In R. C. Barnett, L. Beiner, & G. K. Baruch (Eds.), *Gender & stress* (pp. 257–277). New York: Free Press.

Belle, D. (Ed.). (1989). *Children's social networks and social supports*. New York: Wiley.

Boerner, K., & Silverman, P. R. (2001). Gender differences in coping patterns in widowed parents. *Omega: Journal of Death and Dying, 43*(3), 201–216.

Borkman, T. (1978). Experiential knowledge: A new concept for the analysis of self-help. *Social Service Review,* 445–456.

Brown, L. M., & Gilligan, C. (1992). *Meeting at the crossroads: Women's psychology and girls development*. Cambridge, MA: Harvard University Press.

Campbell, S., & Silverman, P. R. (1996). *Widower: When men are left alone*. Amityville, NY: Baywood.

Caplan, G. (1976). Family as a support system. In G. Caplan & M. Killilea (Eds.), *Support systems and mutual help*. New York: Grune & Stratton.

Cobb, S. (1976). Social support as a moderator of life stress. *Psychosomatic Medicine, 38*(5), 300–314.

Cook, J. A. (1988). Dad's double binds: Rethinking father's bereavement from a men's studies perspective. *Journal of Contemporary Ethnography, 17*(3), 285–308.

Dakoff, G. A., & Taylor, S. E. (1990). Victims, perceptions of social support: What is helpful for them? *Journal of Perspectives in Social Psychology, 58*(11), 80–90.

Eckenrode, J., & Gore, S. (1981). Stressful events and social supports: The significance of context. In B. H. Gottlieb (Ed.), *Social networks and social support* (pp. 43–81). Beverly Hills, CA: Sage.

Folkman, S. (1997). Positive psychological states and coping with severe stress. *Social Science and Medicine, 45,* 1207–1221.

Folkman, S. (2001). Revised coping theory and the process of bereavement. In M. Stroebe, R. Hansson, W. Stroebe, & H. Schut (Eds.), *New handbook of bereavement: Consequences, coping and care* (pp. 563–584). Washington, DC: American Psychological Association.

Folkman, S., & Moskowitz, J. T. (2000a). Positive affect and the other side of coping. *American Psychologist, 55*(6), 647–645.

Folkman, S., & Moskowitz, J. T. (2000b). The context matters. *Personality and Social Psychology Bulletin, 26*(2), 150–151.

Garmezy, N. (1987). Stress, competence, and development: Continuities in the study of schizophrenic adults, children vulnerable to psychopathology, and the search for stress-resistant children. *American Journal of Orthopsychiatry, 57,* 159–185.

Gartner, A., & Riessman, F. (1977). *Self-help in the human services*. San Francisco: Jossey-Bass.

Gilligan, C. (1982). *In a different voice*. Cambridge, MA: Harvard University Press.

Gilligan, C., Ward, J. V., & Taylor, J. M. (1988). *Mapping the moral domain*. Cambridge, MA: Harvard University Press.

Gottlieb, B. H. (Ed.). (1981). *Social networks and social support*. Beverly Hills, CA: Sage.

Gottlieb, B. H. (1990, August). Quandaries in translating support concepts to interviewers. Paper presented at the Annual American Psychological Association Convention, Boston, MA.

Hamburg, D. A., & Adams, J. E. (1967). A perspective on coping: Seeking and utilizing information in major transitions. *Archives of General Psychiatry, 17,* 277–284.

Hughes, E. C. (1971). *The sociological eye.* Chicago: Aldine-Atherton.

Jacobs, S. (1999). *Traumatic grief: Diagnosis, treatment and prevention.* Philadelphia: Bruner/Mazel.

Katz, A. H. (1970). Self-help organizations and volunteer participation in social welfare. *Social Work, 15*(1), 51–60.

Klass, D. (1988). *Parental grief: Solace and resolution.* New York: Springer.

Levinson, D. J. (1978). *The seasons of man's life.* New York: Knopf.

Lieberman, M. A. (1993). Bereavement self-help groups: A review of conceptual and methodological issues. In M. Stroebe, W. Stroebe, & R. O. Hansson (Eds.), *Handbook of bereavement: Theory, research and intervention* (pp. 411–426). New York: Cambridge University Press.

Lieberman, M. A., & Borman, L. D. (1979). *Self-help groups for coping with crisis.* San Francisco: Jossey-Bass.

Lieberman, M. A., & Videka-Sherman, L. (1986). The impact of self-help groups on the mental health of widows and widowers. *American Journal of Orthopsychiatry, 56,* 435–439.

Lopata, H. Z. (1988). Support systems of American urban widowhood. *Journal of Social Issues, 44*(3), 113–128.

Lund, D. A. (Ed.). (1989). *Older bereaved spouses: Research with practical applications.* New York: Hemisphere.

Lyons, N. P. (1989). Listening to voices we have not heard. In C. Gilligan, N. P. Lyons, & T. J. Hammer (Eds.), *Making connections: The relational worlds of adolescent girls at Emma Willard School* (pp. 30–72). Troy, NY: Emma Willard School.

Maddison, D., & Walker, W. L. (1967). Factors affecting the outcome of conjugal bereavement. *British Journal of Psychiatry, 113,* 1057–1067.

Marmar, C. R., Horowitz, M. J., Weiss, D. S., Wilner, N. R., & Katreider, N. B. (1988). A controlled trial of brief psychotherapy and mutual-help group treatment of conjugal bereavement. *American Journal of Psychiatry, 145*(2), 203–209.

Miller, J. B. (1986). *Toward a new psychology of women* (2nd ed.). Boston: Beacon Press.

Miller, J. B., & Stiver, I. P. (1997). *The healing connection: How women form relationships in therapy and in life.* Boston: Beacon Press.

Murphy, L. B. (1974). Coping, vulnerability, and resilience in childhood. In G. V. Coelb, D. A. Hamburg, & J. E. Adams (Eds.), *Coping and adaptation* (pp. ____). New York: Basic Books.

Nadeau, J.(1998). *Families making sense of death.* Thousand Oaks, CA: Sage.

Neimeyer, R.A. (1998). *Lessons of loss: A guide to coping.* New York: McGraw-Hill.

Osterweis, M., Solomon, F., & Greene, M. (1984). (Eds.) *Bereavement: Reactions, consequences, & care.* Washington, DC: National Academy Press.

Pancoast, D. L., Parker, P., & Froland, C. (Eds.) (1983). *Rediscovering self-help: Its role in social care.* Beverly Hills, CA: Sage.

Pearl, A., & Riessman, F. (1965). *New careers for the poor.* New York: Free Press.

Powell, T. (1987). *Self-help organizations and professional practice.* Washington, DC: National Association of Social Workers.

The President's Commission on Mental Health. (1978). *A report to the president from the president's commission on mental health* (Vol. 1). Washington, DC: U.S. Government Printing Office.

Riessman, F. (1965). The "helper-therapy" principle. *Social Work, 10,* 27–32.

Shamgar-Handleman, L. (1986). *Israeli war widows: Beyond the glory of heroism.* Boston: Bergin & Garvey.

Shapiro, E. R. (1994). *Grief as a family process: A developmental approach to clinical practice.* New York: Guilford Press.

Silverman, P. R. (1966). *Services for the widowed during the period of bereavement. Social work practice.* New York: Columbia University.

Silverman, P. R. (1969). *Study of spoiled helping: Clients who drop out of psychiatric treatment.* Unpublished doctoral dissertation, Brandeis University, Waltham, MA.

Silverman, P. R. (1970). A re-examination of the intake procedure. *Social Case Work, 51,* 625–634.

Silverman, P. R. (1976). The widow as caregiver in a program of preventive intervention with other widows. In G. D. Caplan & M. Killilea (Eds.), *Support systems and mutual help* (pp. 233–244). New York: Grune & Stratton.

Silverman, P. R. (1978). *Mutual help groups and the role of the mental health professional.* Washington, DC: U.S. Government Printing Office, NIMH, DHEW Publication No. (ADM) 78-646, Reprinted 1980.

Silverman, P. R. (1980). *Mutual help: Organization and development.* Beverly Hills, CA: Sage.

Silverman, P. R. (1981). *Helping women cope with grief.* Beverly Hills, CA: Sage.

Silverman, P. R. (1982). The mental health consultant as a linking agent. In D. E. Biegel & A. I. Naparstek (Eds.), *Community support systems and mental health* (pp. 238–249). New York: Springer.

Silverman. P. R. (1986). *Widow to widow.* New York: Springer.

Silverman, P. R. (1987). The impact of parental death on college-age women. *Psychiatric Clinics of North America, 10,* 387–404.

Silverman, P. R. (1988a). Research as process: Exploring the meaning of widowhood. In S. Reinharz & G. Rowles (Eds.), *Qualitative gerontology* (pp. 217–240). New York: Springer.

Silverman, P. R. (1988b). In search of selves: Accommodating to widowhood. In L. A. Bond (Ed.), *Families in transition: Primary prevention programs that work* (pp. 200–220). Beverly Hills, CA: Sage.

Silverman, P. R. (1988c). Widowhood as the next stage in the life cycle. In H. Z. Lopata (Ed.), *Widows* (pp. 170–189). Durham, NC: Duke University.

Silverman, P. R. (1999). Widowhood revisited: The next stage in the life cycle. In American Association of Retired Persons, *Widowed Persons Service Participant Manual* (pp. 30–37). Washington, DC: AARP.

Silverman, P. R. (2000). *Never too young to know: Death in children's lives.* New York: Oxford University Press.

Silverman, P. R., Mackenzie, D., Pettipas, M., & Wilson, E. (Eds.). (1975). *Helping each other in widowhood.* New York: Health Sciences.

Silverman, P. R., & Worden, J. W. (1992). Children's reactions to the death of a parent in the early months after the death. *American Journal of Orthopsychiatry, 62*(11), 93–104.

Stephens, S. (1972). *Death comes home* (1st American ed.). New York: Morehouse–Barlow.

Stylianos, S. K., & Vachon, M. L. S. (1993). The role of social support in bereavement. In M. Stroebe, W. Stroebe, & R. O. Hansson (Eds.), *Handbook of bereavement: Theory, research and intervention* (pp. 397–410). New York: Cambridge University Press.

Tracey, T. J., & Toro, P. A. (1989). Natural and professional help: A process analysis. *American Journal of Community Psychology, 17*(4), 443–458.

Vachon, M. L. (1979). *Identity change over the first two years of bereavement: Social relationships and social support.* Unpublished doctoral dissertation, York University, Toronto.

Vachon, M. L., Lyall, W. A., Rogers, J., Freedman-Letofsky, K., & Freeman, S. J. (1980). A controlled study of self-help intervention for widows. *American Journal of Psychiatry, 137,* 1380–1384.

White, B. J., & Madera, E. J. (Eds.). (2002). *The self-help group sourcebook: Your guide to community & online support groups* (7th ed.). Denville, NJ: American Self-Help Group Clearinghouse, Saint Clare's Health Services.

Yalom, I. D., Vinogradov, S., Stone, W. N., & Maclennan, B. W. (1988). Bereavement groups: Techniques and themes. *International Journal of Group Psychotherapy, 38*(4), 419–446.

Thirteen

Helping Children During Bereavement

Elizabeth P. Lamers

Elizabeth Lamers holds a BS cum laude from the State University of New York at New Paltz and a MA in education (reading) from Sonoma State University. She is credentialed as both a classroom teacher and a reading specialist. Mrs. Lamers has worked with terminally ill and bereaved children for the last 20 years. She has conducted workshops and lectured extensively on the dying child and return to the classroom, children and grief, children's literature and death.

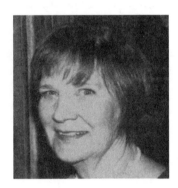

Historical Background

Attitudes regarding children and death have undergone significant change in the past century, especially in the last 30 years. If we hope to be of assistance to children experiencing loss, it is essential that we understand some of the changes regarding children and death that have occurred during this time.

The demographics of dying and death have changed greatly: At the turn of the last century, most deaths in any year occurred in children under 15 years old. Today, most deaths in any year occur in persons older than 65 years. Dying once occurred almost exclusively at home after a short illness; it now occurs almost exclusively in some sort of health care institution, following a prolonged (and often expensive) illness. Although the hospice movement has brought dying back into the home, the majority of elderly persons still die in some type of institution (nursing home or hospital). As a result, today children and even young adults are separated from the reality of death (DeSpelder & Strickland, 1992).

Family structure has also changed. Children once grew up as part of a close "extended" family consisting of parents, grandparents, aunts, and uncles who lived in the same rural area, and sometimes even in the same house. Today, so called "nuclear" families live in cities, often separated by hundreds of miles from relatives. Deaths of relatives were once occasions for family coherence; today, deaths in families may pass unobserved. Many parents today have the attitude that children should be shielded from dying and the facts of death (Lamers, 1986a). Commonly today, children do not attend funeral services (Lamers, 1986b).

Children in rural areas once were exposed to dying and death in their families and among farm animals. They had repeated opportunities to observe dying and death, to ask questions about death, to participate in burials, and also in supportive religious and social bereavement ceremonies and rituals.

Children today are frequently exposed to a different kind of death: the death of a "bad" person or a stranger on television. It has been estimated that children witness hundreds of such unreal, "unsanctioned" deaths by the time they enter high school. Children are exposed to death and violence regularly through TV, and especially through children's cartoons. Cartoons, however, show death as reversible or death of the bad character. As a model to learn about death, cartoons give children a constant and consistently distorted view (Lamers, 1986b).

Books About Death for Children

Children's books reflect some of the changes that have occurred in the larger society. The removal of death and dying from the child's sphere can be easily traced in their literature. *McGuffey's Eclectic Readers* (1920), a series of text books used to teach children to read in the late 1800s and early 1900s, contained many selections and poems pertaining either to the death of a mother or of a child. These deaths were seen as a tragic, but natural part of life. Today, school texts rarely, if ever, contain any references to death or dying. In *Little Women*, Alcott (1869/1947, p. 464) told of Beth's death in a straightforward manner, adding in the next paragraph "Seldom, except in books, do the dying utter memorable words, see visions, or depart with beatified countenances; . . . ," all common elements of a death scene in the literature of the mid-1800s.

In current children's literature, fairy tales have been sanitized; references to death have been removed or glossed over. For example, in the original "Little Red Riding Hood," the wolf ate Grandma and Little Red, and there was no intervening hunter or woodcutter. The hunter/woodcutter was introduced as a way of rescuing Little Red and her grandmother, first by the hunter/woodcutter slicing open the wolf and letting them out. In later versions, the hunter shoots the wolf before he eats either the grandmother or Little Red. In other versions, even the wolf is spared to escape through an open window, or in one version, to become Little Red's pet.

Between 1940 and 1970, only a few children's books contained references to death. Children's books in the late 1960s began to discuss previously taboo subjects: divorce, sex, feelings, and eventually even death. During the 1970s and 1980s, more than 200 fiction books were published for children with death as a major theme. Unfortunately, very few measured up to the standard set by *Charlotte's Web*, *Little Women*, *The Yearling*, or *The Dead Bird*. During the same period, some very good nonfiction books about death were written for children of various ages. (See resource list at the end of the chapter.)

This cornucopia of books on death has helped re-expose children to death. The hospice movement has also helped by reintroducing home care for dying persons, in many communities. Even so, many children are still insulated from death and often are discouraged from attending funerals. As a result, it is not unusual to find adults in their forties who have never attended a funeral (Newton, 1990).

Study of Childhood Loss

After World War II, behavioral scientists started to study the way children reacted to loss. The rise in delinquency following World War II focused attention on the loss experiences in early childhood of the adolescents involved. John Bowlby, a psychiatrist in England, published a three-volume study, *Attachment and Loss* (1980). His study of young children, and their reaction to the loss of their mother figure, was prompted by his finding that many of the delinquents he studied had lost one or both parent(s) before the child was 5 years old. Bowlby described the relationship between the young child's responses to loss of the mother and adult grief. Bowlby divided the young child's response to the loss of a mother figure into three phases: protest, despair, and detachment. Bowlby showed that even very young children do mourn.

Shoor and Speed (1963, p. 540) studied the relationship between early childhood loss of a parent or other close relative and the development of delinquent behavior. They pointed out that parental death could set the stage for at least four possible reactions in the child: (1) normal mourning with resolution of grief, (2) immediate pathological response, (3) delayed reaction leading to a psychiatric syndrome in later life, or (4) delinquent behavior.

Hilgard (1969) and others studied anniversary reactions to a death. They showed that reactions to loss may present as depression (ranging from mild to psychotic level), as physical symptoms (ranging from hysterical conversion reactions to psychophysiological autonomic and visceral responses), or as organic illness (such as ulcerative colitis).

Needs of Grieving Children

There is no automatic grieving mechanism, nor do we automatically handle grief in a successful manner. We learn to survive grief through early loss experiences. The tasks of grieving are multiple, and the process may be complicated by prior experiences with loss and grief, current physical health, the quality of the relationship with the deceased, the impact of the death, the age of the survivor, and a host of other variables. The following are some of the things children need in order to begin to successfully cope with grief. Lamers (1965) states that grieving children need:

1. to know they will be cared for (fed, loved, sheltered);
2. to know they did not cause the death by their anger or shortcomings;
3. to know they will not necessarily die of the same condition or when they reach the same age as the deceased;
4. to know what is happening, if possible, before the death occurs;
5. factual knowledge about the cause of the death;
6. someone who will listen to them—to their questions, their fears, their fantasies; someone who will be consistent and reasonable; someone they can trust;
7. to establish a framework for conceptualizing death;
8. an opportunity, if possible, for honest interaction with the dying person, whether this is a grandparent, parent, or sibling;
9. opportunities for involvement and interaction after death occurs;
10. assistance in dealing with feelings that may seem to be too intense or complex to be put in words.

Children and adults grieve in similar ways. Both may cry, get angry, blame themselves for the death, or have problems eating and sleeping. The greatest difference in the grief process of adults and children is that most adults can separate fact from fantasy. They know that, in most cases, they did not cause the death. Children often cannot tell fact from fantasy, and need to discuss their fears with an adult who can reassure them that they are in no way responsible for the death through their anger or fantasies or short-comings. This particular subject needs to be brought up by the adult, even if the child doesn't mention it. Children may feel anxious, panicky, or guilty. Children may improperly associate, with the death, something they did with or to the deceased. Sometimes the connections children make can be far-fetched, such as believing, as one boy did, that the glass of lemonade he made for his grandmother killed her. Children may deal with the fear that they caused the death through indirect questions, or they may hide their fear in silence. Children can also feel guilty that they were not "good enough" to prevent the death, such as one 8-year-old, who explained to me that she felt that God was angry with her.

How Children Respond to Loss

The spectrum of response to loss is quite variable. To respond successfully to a death, children must verify that a death actually occurred. This takes time and requires support. Death may cause children to feel vulnerable, especially when the death was violent or unexpected. The death of a sibling, classmate, or friend can lead to feelings of anger: anger at death for "taking" the person, at God for letting it happen, at the deceased for going away, and even at themselves for not being able to prevent the death. They may also feel anger at their parents for excluding them from information, or for not being available to talk about their feelings. Children may feel guilty for not having done enough for the person before death or for not being a good-enough person. Children may feel death has cheated them of a long and satisfying relationship. They may feel that, in some way, they must be punished for their shortcomings and their angry feelings. They may assume mannerisms of the deceased or they may even come to idealize the deceased person.

Those who work with grieving children must keep a basic premise in mind: All behavior has meaning (Lamers, 1965). A grieving child may withdraw or become aggressive or destructive. The child may strive to excel in school or may be unable to concentrate on their studies. The child may determine to take up a career in medicine or nursing to help prevent death. Some children may develop thoughts of suicide. In brief, children do react to death, and at a much younger age than has been widely recognized.

Children may react to death with tears or, as one small child (age 3 years) explained to me, "When I'm very, very sad, I laugh." Adults should not conclude that a child is not sad or grieving just because the child is not crying. Children also have an ability to take breaks from their grieving and at times seem to forget the loss. Very small children may not realize the death has occurred, even though informed, until the time for the usual visit to the deceased person arrives. This is more apt to occur when the death occurs at a distance, when the child does not attend the funeral, and when there is a set pattern to the visits, such as a visit to grandparents every summer or every Christmas. The small child may be upset when the visit does not take place or when it does occur and the grandparent is missing. Only then may the reality of the death register with the child.

With proper support, children will ask the necessary questions, perhaps not all at once, but with increasing frequency, as they become more trusting of the adult to whom they are addressing their questions. Children will want to know things, such as: Can the person (or pet) breathe? Are they hungry or will they need to eat? Why are they so still? Can they feel? Will they be cold? When visiting the grave, they will often ask repeatedly where the person is. The younger the child, the more concrete the questions and the more often the same questions will be repeated. Parents need to know that they do not need to have the perfect answer to every question. Some questions have no answers, even from experts, and children can accept this. Children's fears are not always voiced. Parents may be able to determine the existence of these fears by careful questioning. Parents and other adults should try to address any possible fears during these discussions. For example, very few children will admit to the fear that they caused the death, and yet this type of magical thinking is common in children, particularly in very young children. The parent can address the fact that, in spite of our wishes, no one can cause a death through anger or prevent a death that is caused by incurable illness or old age or an accident. To prevent this kind of magical thinking, fears need to be addressed, whether or not the child openly expresses them. Adults also need to be aware that the child will take admonitions, such as "pray for Daddy" very concretely, and will feel responsible if the prayers are not successful.

Adolescents and Bereavement

Adolescents have more difficulty expressing their emotions than younger children do. They may show no immediate grief reaction or may display an exaggerated grief reaction. Adolescents, unlike younger children, often will not discuss their feelings about a death or impending death with their parents. They will instead seek out a trusted adult, "the intimate stranger" (R. Fulton, personal communication, June 10, 1985). This may be an aunt, an uncle, or other relative, a teacher, coach, minister, or other unrelated adult. They usually are able to discuss their feelings more easily with this trusted person than with their mother or father. The adolescent needs to know what can be expected during a funeral. They need to know that the feelings and behaviors that occur during bereavement, which might be considered abnormal at other times, are normal.

Variables Affecting Childhood Grief

Children will react differently to each death, depending on:

1. the family reaction to that death and the particulars of the death;
2. who died;
3. how close they were to the deceased;
4. the circumstances of the death—sudden or over a long period of time;
5. whether or not the child had any unfinished business with the deceased;
6. the age of the deceased; the age of the child at the time of the death; and
7. whether or not the living circumstances of the child will, or have, changed because of the death. (Lamers, 1965)

Each death will have a different impact on the child. Is it the father, whose death will change the economic circumstances of the family? Is it the mother, putting the care of the child in question? A sibling? A beloved pet? Was the person a public figure with whom the child identified, such as John F. Kennedy, Jr. or Princess Diana? Or years earlier President Kennedy, Robert Kennedy, or Christa McAuliffe? With these latter three deaths, it was possible to view the circumstances of the death over and over again on TV. When Robert Kennedy was assassinated, one of his sons, who was with him on the campaign, was found in their hotel room repeatedly viewing the shooting as the TV stations showed the tape of the incident over and over again. With John Jr. and Princess Diana, the scenes of the deaths were shown over and over amid much speculation as to what had happened.

How the death occurred also influences the effect on a child or adult. If the death occurred after a lengthy illness, the child may have had time to adjust to the coming death, time to say good-byes, and in some cases time to grieve before the loss. If some grieving has taken place before the actual death, there may be fewer tears and other signs of grief than we expect at the time of a death. This does not mean that the child does not care or feels no grief at the time of death.

Suicide is particularly stressful on the family, children included. It often results in "unsanctioned grief." Whether or not it is an acknowledged suicide makes a difference to the child. If the family does not acknowledge that a suicide occurred, it can leave the child very confused. The fact that a death was a suicide should never be kept from the child. They eventually learn the truth, and the deception destroys the child's trust. The suicide of a peer can be very upsetting. The child may feel that he or she could have prevented it. The death of someone the same age makes death seem that much more real and possible.

Children base their beliefs and knowledge about death on what they have learned in their family. If parents feel comfortable with their own beliefs and knowledge about death, it is easier for them to talk to their child about death. If a child has grown up with animals that have died, then that child will have a better understanding of death and grief than a child who has not experienced such a loss. A child who has experienced the death of someone close to them will likewise have a different perspective than a child who has experienced no losses or who has been shielded from losses by his or her family.

If death has been a taboo subject, the child may have a very distorted view about death. Most children will at some point in their childhood ask questions about death. If these questions are answered in an open and honest way, it will prepare the child to seek the information and support needed when someone close to them dies. Children whose questions about death have been ignored or who have been told to talk about something more pleasant, or, even worse, have been chastised for bringing up the "morbid" subject, will go elsewhere for their information, most likely to a peer. Adults must keep in mind that children are very curious and have very active imaginations. If a question brings a reaction of horror from the adult questioned, a child may supply his or her own reason as to why this subject is too terrible to talk about. Frequently, a child's own answer is much more frightening than the simple truth. Very small children can become confused by concepts such as heaven and an afterlife. Adults need to remember that small children are very concrete in their thinking. For example, a child hearing that "We lost Grandma" wants to know, "How did we lose her? Where did we lose her? Why aren't we looking for her? Where can we find her?" If a child is told from the beginning of the discussion that the person has died, then misconceptions do not need to be corrected. The discussion can focus on other important things the child may need to ask about, such as: How are they going to breathe in the ground? Won't they become cold or wet? How can they eat?

Needs of Surviving Siblings

Surviving siblings may have special problems in dealing with a brother's or sister's death. The death of a sibling may be a double loss to the surviving siblings. Their parents may become so involved in their own grief that they withdraw from the surviving children. Survivors may feel that they cannot show their grief because it will make their parents sadder. The sadness may be replaced with acting-out, to handle their own fears and anger. Unthinking adults may reinforce this thinking by making remarks such as: "You'll have to be extra good now, because your parents have enough to think about with the death of your brother/sister." The sibling is also grieving, and this statement does not acknowledge or allow the grief of the surviving sibling(s).

Parents can idealize the dead sibling to the point that the surviving sibling(s) can develop a dislike, if not hatred, of the deceased and/or the idealizing parent. Surviving siblings sometimes feel they are expected to follow in the footsteps of the deceased. They may distort their own personality to do this, or they may rebel and strive to be the opposite. Parents may also try to replace the dead child by having another baby and will dote on the new baby more than the surviving sibling(s). Parents may also become overprotective of the surviving siblings.

The surviving sibling(s) need to know that they are as important to the parents as the child who died. Holidays that come soon after a death need to be celebrated as traditionally done in the family. If the holiday celebration is to be curtailed, it should be a family as a whole who decides, not just the parents. Small children can feel that they don't count if, for instance, a holiday celebration is changed or greatly curtailed. I can still remember the feelings of worthlessness, of not counting, when the first Christmas after my brother's death was largely a nonexistent celebration "Because," my grandparents explained, "your parents don't feel much like celebrating since your brother's death." I wanted to scream, "What about me? Don't

I count for anything?" I didn't scream or even say anything, but I was hurt. I also hurt when all my brother's toys and other possessions were disposed of without asking me if there was anything I wanted. It didn't occur to anyone that an 8-year-old sister might want something concrete with which to remember her 10-year-old brother. Surviving siblings should be asked if there are any things something belonging to the dead sibling that they would like to keep as a memento.

If the sibling identified with or idealized the dead sibling while alive, there may be problems, such as intense anniversary reactions or the expectation of dying at the same age or in the same way. The expectation of dying at the same age and/or in the same way may also be part of the reaction to the death of a parent (Hilgard, Newman, & Fisk, 1960). This may not become evident until many years later.

Outcome of Childhood Loss

The outcome of a child's reaction to a death depends upon three major factors:

1. The psychological stability of the child
2. The general stability of the family
3. The availability of opportunities to share feelings about the loss and to receive support from significant persons, especially from parents

When one parent has died, the other parent may not be in a position to give the children all the support they need. Children may seek another adult for support, or they may delay their grieving until the surviving parent can be supportive of their grief.

Children need to know how the death occurred. They may need to ask questions like, "Did it hurt?" "Where is (the deceased) now?" "Can I die of the same thing?" "Will I die at the same age?" Children need to know whether a death was caused by an illness that is contagious or transmissible. In the absence of accurate information, the child may develop a host of needless fears about death and disease. For some questions, there may be more than one answer. Or there may be answers on several levels. The answers from a parent will depend on the family belief system and the age of the child. It is important to ask the child what kind of information he or she is seeking. When the child asks, "Where is Grandma?" are they asking where is the physical body, or are they really asking about heaven and an afterlife? Only by carefully and patiently listening to the child, and asking questions, can an adult be sure that they have answered the real question the child was asking.

Children and Funerals

Children naturally ask questions about the funeral, such as: What will happen at the funeral? What will happen to the body? The child should be encouraged to attend funerals, to say their good-byes to a loved one or friend. This is also another way a child can satisfy the need to determine that the death really occurred. In the time of turmoil following a death, children should be included in the family ceremonies and grieving. One 3-year-old in a family I worked with went to the rosary service for his father, but was deemed too young to attend the funeral and interment. Later, he had a very difficult time understanding that his father was buried in the grave.

Children are curious about the body of the dead person, but frequently suppress their questions. When my father-in-law died, his 8-year-old great-granddaughter had no patience with her mother, who wished to visit with relatives and friends on her way through the rooms at the funeral home, before saying her good-byes to "Pa." Susan wanted to see Pa, and kept tugging at her mother's hand to move on, until I took Susan in to see her Great-Grandpa. She stopped walking and started looking at about two feet from the casket. Gradually she got closer, and then the questions started. Could she touch him? Why was he cold? Why was his skin hard? Susan needed to confirm that he was really dead. Eventually, I helped her place the red carnation lei, which she had brought from Hawaii, around Pa's neck. Once Susan had her questions answered and the death confirmed, she could relax and visit with her aunts, uncles, and cousins. Children who do not get answers to their questions will internalize them and may worry needlessly.

Children's Understandings of Death

The stages at which a child understands death, and the ages when these stages occur, have been described in the literature. Basically, the stages are (Lamers & Lamers, 1987):

1. Death is reversible and not permanent.
2. Death is permanent, but only happens to others not close to me such as old persons, bad persons, and strangers.
3. Death is universal and happens to all living things.

This eventually leads the child to consider the sequence: I could die, I might die, and I will die. These realizations may come slowly in phases or may come all at once.

The very young child (age 0 to 5 years) tends to believe that death is reversible. The very young child who has had someone very close to him die, or a beloved pet die, knows that death is not reversible, that it is permanent. It is difficult to assign ages to the other two stages of understanding death. Generally speaking, the child between the ages of 5 and 9 years knows that death is permanent, and those older than 9 years know that death is inevitable. Again, life experience can change the ages at which a child develops a realistic understanding about death. Dying children of all ages reach a point at which they realize that they will die, and that death is permanent (Bluebond-Langner, 1978). On the other hand, many adults believe that only old persons and bad persons die, but deny the possibility that any one close to them will die.

Life experiences influence a child's understanding of death. Children who learn about the death of pets or family members, and who receive support and reassurance from their parents and other significant adults, can make a gradual and successful adjustment to their growing awareness of death. Death will be accepted as a natural, normal part of life. If they do not receive the support and assurance of parents, they may develop unrealistic fears and behavioral disturbances that reflect their unspoken fears and anxieties.

How to Help a Bereaved Child

For an adult to help a child when a death has occurred, the adult must first determine what the child knows and believes about death. If the lines of communication between the adult and child have always been open, this may be as easy as asking the child directly what he or she believes. Another way could be through reading one of the excellent books about death with the child. Books such as *The Tenth Good Thing About Barney*, by Viorst, or *Badger's Parting*, by Varley, could be used with young children. (See references at the end of the chapter for more suggested books.) Adults must be sure, when using books with children, that the book is consistent with their own beliefs and ideas concerning death. Adults must always be truthful when discussing death with children. Grollman (1977) points out that, to tell a child the deceased has gone on a long, long trip will not be consistent with what the child sees happening around him. If Grandpa has only gone on a trip, then why are people crying and upset, and why didn't he say good-bye? When the child discovers the truth, it is very hard to reestablish trust with the adult. The anecdotal literature has many stories from adults who were deceived about the death or impending death of a loved one (Galle, 1977). Most of the adults were angry and upset over deception when they discovered the truth, in some cases many years later (Gorer, 1965). I can remember when I was 8 years old and my brother died. My first reaction was the realization that I was the only one in the family who had expected him to survive to adulthood and that all my daydreams, about what it would be like to have an older brother as we grew up together, really were pure fantasy. I felt very alone and left out.

When discussing death with children, the subject is best raised sometime before the need arises. Death is a difficult subject and, like sex, should be discussed over a long period of time, in an age-appropriate manner. Unfortunately, this is not always possible. When a death occurs, explanations of what happened should be presented in a calm and careful manner by someone close to the child. It should be done without lurid, gruesome, or terrifying details. Words should be chosen carefully, with attention to their possible meaning to the child. Children tend to be very literal: the younger the child, the more literal. Describing death as being like sleep, or like going to sleep, can be very frightening to children who may assume that they too will die when they fall asleep.

Euphemisms should be avoided when discussing death with children. Words such as "lost" (why don't we find them again?), "passed on," "gone to his/her great reward," "no longer with us," or "departed" have meanings other than death for children and can be needlessly confusing. Even adults can be confused or bothered by euphemisms. When I recently received a letter announcing that a colleague had "expired," I immediately had the urge to rush out and renew her for another month or two, at the very least.

The more discussions and opportunities children have to share their feelings, the less likely it is that there will be problems later from the death. If the adults feel unprepared to discuss death, there are books such as Grollman's *Explaining Death to Children* or Gaffney's *The Seasons of Grief, Helping Your Child Grow Through Loss*, which can help. (See references for additional books.) These books may be available at the local library or for purchase at a bookstore or on the Internet, at such places as amazon.com or barnesandnoble.com.

Professional Responsibilities

The professionals (i.e., nurses, social workers, clergy, funeral directors, etc.) in contact with a family in which there is an impending or recent death, should inquire about the children of the family. The professional's job is not to inform the children, but to gently help those close to the children to do this. Professionals should stress the importance of keeping the children informed and should explain how intuitive children are. Often, children know something is happening without being told, and their imaginations supply the unshared details. Professionals should be aware of resources for families, such as books, counseling centers, hospices, social workers, or psychologists. They can inform the family that children are able to handle death and funerals and that children frequently think about death, even though they may not discuss it with the family members. Professionals can inform concerned parents that many references to death occur in children's games and jump-rope rhymes. References to death show up in children's writing, art work, and poetry. A school assignment to write a poem for an English class will often result in one or two poems that refer to death or grief.

After a death, children instinctively know there should be some ritual for closure. When a pet dies, children often spontaneously arrange a funeral and burial. If an adult is reluctant or even adamant about shielding the children, the professional should take the time to sit and talk with the adult about why he or she feels this way. Often, it is discovered that the adult had an unfortunate and/or unpleasant experience with death during childhood and wants to protect the children from the same type of exposure. The adult may have memories, such as being held up to the casket and being told to kiss the deceased good-bye without any preparation. Through a discussion about such a childhood experience, it may be possible to show the adult that he or she has control and can make the death a positive experience for the children in the family.

Conclusion

Seeing adults grieve is helpful for children. Grieving is not an automatic inborn skill: It is a learned skill. Children learn to grieve through coping with loss and looking to the adults around them for clues. Adults should realize that children often grieve in small increments and return to play or studies in between. The child's grief should not be considered inappropriate just because it is intermittent. Parents and other adults should not underestimate the duration of the child's grieving process.

Children can and do survive grief. With adult support and guidance, children have the opportunity to also grow through grief. Erikson (personal communication to W. M. Lamers, October 10, 1975) has pointed out that "Grief, successfully handled, can serve as the focus for new social and psychological growth."

About the Resources

The resources listed at the end of this chapter are suggestions. In the last 5 years, there have been very few books written about death for children. Most of these are not as well written as the previous books. Adults should read any book they consider using with a child. It is essential to determine whether or not the book fits the child and the particular situation, before presenting the book to the child. I once gave several books to a colleague to use with her own children and did not mention she should read them first. She came back to me very upset. She had read one of the books to her children to help them understand the death of their great-grandmother. In this book, the little boy died of an allergic reaction to a bee sting. It was an unfortunate choice for her children, because they were already afraid of bees, and now they were terrified. I had no way of knowing her children were afraid of bees. Had she read the book first, she would not have read it to her children. It is impossible for the professional to know every child in such detail, making it imperative that the adult using the books read them first.

There are now resources available on the Internet to help both professionals and bereaved persons. Some sites provide information on grief and bereavement; others offer chat rooms for the bereaved, where they can share experiences and feelings with others who have experienced a death. Many chat rooms are specific both for age of the bereaved and type of death. Therefore, it is possible for a teenager to discuss feelings about suicide bereavement or parental death bereavement with other teen participants. As with any resource on the Internet for children, parents need to be aware of what their children are accessing and need to check on the credentials of the sponsor of the Web page. The anonymity of an Internet chat room may make it easier for a teen to share feelings, but a parent still needs to be aware of what their child is accessing on the Internet.

The Internet is also a very fluid medium. This makes it impossible to list specific web pages with any confidence. One approach is to enter "grief" or "bereavement" in one of the many search engines (such as Yahoo, AltaVista, Google, Lycos, or MSN Internet Search), with as many modifiers as needed to narrow the search. The Internet has a great deal of information available, and it is best to make the search as narrow as possible, so that the results are not overwhelming.

Discussion Questions

1. Identify the needs of grieving children.
2. What are some of the variables that affect grief in children?
3. How would you evaluate the appropriateness of children's books about death?

References

Alcott, L. M. (1947). *Little women.* New York: Grosset & Dunlop. (Original work published 1869)

Bluebond-Langner, M. (1978). *The private worlds of dying children.* Princeton, NJ: Princeton University Press.

Bowlby, J. (1980). *Attachment and loss* (Vols. 1–3). New York: Basic Books.

Brown, M. W. (1965). *The dead bird.* Reading, MA: Addison-Wesley.

DeSpelder, L. A., & Strickland, A. L. (1992). *The last dance: Encountering death and dying.* Palo Alto, CA: Mayfield.

Galle, J. E. (1977). The train that never came. *Thanatos, 2*(3), 4–7.

Gorer, G. (1965). *Death, grief and mourning.* New York: Doubleday.

Grollman, E. (1977). Explaining death to children. *Journal of School Health, 47,* 336–339.

Hilgard, J. R., Newman, M. F., & Fisk, F. (1960). Strength of adult ego following childhood bereavement. *American Journal of Orthopsychiatry, 30*(4), 788–798.

Hilgard, J. R. (1969). Depressive and psychotic states as anniversaries to sibling death in childhood. *International Psychiatry Clinics, IV,* 197–211.

Lamers, E. P. (1986). Books, adolescents and death. In C. Corr & J. McNeil (Eds.), *Adolescents and death* (pp. 233–242). New York: Springer.

Lamers, E. P. (1986). The dying child in the classroom. In G. H. Paterson (Ed.), *Children and death* (pp. 175–186). London: King's College.

Lamers, W. M. (1965). *Death, grief, mourning, the funeral and the child.* Milwaukee, WI: Bulfin Press.

Lamers, W. M. (1986). Helping the child to grieve. In G. H. Paterson (Ed.), *Children and death* (pp. 105–119). London: King's College.

Lamers, W. M., & Lamers, E. P. (1987). *Children and their grief.* NFDA Caregivers Manual. Available from: National Funeral Directors Association, 11121 West Oklahoma Ave., Milwaukee, WI 53227.

McGuffey's Eclectic Readers (Vols. 2–6) (1920). New York: Van Nostrand Reinhold.

Newton, F. I. (1990). *Children and the funeral ritual: Factors that affect their attendance and participation.* Master's Thesis, California State University, Chico. Unpublished.

Parnass, E. (1975). Effects of experiences with loss and death among preschool children. *Children Today, 4,* 2–7.

Shoor, M., & Speed, M. H. (1963). Delinquency as a manifestation of the mourning process. *Psychiatric Quarterly, 37*(3), 540–558.

Resources

Children's Books About Death

All of the books listed below are available from the public library in Los Angeles (unless noted with *), and should be available at other public and/or school libraries. Some of these books can be located through the Internet sites that deal in used books, such as amazon.com, abebooks.com, alibris.com, or bibliofind.com. Amazon.com and barnesandnoble.com are sources for new books. New books are also available from the Centering Corporation and Compassion Books. Many books that are no longer available in hardcover are available in paperback.

Nonfiction

Bernstein, Joanne. *Loss and how to cope with it.* New York: Houghton Mifflin, 1977.

Bernstein, Joanne, & Gullo, Stephen J. *When people die.* New York: Dutton, 1977.

*Brown, Laurie K. *When dinosaurs die: A guide to understanding death.* Boston: Little Brown, 1996.

Le Shan, Eda J. *Learning to say good-by: When a parent dies.* New York: Macmillan, 1976.

Langone, J. *Death is a noun.* Boston: Little, Brown, 1972.

Richter, Elizabeth. *Losing someone you love. When a brother or sister dies.* New York: Putnam, 1986.

Rofes, Eric E. & The Unit at Fayerweather Street School. *The kids' book about death and dying.* Boston: Little, Brown, 1985.

Segerberg, Osborn, Jr. *Living with death.* New York: Dutton, 1976.

Stein, Sara B. *About dying.* New York: Walker, 1974.

Fiction

Alcott, Louisa M. *Little women*. New York: Grosset & Dunlop, 1947. (originally pub. 1869) (sister—illness)

Alexander, Sue. *Nadia the willful*. New York: Pantheon, 1983. (brother—accidental)

*Aliki. *Two of them*. New York: Greenwillow, 1979. (grandfather—old age)

Bartoli, Jennifer. *Nonna*. New York: Harvey House, 1975. (grandmother—natural death)

Blume, Judy. *Tiger eyes*. Scarsdale, NY: Bradbury, 1981. (father—murdered in robbery)

Brown, Margaret W. *The dead bird*. Reading, MA: Addison-Wesley, 1965. (wild bird—natural death)

Bunting, Eve. *The empty window*. New York: Frederick Warne, 1980. (friend—illness)

Bunting, Eve. *The happy funeral*. New York: Harper & Row, 1982. (grandfather—Chinese-American customs)

Bunting, Eve. *A sudden silence*. New York: Harcourt Brace Jovanovich, 1988. (brother—accidental)

Carter, Dorothy. *Bye, Mis' Lea*. New York: Farrar, Strauss & Giroux, 1996. (caretaker—old age)

Cohn, Janice. *I had a friend named Peter: Talking to children about the death of a friend*. New York: Wm. Morrow, 1987.

Coutant, Helen. *First snow*. New York: Knopf, 1974. (grandmother—old age—Vietnamese)

de Paola, Tomie. *Nana upstairs and Nana downstairs*. New York: Putnam, 1973. (great-grandmother and grandmother—natural death)

Deaver, Julie Reece. *Say goodnight, Gracie*. New York: Harper & Row, 1988. (friend—accidental)

*Douglas, Eileen. *Rachel and the upside down heart*. Los Angeles: Price, Stern, Sloan, 1990. (father—heart attack)

Gerstein, Mordicai. *The mountains of Tibet*. New York: Harper & Row, 1987. (reincarnation)

Hermes, Patricia. *You shouldn't have to say good-bye*. New York: Harcourt, 1982. (mother—illness)

Hoopes, Lyn L. *Nana*. New York: Harper & Row, 1981. (grandmother—natural death)

Little, Jean. *Mama's going to buy you a mockingbird*. New York: Viking Kestrel, 1984. (father—cancer)

Miles, Miska. *Annie and the old one*. Boston: Little, Brown, 1971. (Navajo Indians—grandmother—natural death)

Newman, Lesléa. *Too far away to touch*. New York: Clarion, 1995. (uncle—AIDS)

Orgel, Doris. *Mulberry music*. New York: Harper & Row, 1971. (grandmother—illness)

Paterson, Katherine. *Bridge to Terabithia*. New York: Crowell, 1977. (friend—accidental death)

Pfeffer, S. B. *About David*. New York: Delacorte, 1980. (friend—suicide)

Smith, Doris B. *A taste of blackberries*. New York: Crowell, 1973. (friend—bee sting allergy)

Stevens, Carla. *Stories from a snowy meadow*. New York: Seabury, 1976. (personified animals—natural death)

*Tiffault, Benette W. *A quilt for Elizabeth*. Omaha, NE: Centering, 1992. (father, Elizabeth, and her grandmother make a quilt from her father's clothes while remembering him)

Tobias, Tobi. *Petey*. New York: Putnam, 1978. (pet gerbil—illness)

Varley, Susan. *Badger's parting gifts*. New York: Lothrop, Lee & Shepard, 1984. (personified animals—remembering someone after death)

Viorst, Judith. *The tenth good thing about Barney*. New York: Atheneum, 1971. (pet cat—natural death)

White, E. B. *Charlotte's web*. New York: Harper & Row, 1952. (death as a natural consequence of life)

Wilhelm, Hans. *I'll always love you*. New York: Crown, 1985. (pet dog—natural death)

Williams, Margery. *The velveteen rabbit*. New York: Holt, Rinehart & Winston, 1983 edition. (life and death—general)

Wood, Douglas. *Grandad's prayers of the earth*. Cambridge, MA: Candlewick, 1999. (grandfather—old age)

Yolen, Jane. *Grandad Bill's song*. New York: Philomel, 1994. (grandfather—old age)

Books and Articles for Adults

Bernstein, J., & Rudman, M. K. (1989). *Books to help children cope with separation and loss*. New York: R. R. Bowker.

Bowlby, J. (1961). Childhood mourning and its implications for psychiatry. *American Journal of Psychiatry, 118*(6), 481–489.

Cain, A. C., Fast, I., & Erickson, M. E. (1964). Children's disturbed reactions to the death of a sibling. *American Journal of Orthopsychiatry, 34*, 741–752.

Carey, A. (1977). Helping the child and the family cope with death. *International Journal of Family Counseling, 5*, 58–63.

Cavenar, J. O., Nash, J. L., & Maltbie, A. A. (1978). Anniversary reactions presenting as physical complaints. *Journal of Clinical Psychiatry, 134*(11), 369–374.

Corr, C. A., & McNeil, J. N. (Eds.). (1986). *Adolescence and death*. New York: Springer.

Crase, D., & Crase, D. (1983). Communication with children about death and dying. *Thanatos, 8*(1), 15–16.

Davies, B. (1999). *Shadows in the sun: The experiences of sibling bereavement in childhood*. Philadelphia: Brunner/Mazel.

Fassler, J. (1978). *Helping children cope*. New York: The Free Press.

Feinberg, D. (1970). Preventive therapy with siblings of a dying child. *Journal of American Academy of Child Psychiatry, 9*, 644–668.

Fredlund, D. (1978). The lemonade story. *Thanatos, 3*(3), 9–11.

Furman, E. (Ed.). (1974). *A child's parent dies: Studies in childhood bereavement*. New Haven, CT: Yale University Press.

Gaffney, D. A. (1988). *The seasons of grief, helping your children grow through loss*. New York: New American Library.

Gogan, J. L., Koocher, G. P., Foster, D. J., & O'Malley, J. E. (1977). Impact of childhood cancer on siblings. *Health and Social Work, 2*(1), 41–57.

Grollman, E. (Ed.). (1967). *Explaining death to children.* Boston: Beacon.

Harrison, S. I., Davenport, C. W., & McDermott, J. F. (1967). Children's reactions to bereavement: Adult confusions and misperceptions. *Archives of General Psychiatry, 17,* 593–597.

Klagsbrun, F. (1976). *Too young to die: Youth and suicide.* Boston: Houghton Mifflin.

Koocher, G. P. (1973). Childhood, death, and cognitive development. *Developmental Psychology, 3,* 369–375.

Lamers, W. M. (1986). Helping the child to grieve. In G. H. Paterson (Ed.), *Children and death* (pp. 105–119). London: King's College.

Lindemann, E. (1944). Symptomatology and management of acute grief. *American Journal of Psychiatry, 101,* 141–148.

Lonetto, R. (1980). *Children's conceptions of death.* New York: Springer.

Rosen, H. (1984). *Unspoken grief: Coping with childhood sibling loss.* Lexington, MA: D. C. Heath (Lexington Books).

Rudolph, M. (1978). *Should the children know?* New York: Schocken Books.

Sahler, O. J. Z. (1978). *The child and death.* St. Louis, MO: Mosby.

Scott, F. (1981). When a student dies . . . *English Journal, 70,* 22–24.

Siegel, B. S. (1986). Helping children cope with death. *Research Record, 3*(2), 53–63.

Silverman, P. (2000). *Never too young to know: Death in children's lives.* New York: Oxford University Press.

Sternberg, F., & Sternberg, B. (1980). *If I die and when I do.* Englewood Cliffs, NJ: Prentice-Hall.

Wass, H., & Corr, C. A. (1984). *Helping children cope with death: Guidelines and resources.* New York: Hemisphere.

Wass, H., & Corr, C. A. (1984). *Childhood and death.* New York: Hemisphere.

Williams, Y. (1988, March–April). Grief work is play: Dealing with children's grief. *The Forum Newsletter, 12*(2), 7–8.

Wolfelt, A. (1989). What bereaved children want adults to know about grief. *Bereavement, 3*(9), 34–45.

Worden, J. W. (1996). *Children and grief: When a parent dies.* New York: Guilford Press.

Fourteen

The Study of Sibling Bereavement: An Historical Perspective

Betty Davies

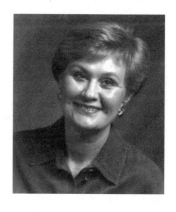

Betty Davies earned her B.Sc.N. from the University of Alberta, her M.S.N. from the University of Arizona, and her Ph.D. in nursing science from the University of Washington. Dr. Davies was postdoctoral fellow at the University of California, San Francisco, being the first nurse awarded a postdoctoral fellowship from the American Cancer Society, California Division. Dr. Davies is a professor in the School of Nursing, University of British Columbia, Vancouver, Canada, and an investigator in the Research Division, British Columbia's Children's Hospital. Dr. Davies is the first nurse and the first psychosocial researcher to be awarded an investigatorship.

Dr. Davies has worked in the area of death, dying, and bereavement for more than twenty years. She has given numerous workshops related to coping with loss, particularly for families following the death of a child. Her seminal work pertaining to bereavement in siblings forms the basis for many presentations and publications. Dr. Davies has recently completed two collaborative research projects, which include exploring the experience of families caring for a terminally ill person and investigating the experience of nurses caring for chronically ill children during the terminal phase. Dr. Davies is a founding member of HUGS Children's Hospice Society, the driving force behind establishing Canuck Place, North America's first freestanding hospice for children. In recognition of her contributions to the field, Dr. Davies has been awarded the YWCA Woman of the Year Award in British Columbia, the Excellence in Nursing Research and the Award of Merit from the British Columbia Registered Nurses Association.

Despite the potential significance of sibling loss, sibling bereavement has been an ignored phenomenon until recent decades. When I began my exploration of the topic in the early 1980s, very little literature was available. During the intervening years, the study of sibling bereavement has grown considerably. A description of the evolution of this field of study is the focus of this chapter.

The Sibling Relationship

Siblings are brothers and sisters, children who have parents in common. Siblings are related to one another, but they are so much more. Siblings share a bond of relationship that is unique: It begins early in the life of the second child. Indeed, the relationship between siblings may begin early in the mother's pregnancy. As the children grow and develop, the relationship between them changes. Moreover, the sibling relationship exists within, and is influenced by, relationships with other family members, peers, and members of the larger community. And, the sibling bond does not end in childhood, but continues throughout life. In fact, Cicirelli (1988) states that relationships between siblings assume considerable importance in old age, with feelings of closeness and affection increasing with age. Kahn (1983) regarded trust and interdependence between siblings in later years to be one of the most important of human relationships. Thus, to experience the death of a sibling in childhood means not only losing a companion during childhood and youth, but also losing the potential of a lifelong companion who can offer something that no one else can.

Sibling relationships share common attributes with all interpersonal relationships, but they are also characterized by certain unique features. First, sibling relationships last a long time, often for a lifetime. In fact, siblings spend 80–100% of their lifetimes with each other (and only 40–60% of their life-spans with their parents). Second, the sibling relationship is ascribed by birth or legal action (e.g., adoption), rather than earned. Once ascribed, it never ends. One cannot divorce a sibling. When a sibling dies, the remaining children continue to think of the deceased child as a sibling.

Sibling relationships are more or less egalitarian. Siblings think of themselves as equal, and expect to be treated by others (especially by their parents) as equals. Although perceived as equal by themselves and others, siblings are not necessarily the same. Their individual experiences within their families and in the world make them different from one another.

Consequently, when a child dies, the surviving children each respond in their own unique ways.

Children see themselves as teachers, friends, comforters, competitors, and companions, although it is most often younger siblings who regard their older brothers and sisters as teachers and comforters. Despite these positive aspects of the sibling relationship, siblings also quarrel, tattle on one another, tease, and antagonize each other. As a result, sibling relationships are complex and complicated, and, when a sibling dies, the grief of the remaining children can be profound.

Investigations of the impact of a child's death once focused primarily on the parents. Much less was written on the impact of such a loss on siblings, even though the child's response to major loss became a source of growing interest and considerable study in the 1960s and 1970s. For example, there were clinical and theoretical considerations of the younger child's capacity to mourn (Bowlby, 1963; Wolfenstein, 1966), epidemiological studies attempting to link adult depression to childhood loss (Birtchnell, 1970; Blinder, 1972; Brown, Harris, & Copeland, 1977; Hilgard, 1969), and descriptive studies of children's bereavement responses to the death of parents (Furman, 1974).

Few studies focused on siblings (Cain, Fast, & Erickson, 1964; Kaplan, Grobstein, & Smith, 1976; Lewis, 1967; Payne, Goff, & Paulson, 1980; Stehbens & Lascari, 1974). Close scrutiny of a bibliographic compilation written over 20 years ago, entitled *Death, Grief and Bereavement: A Bibliography 1845–1975* (Fulton, 1977), indicates how little work pertained to sibling bereavement. Fulton's bibliography contains a total of 309 citations classified under the general heading of "children." Of these, only 15 are listed under the subheading of "reactions to the death of siblings." Of these 15 references, only 5 were written during the period 1970–1975; the remaining 10 references were written before 1970, and, of these, 3 were written in the 1940s. A novel written in German was one of the resources listed. Other entries focused on adults: 3 cited articles about the death of adult siblings, and an additional 4 were about adult psychiatric problems associated with childhood experiences of sibling death. Only 7 resources referred to bereavement experience by the child at the time of his or her sibling's death. A few years later, a major Institute of Medicine report (Osterweis, Solomon, & Green, 1984) stated that a lack of information on sibling bereavement precluded incorporating a section devoted to sibling grief. Fortunately, the field has expanded considerably during the intervening 20 years.

The Evolution of the Study of Sibling Bereavement[*]

The earliest publication that specifically addresses sibling bereavement was written by Rosenzweig in 1943.[**] His paper discussed the relationship between sibling death and schizophrenia. No other articles appeared until the 1960s, when four were written (Pollock, 1962; Cain et al., 1964; Rosenblatt, 1969; Hilgard, 1969). Two of these papers (Pollock, 1962; Hilgard, 1969) followed a theme similar to Rosenzweig's paper: the effect of childhood bereavement on adult patients being treated for psychiatric disturbance. Cain et al. reported on their observations of disturbed reactions in children following the death of a sibling. Similarly, Rosenblatt described the disturbed reactions of a young boy to his sister's death. All authors were psychiatrists, and published their work in psychiatric journals. A strong psychiatric orientation was obvious in the focus on *disturbance* or *psychopathology*. This is not surprising, however, because the subjects of all papers were individuals undergoing psychiatric treatment.

During the next decade, of the six publications located, four were published in psychiatric journals, and were authored by psychiatrists. Blinder (1972) presented three case studies to illustrate the potentially profound effects of sibling death in childhood. Binger (1973), based on children in 20 families in which a sibling had died from leukemia, focused on the aftermath of such an experience. Tooley (1973), although focusing on maternal bereavement, addressed the possibility of surviving siblings becoming scapegoats in maternal bereavement. Pollock (1978), building on his earlier work, discussed sibling loss and creativity, and he was the first to consider that sibling bereavement may have creative outcomes, not just be the source of pathology. In Australia, Nixon and Pearn (1977) looked at the emotional sequelae on parents and siblings of the drowning or near-drowning of a child. The decade's publications concluded with a paper by Krell and Rabkin (1979), in which they introduced the effects of sibling death on surviving children, from a family perspective.

The publications of the 1980s began with a paper entitled, "Sibling: The forgotten grievers" (Zelauskas, 1981), a title which reflected the situation up until that time. The ensuing decade provided a dramatic increase in the number of publications pertaining to sibling bereavement. Thirty-two publications were located. Shifts were noted in the authors' disciplines and

---

[*]This discussion is adapted from Davies, B. (1999). *Shadows in the sun: The experiences of sibling bereavement in childhood.* Philadelphia: Taylor and Francis. Chapter 2, pp. 15–18.
[**]References that explicitly referred to the concept of sibling bereavement in the title were selected for categorizing into chronological order.

in the range of journals in which papers were published. Authors now included other health care professionals who were interested in the well-being of children, particularly nurses and psychologists. Publications no longer appeared solely in psychiatric journals. Instead, papers were in journals focusing on death and dying (*Death Studies, Death Education,* and *Omega*), social work and school health (*School Health* and *Child and Adolescent Social Work Journal*), pediatric medicine (*Pediatric Annals* and *Archives of Diseases in Childhood*), nursing (*Issues in Comprehensive Nursing, Cancer Nursing, Archives of Psychiatric Nursing, Recent Advances in Nursing,* and *Pediatric Nursing*), and children's health (*Children's Health Care*). The focus had turned from examining sibling bereavement primarily as a psychiatric concern to looking at childhood bereavement as the concern of many disciplines interested in promoting children's health.

Four of the publications during this decade were doctoral dissertations (Balk, 1981; McCown, 1982; Davies, 1983; Hogan, 1987). These dissertations and the publications that derived from them account for 50% of the publications during the decade. An additional five publications (Lauer, Mulhern, Bohne, & Camitta, 1985; Birenbaum, 1989a, 1989b; Birenbaum, Robinson, Phillips, Stewart, & McCown, 1990; Martinson, Davies, & McClowry, 1987) resulted from the implementation of models of care for children dying of cancer and their families. Some other papers focused on the bereavement responses of a particular age group, heretofore not specifically mentioned—adolescents (Balk, 1983a, 1983b; Mufson, 1985; Hogan, 1988). Publications of this decade reflected an expanded conceptualization of sibling bereavement, including an examination of various factors that affected bereavement outcome: location of death (Lauer et al., 1985), funeral attendance (McCown, 1984), closeness between siblings (Davies, 1988a), family environment (Davies, 1988b), cause of death (Adams & Deveau, 1987), parental grief (Demi & Gilbert, 1987), time (Hogan, 1988), and parent communication (Birenbaum, 1989a, 1989b; Birenbaum et al., 1990). In addition, outcomes of bereavement were reported, notably in relation to self-concept (Balk, 1983b; Martinson et al., 1987).

Some papers continued to focus on deaths from cancer (Davies, 1988a, 1988b; Birenbaum, 1989a; Birenbaum et al., 1990; Lauer et al., 1985; Martinson et al., 1987). Other papers were derived from situations in which the deaths occurred from sudden and unexpected deaths, as well as cancer. Mandell, McAnulty, and Carlson (1983) were the first to describe sibling bereavement responses when the death had resulted from sudden infant death syndrome (SIDS).

Interest in sibling bereavement continued into the 1990s, including accounts by bereaved siblings themselves (Romond, 1990; Van Riper,

1997), and clinical descriptions continue to offer insight into the experiences of this group of children and adolescents (Heiney, 1991). A focus on adolescent bereavement continued, with additional papers by Balk (1990, 1991), Fanos and Nickerson (1991), Hogan and Balk (1990), Hogan and Greenfield (1991), and Hogan and DeSantis (1992, 1994). Batten and Oltjenbruns (1999) explored relationships between bereaved adolescents' search for meaning and spirituality. Hogan contributed the first description of a measurement tool for assessing sibling bereavement (Hogan, 1990).

Effects of sibling bereavement on younger children were described (McCown & Davies, 1995), and differences between twin and singleton adjustment to loss in adolescents were examined (Wilson, 1995). In addition to looking at the immediate response of bereaved siblings, the long-term effects of sibling bereavement were noted (Davies, 1991; Martinson & Campos, 1991; Hogan & DeSantis, 1992). Explorations into sibling bereavement following death from various causes continued. Brent et al. (1993) explored the psychiatric impact of the loss of an adolescent sibling to suicide on surviving adolescent siblings. Wright (1999) investigated the impact of suicide during childhood on the mourning process of child and sibling survivors. Juhnke and Shoffner (1999) tested a family-level intervention in cases of adolescent suicide. Hutton and Bradley (1994) investigated sibling reactions to a brother's or sister's death from SIDS; and Mahon (1993) explored children's concepts of death in relation to sibling death from trauma. These last two studies used comparison group—a step forward in research design. For the first time, research focused on sibling responses to death of a brother or sister who had been murdered (Udell, 1995; Lohan, 1998).

Theoretical articles also appeared in the literature. Robinson and Mahon (1997) described the results of their concept analysis of sibling bereavement. Hogan and DeSantis (1996a, 1996b) proposed a theory of adolescent bereavement. Research was reported that focused on comparisons of parents' and siblings' grief (Mahon & Page, 1995; Worden, Davies, & McCown, 1999). Research-based guidelines were suggested for nurses working with bereaved siblings (Davies, 1993). Finally, in this decade, publications began to describe intervention programs for siblings (Gibbons, 1992). A weekend intervention for children whose sibling had died in a children's hospice program was described by Potts, Farrell, and O'Toole (1999). Some programs focused on family members, not specifically on siblings; for example, Juhnke and Shoffner (1999) tested the use of the Family Debriefing Model, a solution-focused intervention designed to facilitate treatment of parents and siblings who survive a family member's suicide. Other interventions

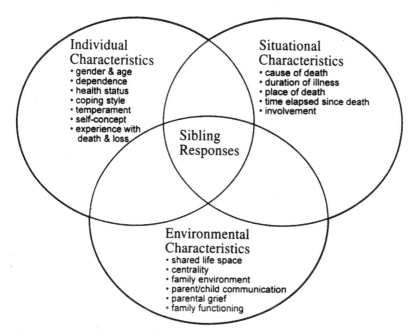

FIGURE 14.1   Conceptualization of the mediating variables that impact the phenomenon of sibling bereavement.

focused on bereaved children, not solely bereaved siblings. Tonkins and Lambert (1996), for example, tested the effectiveness of an 8-week children's psychotherapy group.

Finally, two books on sibling bereavement were published during the 1990s (Fanos, 1996; Davies, 1999). Fanos highlights the issues facing siblings of children who have died following a chronic illness. Davies's book shares the knowledge of sibling bereavement accumulated from a long-standing program of research that includes siblings of all ages whose brother or sister died from a variety of causes. Her program includes exploration of immediate and long-term effects and examines the influence of contextual variables on sibling bereavement (see Figure 14.1). The book synthesizes these research findings with her own clinical experiences in working with bereaved children and their families, and concludes with a conceptualization of sibling bereavement that identifies the relationships among the variables that impact siblings' experience and their responses. The model provides a comprehensive understanding of childhood sibling bereavement and provides guidance for professional caregivers, parents, and other adults who seek to help children who have experienced the death of a brother or sister.

The new millennium has thus far offered only a few publications pertaining to sibling bereavement (Birenbaum, 2000). A literature review and an exploratory secondary analysis from a prospective longitudinal design were used to develop the empirical criteria for behavioral items indicative of bereavement. Discussion focuses on the beginning development of a screening tool for childhood bereavement services.

Literature Reviews Pertaining to Sibling Bereavement

During the past 15 years, as sibling bereavement has become a topic deemed worthy of study, six literature reviews have been published. Waechter's was the first, originally written in 1964 with limited availability, then published in a book that was edited as a tribute to Waechter (Krulik, Holaday, & Martinson, 1987). Waechter's review provided a broad overview of the literature pertaining to death, dying, and bereavement. She did not specifically address the needs of grieving children; however, she indicated that the death of a parent or sibling "is a shattering experience for the child and may have far reaching effect" (p. 10). She explained these effects in relation to children's understanding of death at various ages. Doing so was part of her argument for talking directly to terminally ill children about their experience; until this time, talking to a child about his diagnosis and prognosis was thought to cause irreparable psychological damage to the child.

Betz (1987) contributed a review that followed up on Waechter's. Betz reviewed the research and theory generated in the field of pediatric thanatology during the years 1970–1985. She concentrated on four major areas of inquiry: children's conceptions of death, the fatally ill child, and child and parental bereavement responses. In the section about children's bereavement responses, Betz includes discussion of bereavement responses following the death of both parents and siblings. In this latter section, Betz briefly discusses nine studies pertaining to the study of sibling bereavement, and concludes with suggestions for future research.

Stephenson (1986) reviewed the literature on grieving children, with special emphasis on those who have lost a sibling. Instead of summarizing or critiquing the literature, he based recommendations for helping grieving children on the review.

More recently, Opie (1992) and Walker (1993) published critical reviews. Opie concentrated on nursing studies, identifying limitations of small sample sizes and designs that include nonrepresentative samples, lack of control groups, and unclear definitions. These limitations, of course, are relevant and pertinent, but are characteristic of many new fields of study. Walker categorized the literature into early studies identifying pathological grief responses (1950–1985) and late studies identifying grief responses (1985–present). In this latter grouping, she categorized studies into developmental age-specific studies, impact of family environment on grief responses, and intervention studies. Her review encompassed a final sample size of 24 research reports and 15 clinical papers obtained from a Medline computer search from 1982 to 1992, and searching the reference lists from articles found to locate related works. Even with this extensive search, however, significant research papers published during this time frame were excluded from Walker's review. She provided a concise summary of each paper reviewed, and offered conclusions about the future research, similar to those put forth by Betz (1987).

The sixth review (Davies, 1995) provided a comprehensive review of the "state of the art" of sibling bereavement research, according to behavioral responses (both problem and positive responses) and mediating variables, which include individual, situational, and environmental characteristics. For a comprehensive listing of literature pertaining to sibling bereavement, see Davies (1999). As a reference for other researchers, clinicians, and educators, summaries of journal articles that refer explicitly to "sibling bereavement" in their titles are included in two appendices in Davies' book. One appendix includes research articles; the second includes anecdotal or clinical accounts of sibling bereavement and literature reviews that pertain to some aspect of the topic.

As a group, these literature reviews indicate that the field of sibling bereavement research continues to evolve. As stated earlier, the first studies of sibling bereavement (1960s to mid-1970s) focused on the psychiatric implications for adults who experienced a sibling's death in childhood. Even the first studies of bereaved siblings focused on problematic outcomes among bereaved children undergoing psychiatric treatment. From the middle of the 1970s to the middle of the next decade, oncology, instead of psychiatry, provided the setting for many studies. In the early 1970s, Martinson and her colleagues initiated the first home care program for dying children, representing the beginning of a changed emphasis to intervention programs for children with cancer (Martinson, 1980). This allowed some investigation of the impact of such programs upon the siblings. During the 1980s, attention was given to sibling bereavement associated with a child's death from diseases other than cancer, including cystic fibrosis and SIDS, and from other causes, such as suicide. The focus also was directed to specific age groups, especially adolescents. The literature conveyed the difficulty that exists in attempting to isolate factors that affect sibling adjustment and bereavement outcome, and acknowledged the contribution of environmental factors, such as the family, to bereavement outcome. During the past decade, the focus on adolescent sibling bereavement continued. Cause of death not only continued to address suicide, but also began to explore sibling bereavement following violent death (i.e., murder). The development of measurement tools appeared, and the testing of interventions for bereaved siblings also took a small step forward.

It is enlightening to look back over the published research pertaining to families and sibling bereavement. Cobb's (1956) was the first published paper that addressed the effects on the family of a child's death. Cobb's paper, a clinical description, derived from her own experience as a pediatrician caring for families in which a child was dying. In the next decade, the titles of three papers specifically mentioned the effects on families of having a child with leukemia (Natterson & Knudson, 1960; Lewis, 1967; Binger et al., 1969). None of the papers focused specifically on the siblings, but did mention the special needs of siblings.

The family focus broadened during the 1970s: Five publications referred specifically to family functioning following the death of a child. As with publications directly related to sibling bereavement, publications pertaining to families reflected the ongoing interest in childhood cancer and leukemia, but two papers with a family focus introduced deaths from other causes: suicide (Rudestam, 1977) and cystic fibrosis (Kerner, Harvey, & Lewiston, 1979). The focus on family functioning and childhood cancer prevailed into the 1980s as well (Davies, Spinetta, Martinson, McClowry, & Kulencamp, 1986). The focus on families following the death of a child seems to have lost some momentum during the first part of the 1990s: Only one paper was located that addressed the needs of families after a child dies (Parkman, 1992). Later, however, Juhnke and Shoffner (1999) report on the use of a family-based intervention for assisting family members, including siblings, deal with the aftermath of death from suicide. Davies (1999) emphasizes the importance of family, particularly parents, on sibling bereavement outcome. This trend toward including the family is probably part of the ongoing evolution of sibling bereavement research. The focus now needs to turn to assessing the complex interactions of multiple factors affecting sibling bereavement, to assessing bereavement interventions for siblings, and to continue to document the long-term outcomes of sibling bereavement. In addition, the focus needs to broaden beyond the boundaries of our own Western world, to include the experiences of siblings of various cultural backgrounds. We have progressed substantially during the past several decades in the study of sibling bereavement, and we still have much to learn.

Discussion Questions

1. What factors contributed to the development of interest in sibling bereavement occurring only in relatively recent years?
2. What dimensions of sibling bereavement should be addressed in future sibling bereavement research?

References

Adams, D. W., & Deveau, E. J. (1987). How the cause of a child's death may affect a sibling's grief. In M. A. Morgan (Ed.), *Bereavement: Helping the survivors* (pp. 67–77). Proceedings of the 1987 King's College Conference. London, Ontario: King's College.

Balk, D. (1981). *Sibling death during adolescence: Self concept and bereavement reactions.* Unpublished doctoral dissertation, University of Illinois at Urbana-Champaign.

Balk, D. (1983a). Adolescents' grief reactions and self-concept perceptions following sibling death: A study of 33 teenagers. *Journal of Youth and Adolescents, 12*(2), 137–161.

Balk, D. (1983b). Effects of sibling death on teenagers. *Journal of School Health, 1*(53), 14–18.

Balk, D. (1990). The self-concepts of bereaved adolescents: Sibling death and its aftermath. *Journal of Adolescent Research, 5,* 112–131.

Balk, D. (1991). Death and adolescent bereavement: Current research and future directions. *Journal of Adolescent Research, 6,* 7–27.

Batten, M., & Oltjenbruns, K. A. (1999). Adolescent sibling bereavement as a catalyst for spiritual development: A model for understanding. *Death Studies, 23*(6), 529–546.

Betz, C. L. (1987). Death, dying, and bereavement: A review of literature, 1970–1985. In T. Krulik, B. Holaday, & I. M. Martinson (Eds.), *The child and family facing life-threatening illness* (pp. 32–49). New York: J. B. Lippincott.

Binger, C., Ablin, A., Feuerstein, R., Kushner, J., Zoger, S., & Mikkelsen, C. (1969). Childhood leukemia: Emotional impact on patient and family. *New England Journal of Medicine, 280*(8), 414–418.

Binger, C. M. (1973). Childhood leukemia—emotional impact on siblings. In J. E. Anthony & C. Koupernik, *The child and his family: The impact of disease and death* (Vol. 2). New York: Wiley & Sons.

Birenbaum, L. K. (1989a). The relationship between parent-siblings' communication and siblings' coping with death experience. *Journal of the Association of Pediatric Oncology Nurses, 6*(2), 26–27.

Birenbaum, L. K. (1989b). The relationship between parent–sibling communication and coping of siblings with death experience. *Journal of Pediatric Oncology Nursing, 6*(3), 85–91.

Birenbaum, L. K. (2000). Assessing children's and teenagers' bereavement when a sibling dies from cancer: A secondary analysis. *Child: Care, Health and Development, 26*(5), 381–400.

Birenbaum, L. K., Robinson, M. A., Phillips, D. S., Stewart, B. J., & McCown, D. E. (1990). The response of children to the dying and death of a sibling. *Omega, 20,* 213–228.

Birtchnell, J. (1970). Depression in relation to early and recent parent death. *British Journal of Psychiatry, 116,* 299–306.

Blinder, B. (1972). Sibling death in childhood. Child Psychiatry and Human Development, 2, 169–175.

Bowlby, J. (1963). Pathological mourning and childhood mourning. *Journal of American Psychoanalytic Association, 11,* 500–541.

Brent, D. A., Perper, J. A., Moritz, G., Liotos, L., Schweers, J., Roth, C., et al. (1993). Psychiatric impact of the loss of an adolescent sibling to suicide. *Journal of Affective Disorders, 28,* 249–256.

Brown, G., Harris, T., & Copeland, J. (1977). Depression and loss. *British Journal of Psychiatry, 130,* 11.

Cain, A. C., Fast, I., & Erickson, M. E. (1964). Children's disturbed reactions to the death of a sibling. *American Journal of Orthopsychiatry, 34,* 741–752.

Cicirelli, V. G. (1988). Interpersonal relationships among elderly siblings: Implications for clinical practice. In M. Kahn & K. G. Lewis (Eds.), *Siblings in therapy* (pp. 435–456). New York: W. W. Norton.

Cobb, B. (1956). Psychological impact of long illness and death of a child on the family circle. *Journal of Pediatrics, 49*(6), 746–751.

Davies, E. M. B. (1983). *Behavioral responses of children to a siblings's death.* Unpublished doctoral dissertation. University of Washington, Seattle, WA.

Davies, B. (1988a). Shared life space and sibling bereavement responses. *Cancer Nursing, 11,* 339–347.

Davies, B. (1988b). The family environment in bereaved families and its relationship to surviving sibling behavior. *Children's Health Care, 17*(1), 22–30.

Davies, B. (1991). Long-term outcomes of adolescent sibling bereavement. *Journal of Adolescent Research, 6*(1), 83–96.

Davies, B. (1993). Sibling bereavement: Research-based guidelines for nurses. *Seminars in Oncology Nursing, 9*(2), 107–113.

Davies, B. (1995). Sibling bereavement research: State of the art. In I. B. Corless, B. Germino, & M. Pittman (Eds.), *A challenge or living: Dying, death and bereavement* (pp. 173–202). Boston: Jones & Bartlett.

Davies, B. (1999). *Shadows in the sun: The experience of sibling bereavement in childhood.* Philadelphia: Brunner/Mazell.

Davies, B., Spinetta, J., Martinson, I., McClowry, S., & Kulenkamp, E. (1986). Manifestations of levels of functioning in grieving families. *Journal of Family Issues, 7*(3), 297–313.

Demi, A. S., & Gilbert, C. M. (1987). Relationship of parental grief to sibling grief. *Archives of Psychiatric Nursing, 1,* 385–391.

Fanos, J. H. (1996). *Sibling loss.* Hillsdale, NJ: Lawrence Erlbaum.

Fanos, J. H., & Nickerson, B. G. (1991). Long-term effects of sibling death during adolescence. *Journal of Adolescent Research, 6,* 70–82.

Fulton, R. (1977). *Death, grief and bereavement: A bibliography 1845–1975.* New York: Arna Press.

Furman, E. (1974). *A child's parent dies: Studies in childhood bereavement.* New Haven, CT: Yale University Press.

Gibbons, M. B. (1992). A child dies, a child survives: The impact of sibling loss. *Journal of Pediatric Health Care, 6,* 65–72.

Heiney, S. P. (1991). Sibling grief: A case report. *Archives of Psychiatric Nursing, 5,* 121–127.

Hilgard, J. R. (1969). Depressive and psychotic states as anniversaries to sibling death in childhood. *International Psychiatry Clinics, 6,* 197–207.

Hogan, N. S. (1987). An investigation of the adolescent sibling bereavement process and adaptation (Doctoral dissertation, Loyola University of Chicago, 1987). *Dissertation Abstracts International,* 4024A.

Hogan, N. (1988). The effects of time on the adolescent sibling bereavement process. *Pediatric Nursing, 14*(4), 133–335.

Hogan, N. (1990). Hogan sibling inventory of bereavement. In J. Touliatos, B. Perlmutter, & M. Straus (Eds.), *Handbook of family measurement techniques* (p. 24). Newbury Park, CA: Sage.

Hogan, N., & Balk, D. (1990). Adolescent reactions to sibling death: Perceptions of mothers, fathers, and teenagers. *Nursing Research, 39*(2), 103–106.

Hogan, N., & Greenfield, D. B. (1991). Adolescent sibling bereavement: Symptomatology in a large community sample. *Journal of Adolescent Research, 6,* 97–112.

Hogan, N., & DeSantis, L. (1992). Adolescent sibling bereavement: An ongoing attachment. *Qualitative Heath Research, 2,* 159–177.

Hogan, N., & DeSantis, L. (1994). Things that help and hinder adolescent sibling bereavement. *Western Journal of Nursing Research, 16,* 132–153.

Hogan, N., & DeSantis, L. (1996a). Basic constructs of a theory of adolescent sibling bereavement. In D. Klass, P. R. Silverman, & S. L. Nickman (Eds.), *Continuing bonds: New understandings of grief* (pp. 235–254). Philadelphia: Taylor & Francis.

Hogan, N., & DeSantis, L. (1996b). Adolescent sibling bereavement: Toward a new theory. In C. A. Corr & D. E. Balk (Eds.), *Handbook of adolescent death and bereavement* (pp. 173–195). New York: Springer.

Hutton, C. J., & Bradley, B. S. (1994). Effects of sudden infant death on bereaved siblings: A comparative study. *Journal of Child Psychology and Psychiatry, 35,* 723–732.

Juhnke, G. A., & Shoffner, M. F. (1999). The family debriefing model: An adapted critical incident stress debriefing for parents and older sibling suicide survivors. *Family Journal: Counseling & Therapy for Couples & Families, 7*(4), 324–384.

Kahn, M. D. (1983). Sibling relationships in later life. *Medical Aspects of Human Sexuality,* *17,* 94–103.

Kaplan, D., Grobstein, R., & Smith, A. (1976). Predicting the impact of severe illness in families. *Health and Social Work, 1,* 71–82.

Kerner, J., Harvey, B., & Lewiston, N. (1979). The impact of grief: A retrospective study of family function following loss of a child with cystic fibrosis. *Journal of Chronic Disease, 32,* 221–225.

Krell, R., & Rabkin, L. (1979). The effects of sibling death on the surviving child: A family perspective. *Family Process, 18,* 471–477.

Krulik, T., Holaday, B., & Martinson, I. M. (Eds.). (1987). *The child and family facing life-threatening illness: A tribute to Eugenia Waechter.* Philadelphia: Lippincott.

Lauer, M. E., Mulhern, R. K., Bohne, J. B., & Camitta, B. M. (1985). Children's perceptions of their siblings' death at home or hospital: The precursors of differential adjustment. *Cancer Nursing, 8,* 21–27.

Lewis, I. C. (1967). Leukemia in childhood: Its effects on the family. *Australian Paediatric Journal, 3,* 244–247.

Lohan, J. A. (1998). Parents' perceptions of family functioning and sibling grief in families who have experienced the violent death of an adolescent or young adult child. *Dissertation Abstract International: Section B: The Sciences & Engineering, 59*(6-B), 2682.

Mahon, M. M. (1993). Children's concept of death and sibling death from trauma. *Journal of Pediatric Nursing, 8,* 335–344.

Mahon, M. M., & Page, M. L. (1995). Childhood bereavement after the death of a sibling. *Holistic Nursing Practice, 9*(3), 15–26.

Mandell, F., McAnulty, E., & Carlson, A. (1983). Unexpected death of an infant sibling. *Pediatrics, 72,* 652–657.

Martinson, I. M. (1980). Home care for the child with cancer. Final report (National Cancer Institute Grant CA 19490). Minneapolis, MN: University of Minnesota.

Martinson, I. M., Davies, E. B., & McClowry, S. G. (1987). The long-term effects of sibling death on self-concept. *Journal of Pediatric Nursing, 2*(4), 227–235.

Martinson, I. M., & Campos, R. G. (1991). Adolescent bereavement: Long-term responses to a sibling's death from cancer. *Journal of Adolescent Research, 6,* 54–69.

McCown, D. E. (1982). *Selected factors related to children's adjustment following sibling death.* Unpublished doctoral dissertation, Oregon State University, Portland, OR.

McCown, D. (1984). Funeral attendance, cremation and young siblings. *Death Education, 8,* 349–363.

McCown, D. E., & Davies, B. (1995). Patterns of grief in young children following the death of a sibling. *Death Studies, 19*(1), 41–53.

Mufson, T. (1985). Issues surrounding sibling death during adolescence. *Child and Adolescent Social Work Journal, 2,* 204–218.

Natterson, J. M., & Knudson, A. G. (1960). Observations concerning fear of death in fatally ill children and their mothers. *Psychosomatic Medicine, 22,* 456–465.

Nixon, J., & Pearn, J. (1977). Emotional sequelae of parents and sibs following the drowning or near-drowning of a child. *Australian and New Zealand Journal of Psychiatry, 11,* 265–268.

Opie, N. D. (1992). Childhood and adolescent bereavement. *Annual Review of Nursing Research, 10,* 127–141.

Osterweis, M., Solomon, F., & Green, M. (Eds.). (1984). *Bereavement: Reactions, consequences, and care.* Washington, DC: National Academy Press.

Parkman, S. E. (1992). Helping families say good-bye. *American Journal of Maternal Child Nursing, 7,* 14–17.

Payne, J. S., Goff, J. R., & Paulson, M. A. (1980). Psychosocial adjustment of families following the death of a child. In J. L. Schulman & M. J. Kupst (Eds.), *The child with cancer: Clinical approaches to psychosocial care—research in psychosocial aspects* (pp. 183–193). Springfield, IL: Charles C Thomas.

Pollock, G. (1962). Childhood parent and sibling loss in adult patients. *Archives of General Psychiatry, 7,* 295–305.

Pollock, G. (1978). On siblings, childhood sibling loss and creativity. *Annual of Psychoanalysis, 6,* 443–481.

Potts, S., Farrell, M., & O'Toole, J. (1999). Treasure weekend: Supporting bereaved siblings. *Palliative Medicine, 13*(1), 51–56.

Robinson, L., & Mahon, M. M. (1997). Sibling bereavement: A concept analysis. *Death Studies, 21*(5), 477–499.

Romond, J. L. (1990, Fall). "It's sad and you hurt a lot": Letters from bereaved brothers and sisters. *Journal of Christian Nursing,* 4–8.

Rosenblatt, B. (1969). A young boy's reaction to the death of his sister. *Journal of the American Academy of Child Psychiatry, 8,* 321–335.

Rudestam, K. E. (1977). Physical and psychological response to suicide in the family. *Journal of Consulting and Clinical Psychology, 45*(2), 167–170.

Stehbens, J. A., & Lascari, A. D. (1974). Psychological follow-up of families with childhood leukemia. *Journal of Clinical Psychology, 30,* 394–397.

Stephenson, J. (1986). Grief of siblings. In T. A. Rando (Ed.), *Parental loss of a child* (pp. 321–338). Champaign, IL: Research Press.

Tonkins, S. A. M., & Lambert, M. J. (1996). A treatment outcome study of bereavement groups for children. *Child & Adolescent Social Work Journal, 13*(1), 3–21.

Tooley, K. (1973). The choice of a surviving sibling as "scapegoat" in some cases of maternal bereavement—A case report. *Journal of Child Psychology and Psychiatry, 16,* 331–339.

Udell, M. E. (1995). Surviving sibling murder: An analysis of eight mental health interventions for inner-city youth. *Dissertation Abstract International: Section B: The Sciences & Engineering, 56*(6-B), 3467.

Van Riper, M. (1997). Death of a sibling: Five sisters, five stories. *Pediatric Nursing, 23*(6), 587–593.

Walker, C. L. (1993). Sibling bereavement and grief responses. *Journal of Pediatric Nursing, 8*(5), 325–334.

Wilson, L. R. (1995). Differences between identical twin and singleton adjustment to sibling death in adolescence. *Journal of Psychological Practice, 1*(2), 100–104.

Wolfenstein, M. (1966). How is mourning possible? *Psychoanalytic Study of the Child, 21,* 93.

Worden, J. W., Davies, B., & McCowen, D. (1999). Comparing parent loss with sibling loss. *Death Studies, 23*(1), 1–15.

Wright, T. R. (1999). The impact of suicide during childhood on the mourning process and psychosocial functioning of child and sibling survivors. *Dissertation Abstract International: Section B: The Sciences & Engineering, 59*(10-B), 5591.

Zelauskas, B. (1981). Siblings: The forgotten grievers. *Issues in Comprehensive Pediatric Nursing, 5,* 45–52.

Fifteen

Loss of a Pet

Morris A. Wessel

Morris A. Wessel, MD, received his BA from Johns Hopkins in 1939 and his MD from Yale in 1943. Dr. Wessel entered pediatric practice in 1951 and retired recently, after 42 years of serving parents and children in the New Haven, CT, area. A study that Dr. Wessel and colleagues entitled "Paroxysmal Fussiness in Infancy Sometimes Called Colic," published in 1954, is regarded as a classic in the field.

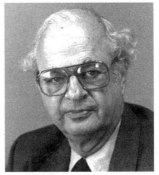

In 1969, Dr. Wessel joined Dean Emeritus Florence Wald of the school of nursing, the Reverend Edward Dobihal, chaplain of Yale New Haven Hospital, and Dr. Ira Goldenberg, professor of surgery at Yale Medical School, in a study of patients experiencing terminal illness. This group concluded, in 1971, that there was need for a separate facility for terminally ill patients in the New Haven community. This decision led the group to intensive planning and eventually to establish what is now the Connecticut Hospice, in Branford, CT.

Dr. Wessel became particularly interested in bereavement in children and adolescents. In 1993, he received the American Academy of Pediatrics Practitioner Research Award.

A Bit of History

Twenty-five years ago I was invited by Florence Wald, formerly dean of the Yale University School of Nursing, to participate in a study concerned with the care of terminally ill patients at the Yale New Haven Hospital. The observations and deliberations of this group, over a period of several years, led to the conclusion that there was definite need for a specific program and institution to provide home care and inpatient care for terminally ill patients. This led to the planning for what is now the Connecticut Hospice in Branford, CT.

Participation in these discussions alerted me to consider the bereavement process as family members experienced the loss of a beloved individual. I became aware of how little attention I focused on the needs of children at these tragic moments. I wondered how I, as a primary pediatrician, might support and enhance the capacity of parents and children to deal with significant losses. My interest in this sphere soon was recognized by parents and children in my practice, and by my colleagues. I am pleased that, as I reflect on the past 30 years, I can report that discussions of tragic losses became accepted in my role as a primary pediatrician. Many parents found it as appropriate to seek my advice when a death occurred as it was when a child presented symptoms of an upper respiratory infection.

I assumed that my experiences in handling tragic losses in families I served would enable me to adapt with equanimity when my dog, Dobisch, suffered inoperable cancer of the jaw. After much deliberation and soul searching, her increasing weakness, apathy, and poor appetite motivated me to take her to the veterinarian to be put to sleep. I was unprepared for the intensity of my grieving over the death of my companion of 14 years. The preparation and publication (*New Haven Register,* June 29, 1990) of this article eased considerably my mourning process.

An Unexpected Grief

Dobisch, our 14-year-old Siberian Husky–German Shepherd died a few weeks ago. This loss is far more painful than I ever imagined. I miss our walks, which she demanded at 10:15 each evening. I now become restless at this hour—I try to read the newspaper, or a novel, or watch television, but to no avail. Nothing relieves the empty feelings that well up as I realize that the evening jaunts, which we took for many years, are no longer possible.

What is it about my relationship with Dobisch that produced joy, comfort, and relaxation for the 14 years she was a member of our family? For me, owning a dog meant the anticipation, upon entering my home, of having Dobisch rise from her slumbers, wander to the front door, and greet me warmly—jumping up, barking, and wagging her tail. I took great comfort in knowing that she always would be there to offer this royal greeting. I continue now, as I open the door, to call her name, still hoping she might appear from somewhere.

Brisk walks or meandering strolls in the evening were more than valuable healthful exercises. Our nightly excursions possessed a deeper meaning. One satisfaction was the lack of demands in the relationship. True, when Dobisch wanted to go for a walk, she would bark and even rub against my body, until I roused myself from the television or the newspaper. But once out the door, we could walk in utter silence, or I could talk aloud and she would look up at me with an approving expression. I have organized many speeches and articles by talking aloud to Dobisch as we wandered through the neighborhood.

On other occasions, when things weren't going well, I bitterly cursed the world, shouting in anguish or in anger. I have cried aloud during these jaunts. Dobisch would look up, rub against my legs, communicating that she cared and wished to comfort me during these stressful moments. She demanded little in return. A pat on the head and a kind word were all she sought to let her know that I appreciated her efforts.

As a pediatrician, my days are full of demands. Each encounter with a child, parent, or colleague, important and satisfying as it may be, does drain one's energy. The limited demands of a dog, who gives much and expects little, provides a welcome relief from an exhausting day filled with intense interpersonal experiences.

On our evening strolls, we met an astonishing number of neighbors, and, over the years, I developed great respect for my neighborhood. On any evening, I have met a virologist, neurologist, surgeon, psychologist, teacher, my own rabbi and cantor, a Protestant minister at one of the churches on the green, and a Nobel Prize economist, to mention only a few friends who also took evening jaunts with their dogs. Conversations, which usually began with talk of the dog's health, what veterinarian they used, or what food they gave their pets, soon led into discussions of the daily events in the medical and university community, or to city, national, and international politics. I would rarely meet these friends, if not for our dogs.

Those evening walks with Dobisch were rejuvenating and relaxing moments, offering time for soul-searching, friendly conversations, introspection, and an opportunity to put the tensions of daily living aside. I miss those nightly jaunts a great deal.

Questions

1. What functions did the nightly jaunts with "Dobisch" serve?
2. Do you think it's valid to remark about the death of a pet, "It's only an animal"?
3. How would you ascertain the role a pet plays in the life of a person?

Part Four

Related Issues

Take Me Home

Bin Yao

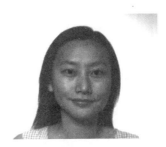

Bin Yao graduated in May 2002 from the MGH Institute of Health Professions at the Massachusetts General Hospital, and received her Masters degree in nursing. She is now working at South Cove Manor Nursing Home in Boston. She was born and raised in Tianjin, China. Before she moved to the United States with her husband, she worked as a dentist for 4 years in China.

In the summer of 1996, I finally decided to move to the United States with my husband. I was not afraid of facing a new environment—I just felt sad about leaving my hometown and my country. I quit my job, said good-bye to my friends, and went one last time to Hangchou, my mother's birthplace.

I could have afforded a plane ticket for that trip, but I decided to take the train, instead. There were too many interesting things I wanted to recall.

Hangchou was more than 1,000 miles from Tianjin, where I grew up. I remembered back to earlier trips to Hangchou as a child. Travel wasn't an easy thing when I was young, but back then, the railroads were the only means of long distance traveling. One round trip ticket to Hangchou cost 1 month of my mom's salary. The whole family had to save a lot before we could make a trip. By how much we spent on the tickets, I could tell how important it was to my mom, and to my family.

Since there were so many people traveling by train, we were lucky that we could always get seats. Still, we had to sit for more than 24 hours, before getting to Hangchou. That wasn't easy for a little girl. I remember one time when the train was so stuffed that we couldn't even move to the door. My dad had to open the window, dropped me out, and then climbed out himself.

Hangchou is a big city in Southern China. There is a huge lake inside the city, called "the West Lake." This ancient capital is famous partly because of this beautiful lake. People often call this place "heaven on earth."

I never enjoyed the trip when I was young, or understood why the family wanted to visit there every year. The first time, in my memory, I visited there with my dad was a winter when I was 5 years old. I was wearing my red leather shoes. The shoes were very pretty, but couldn't keep my feet warm in such a very cold place. I didn't know the South could be that cold. But I was told that they never used a stove to keep the rooms warm. They must have gotten used to it. My little feet suffered with cold, and my toes were stiffened and swollen like baby carrots—very sore.

As a kid, I sometimes did want to go there, to stay with my relatives, and to play with my cousins. People there were so nice. Once my uncle brought me to their rehearsal of a show. When they had a break, I went up on the stage. I didn't know where I got my courage, but I started singing on the stage. The whole stadium went quiet, and then, somebody started to play the piano. They even applauded after I finished. I felt I was a precious flower, being discovered for the first time. Quietly, I stayed there and enjoyed all the appreciation.

In the eyes of my relatives, I was always better and cleverer than my cousins were. They never hid that from me. I think that was part of the reason I wanted to be there. My grandpa liked me the most, because I could always answer the trivial questions he asked.

The railway didn't charge a child who was shorter than one meter, so I was able to get free rides several times. After talking to my other uncle, who also visited there periodically, they knew that my cousin had to pay half-price for a child's ticket for that trip. I told them that I bent my knees a little bit and was able to get another free ticket. (My long winter coat covered me so well that nobody ever noticed, not even my mom.) My cousin jumped out, laughed, and said that she finally was able to be better and worth more than I was. Everybody laughed. I did too.

As I grew up, I started to like the view of this city. I liked to walk along the West Lake in the early morning with my grandpa. He would tell me a lot of stories about the places we walked past. The lake was covered by light mist, like a beautiful bride hiding behind her veil. Willows waved their long arms, saying "Good morning" to a full pond of lotus. Bridges and buildings perfectly outlined the background of this quiet picture. It was like a dream, as pretty as my grandpa's stories.

One night, grandpa brought us to see the full moon by the lake. The moon, coming from the shadow of the nearby mountain, made the lake silver in front of us. Decorated by pieces of indistinct songs from faraway boats, the lake was so peaceful. Breezes, flying across the lake, touched my face with their warm hands, gently, like a mother touches her newborn baby. Tears came out from nowhere. This is my hometown.

I knew by then why, for 5,000 years, literati came here and never went back. There was also an emperor, defeated by intruders from the North, who had to move the capital to the South. He chose Hangchou as the new capital. Before he moved, he swore to the nation that he would come back. But half a year later, he even forgot he needed an army. He wasn't able to rebuild his nation, because of his love for this city.

My grandpa knew so many stories. I could never hear them all. He also taught me secrets about how to be successful. One day, he decided to take me on a hike. He said the lake was too big for a full cycle, but we could take bridges and islands that linked the two banks, and do a half-cycle. I had never done that before, and was very excited, but, after two bridges, I was tired already. I wanted to give up, but dared not speak out. Grandpa seemed to know what I was thinking. He asked me to take a break after each bridge, and offered one story for each break. Some of the bridges had really nice curved figures, while other places were named after very fascinating stories. After that, he told me that once we set a goal, we should never give up. He was 76 years old that year. I knew he should be more tired than I was, but he set a very good example for me.

Grandpa came to visit us the first time in my sophomore year. Mother invited him, because grandma had just passed away, and mother did not want him to be alone. Grandpa still told me stories, but he was not as happy as he was before. I knew he must miss grandma all the time. A few months later, he had a stroke; after a week of coma in the hospital, he passed away.

The last time I went to Hangchou, I visited my grandparents' cemetery in the drizzling rain. I didn't use an umbrella. I wasn't trying to hide my crying from others, but I really wanted the rain to wash my memory and make it clearer. I planted a flower in front of their grave to keep them company, and wished my flower could be as pretty as the stories they told me.

Visiting Hangchou became one of my family's traditions. But even now, I feel sad because the whole family never had a chance to visit there together. Last week, I called my mother, and she told me that they were planning another trip to Hangchou, and were going to take my 5-year-old nephew there this time. That's about the age I was when I first visited. That night, I had a dream. I went to a strange place, and was a little scared.

I started to walk. Things were getting brighter, and more familiar. I suddenly realized that I was in Hangchou again. Then I saw my parents, my relatives, and my grandpa. . . . Tears broke my dream apart.

After my last visit to my grandparents' cemetery, I moved to the States. Now I realize how far away I am from my hometown. I understand why my family visited Hangchou so often. The stories from my grandpa and the beautiful memories of my visits to Hangchou will be my comfort now, in this new and mysterious country.

Sixteen

The Role of the Social Worker

Kay Davidson and Zelda Foster

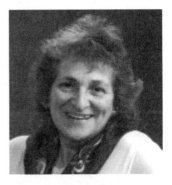

Kay Davidson is dean of the School of Social Work at the University of Connecticut. Prior to her career in graduate social work education and administration, Dr. Davidson was a social worker and social work administrator in health care settings in Britain and the United States. She worked with many cancer patients and conducted a national training program for social workers, based at Memorial Sloan Kettering Cancer Center. She is a graduate of the London School of Economics and the Columbia University School of Social Work. Her DSW degree is from the City University of New York. She co-ed- ited with Sylvia Clarke, Social Work in Health Care: A Handbook for Practice, *a two-volume compendium used by social work practitioners, teachers, and scholars.*

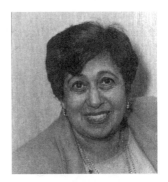

Zelda Foster, MSW, is the former director of a large social work department at the Brooklyn Veterans Affairs Medical Center. She is a cofounder and first president of the New York State Hospice Association. For more information on her background, see p. 79 of this book.

Authors' Note. This paper represents the practice wisdom of two social workers who worked with the dying for many years. It is presented from the social work viewpoint, but the ideas, the stresses, and the satisfactions are not those only of social workers. Their particular responsibility to patient and family may lead social workers to see many of these needs earlier and from a different perspective from other caregivers.

More than 35 years ago, on a hospital ward for veterans with Hodgkin's disease and leukemia, a young social worker felt alone and awed by what was taking place around her. She was participating in a ward culture where life-and-death events were unspoken and unshared, and young men were dying lonely and isolated. No one told them they were dying. Yet beneath the silence was turmoil and chaos; the terror of nightmares. This milieu conflicted with her feelings and her understanding of human need. This was the "conspiracy of silence" that prevailed until the 1960s. Patients and health care providers were becoming less able to repress the terror and pain of separateness the silence tried to cover (Foster, 1965).

Across the country, health care professionals were becoming attuned to what dying patients were experiencing alone, and what they as helpers were also experiencing. Their recognition grew, and they faced their own feelings. The conspiracy of silence and expectations of professional distance were challenged and overturned. Leaders in this revolution in dealing with dying were Dame Cicely Saunders in England and Elisabeth Kübler-Ross in the United States, both involved in treating, speaking, and writing. The influence of these charismatic women and the tenor of the times reshaped professional roles, fostered patients' rights, and placed value on emotional openness and sensitivity. Hospice evolved as a health care reform, growing separately from mainstream medical treatment, over the next two decades. Although increasingly accepted as a legitimate health care option and benefit, hospice often remained apart in structure, values, and supporters. Established medical care continued on a path of cure-oriented treatment, offering scant attention to symptom management and quality of life.

More recently, much needed attention has been paid to the values and effectiveness of hospice and palliative care. There is broader recognition of the holistic care needed by the dying and of deficiencies in end-of-life care (Hallenbeck, 2001). The Institute of Medicine has concluded that there exists a "combination of public fear, misinformation, and oversimplification that views misery as inescapable, pain as unavoidable, and public spending misdirected for people who are approaching death" (Committee on Care at the End of Life, 1997). The rapidly evolving discourse on palliative care in public and professional arenas is having a widespread impact. Palliative care is becoming a mainstream medical approach and is serving as a link between curative care and hospice care (Connor, 1999). As significant gaps in end-of-life care are noted, the call for reform is voiced by diverse practitioners, organizations, and foundations. Improving the quality of care available to the dying has expanded to become the province of all health professions.

The need for change in how care of the dying is administered is not new to social workers, who see the day-to-day absence of services, poor communication, and avoidance of physical and emotional pain on the part of health care providers. Ironically, this new climate of awareness of the needs of patients and families, and the concerted and effective voice of other professional groups, reduce the imperative for social workers to take a lead in encouraging greater attention to quality of life and the psychosocial component of health care. Because this shift in emphasis toward improved management of pain and broader psychosocial responsibility coincides with constraints on social work practice in some settings, social workers need to reestablish their roles in interdisciplinary work with dying patients.

The Contemporary Role of Social Work: Where Do We Find Social Work for the Dying?

At the beginning of the twenty-first century, roles of patients and their health care providers have become increasingly complex and challenging. Social workers continue to provide services in all the settings in which patients die: hospitals, hospice programs, and at home. The specific setting influences the nature of the service, but does not change the basic responsibility and mission. Commitment to help dying patients and their families is based on knowledge and skills in helping them cope with uncertain and often dreadful futures. Valuable services are provided when people are guided or accompanied on their journey.

For more than a decade, health care professionals have experienced constraints on their roles as helpers within complex institutions. The cultures of institutional settings and of acute care settings, with prescribed short stays for inpatients, may press heavily on staff and cause them value conflicts. Mixed institutional messages, seeking both quality and economy, place the health care worker between the needs of the patient and those of the institution, creating both stress and challenge. Fiscal restraints, regulations, narrowly defined roles and functions, and unrelenting work-loads have a broad impact on the capacity of hospital social workers to play their traditional role as psychosocial counselor, offering meaningful service to dying patients. In setting priorities, the social worker may feel pushed to attend more closely to obstacles to discharge, and may lose sight of stressful family relationships and impaired coping in the face of loss and life transitions. The discharge planning process, with an exploration of feelings, assessment of needs, review of options, and resolution through counseling, advocacy, and teamwork, is essential to the patient and the family.

Many traditional social work functions are subject to reconsideration, or are in actual jeopardy, in current hospital practice. Patients generally are admitted to medical and surgical units for very short stays, in a climate where discharge planning is the core of the institutional view of social work's domain. Pressure for early discharge requires the social worker to make a short-term care plan. The patient and family, however, are dealing with a long-term problem and need longer follow-up care and service. This is an item that has slipped from the institutional agenda. Continuity of care during the downward cycle and terminal phase of illness has not been a priority for acute care institutions. Consequently, the worker on a medical service, as a result of this institutional priority, has not followed dying patients or offered the continuity of care needed during terminal illness. The new attention to palliative care may create opportunities for social workers to offer less fragmented care, despite shortcomings of insurance coverage and home care services.

Whether in hospice or palliative care settings, social workers must now respond to new standards and imperatives, carving out their role in pain management, implementation of advance directives, and changes in education of health professionals. In social work programs in nursing homes, community agencies, residential care homes, and home care, there are new challenges and opportunities to join interdisciplinary efforts to improve quality of life. Social workers, who have long supported interdisciplinary collaboration, need to continue their participation in staff support groups and teamwork, as health care professionals face ethical challenges. Social workers can share with colleagues the professional skills that prepare them to influence social policy within or outside the institution, to recognize areas of unmet patient needs, and to advocate for change. Clinical work with clients cannot be separated from influencing the organization of the health care institution. Social workers can help to engage the institution in its efforts to respond to patient needs.

Institutional Responsiveness to Dying Individuals and Their Loved Ones

Although institutions have many biases and barriers to appropriate pain management for patients with advanced cancer or other terminal illness (Glajchen, Blum, & Calder, 1995; Melzack, 1990; Rhymes, 1996), there is growing recognition of the trauma of illness and acceptance of the opportunity to simultaneously offer aggressive treatment and to focus on the quality of life available to patient and family. As palliative care moves into the forefront and commands a new focus, social workers can help patients and families, earlier in their illness, to review care options and make decisions. As advocates, social workers can bring their influence to bear at multiple levels, using technical knowledge and interdisciplinary leadership skills related to pain management and palliative care.

In the past decade, social workers have moved into management roles in organizational development, human services, and staff training. They bring their professional knowledge to provide leadership in the new patient-focused care environment, calling attention to service gaps and offering ways for the institution to meet them. At the same time, social work departments in many health care institutions have been diminished by staff reductions and loss of supervisory personnel. To facilitate their full participation in improving care of the dying, social workers need to develop their own institutional voice and form effective liaisons with community-based agencies, such as Cancer Care Inc. and new community networks. Through these connections, social workers can play pivotal roles, with a wide range of services to help patient and family cope with the effects of illness. These include supportive counseling based on "tuning in," listening, and using educational skills and therapeutic interventions in complex interpersonal conflicts, family upheavals, situations of stress, and role changes. Some patient needs are created by the illness, but many are precipitated by the treatment imperative.

Social workers are developing an important place in pain and symptom control for dying patients. They may provide direct treatment of symptoms through hypnosis or imagery techniques. Others are integral members of interdisciplinary pain control teams. There is a significant body of knowledge about pain and its emotional and social contexts (Glajchen, 2001; Saunders & Baines, 1989). Social workers also contribute to the treatment team's effectiveness, by assessing the psychosocial aspects of pain and helping to plan individualized interventions (Altilio, 1999; Loscalzo & Bucher, 1999; Glajchen et al., 1995). Social workers often find their major role in activities that educate and change attitudes of health care professionals. This is achieved both by assuming institutional leadership in training, and through participation in the work of individual care teams.

Examples of such leadership may currently be seen at Beth Israel Hospital in New York, where Myra Glajchen, DSW, is a director of the Palliative Care Institute, or at Johns Hopkins, in the work of Matthew Loscalzo, codirector of the Center for Cancer Pain Research at Johns Hopkins Oncology Center. Zelda Foster co-edited *The Hospice Heritage,* published by Haworth Press, and Grace Christ and Mary Sormanti, of Columbia University School of Social Work, are principal investigators of the Soros Foundation's Project on Death in America (PDIA), providing resources to advance social work practice related to death and dying. More than 20 social work leaders already have been selected for these PDIA awards. Karen Davie brought her social work background to the presidency of the National Hospice and Palliative Care Organization (NHPCO). These are only a few of the numerous social workers making important contributions to new initiatives (Project on Death in America, 2000).

Hospice as Model for End-of-Life Care

One reason for social workers' involvement in the work of death and dying and palliative care is their knowledge and respect for the hospice form of treatment. Some social workers joined other health professionals and clergy to promote the hospice approach to care early in its development (Foster, 1979). By 1996, more than 3,000 hospice programs across the United States served 450,000 dying patients (Beresford & Connor, 1999). Hospice programs, modeled on Saunders's work, focus on providing opportunity for dignity, freedom from physical pain, and support in emotional pain, to provide compassionate care (Saunders, 1999).

The work of social workers in hospice is more clearly defined, because hospice legislation assures their inclusion. They carry out functions that deepen the connections between patients and their families, promoting closeness and opening up relationships between patients and staff. Such health care professionals encourage intimacy, meaningful communication, problem solving, and resolution. Closeness to the emotional pain of patients and families, and continuous exposure to death and loss, are consequences of this work. Rusnack, Schaefer, and Moxley define the generic foundation of social work there as ecological, enabling "social workers to coordinate the transaction of the terminally ill patient with his or her family and with the hospice staff as well as to coordinate transactions between the hospice and its service network" (1988, p. 18).

Hospice care is noted for providing comfort and support, as well as advocating a flexible approach to terminal care that responds to individual situations. The hospice approach also helps to reduce barriers to talking about dying (Kastenbaum, 1999). A similar philosophy permeates palliative care programs in general hospitals, where a team approach to pain and suffering requires coordination and attention to patient and family alike. Sherman (1999) suggests that palliative care emphasizes "the humanistic qualities of the patient, the family and the care providers and alleviates suffering within the context of these intrapersonal and interpersonal relationships."

Satisfactions and Problems in the Social Work Role

From their earliest days in health care, social workers have known it was important to focus on feelings experienced by patients about their illness. Nevertheless, emphasis has often gone to other aspects of biopsychosocial needs (Johnson et al., 1990; Davidson & Clarke, 1990). More time and effort may be invested in locating resources, advocacy, and interdisciplinary activities, than in direct, one-to-one supportive counseling with sick patients or their emotionally stressed family members. Social workers experience strain between the needs of patients for help with their reactions to their illness, especially in life-threatening situations, and the needs of the caring institution and its staff. The work of a social worker on a medical service may actually involve extensive counseling with patients and families who are facing impending death, but that work may go mostly unrecognized by the broader public (Davidson, 1983). The social worker assigned to an AIDS or oncology program can develop a population approach attuned to meeting a range of needs, because the psychosocial component of care is more broadly understood by the clients, families, hospital administrators, and relevant government agencies (Clarke, 1983).

Throughout the 1990s, those groups able to capture public attention and funding were empowered, but less dramatic work was underfunded. Currently, social workers in AIDS programs, hospice programs, palliative care, and oncology services have opportunities to undertake more extensive counseling with patients and families than those in other parts of the health care system. The social worker assigned to a medical or surgical service has always worked with dying patients, but may have had limited professional support for such work, and consequently, limited satisfaction (Davidson, 1985). The demands are heavy, but, since services are acute rather than "death and dying," the health care worker's emotional stress goes unrecognized. Social workers need the support of colleagues who understand the commonality of the work and the disparity of support.

Social workers, like other health care professionals, may lack explicit education or training in work with the dying (Christ & Sormanti, 1999;

Committee on Care, 1997). The MSW, the practice degree, has a full curriculum to deliver broad-based knowledge and skill for the gamut of social work roles and may offer only limited elective work on death and dying. Social work graduates may find themselves caught in avoidance of in-depth attention to the physical and emotional pain that their patients or their families wish to express or discuss (Davidson, 1985; Christ & Sormanti, 1999). There is a great need for postgraduate education and training, and a host of new educational technologies to deliver content on death and dying. Online teaching of social work and interdisciplinary courses related to death and dying, such as those at Cancer Care Inc., could be readily available with limited funding. Intensive training courses, modeled on the social work with cancer program at Memorial Sloan Kettering Cancer Center, need to be widely accessible and connected to hospice and palliative care programs. Availability of postgraduate courses, some funded by the Soros Foundation, can provide support for social work practitioners to apply their expertise and take leadership roles in the continuing development of end-of-life care.

Social workers coordinate a broad range of services to patients coping with serious illness. The profession is committed to systemic change and mediation, to assure organizational responsiveness to individual needs. Humanizing the care of the dying and bereaved, and concern for underserved and vulnerable populations, are essential to sound social work practice. This assures the long-range alliance of the profession with values held by enlightened, humane public opinion.

Pressures Affecting Priorities

In most hospitals, the time available is short for providing services to patients being transferred home or to other facilities. How do social workers and other professional staff handle the conflict between agency demands and the needs of patients? In some situations, workers use the time pressures, along with finding the painful situations of their clients hard to bear, to rationalize cutting time spent with patients (Davidson, 1983). Desperate pressures of time and avoidance of dying contribute to the gaps in social work services to dying patients. A study by Christ and Sormanti found that, although social workers were aware of new techniques and interventions that might help patients with symptoms of terminal illness, they lacked "time and training to master some of these new skills" (1999, p. 89).

Staff other than social workers also experience the stress of working with patients who die, and may be subject to loss and grief. Recognition of personal mortality is inevitable for social workers and others involved with dying patients and their families (Dunkel & Hatfield, 1986). How can it be handled better? Avoidance or withdrawal have been common practices. We have known for years that workers may be caught between the two powerful forces of professional commitment to the client and very human personal reactions (Reid, 1977). Literature on death and dying, and the establishment of organizations devoted to the care and study of the dying, focus attention on the needs of health professionals, as well as patients, for support and encouragement in their efforts (Committee on Care, 1997; Taylor-Brown, Johnson, Hunter, & Rockwitz, 1981). Workshops and publications on dying and bereavement have proliferated, and there is a reduction of taboos about discussing death, as evident in the publication of multiple books and such journals as *Illness, Crisis and Loss, The Hospice Journal,* and *The Journal of Psychosocial Oncology.*

Practice wisdom suggests that helping patients put their affairs in order, grieve, and face separation from their loved ones and their unfulfilled hopes can bring workers satisfaction (Pilsecker, 1979; Macks, 1988). The profession continues to move in that direction, but it is difficult work. Workers know they have time pressures, but is that the basis for reluctance to become involved in this painful work? The social worker, in considering the outcome of his or her work, may reflect on ways in which he or she may have failed the dying client. This process can cause discomfort and doubts about competence. All too often, the worker has to live with uncertainty about the efficacy and value of work with a client who dies (Pilsecker, 1987; Dunkel & Hatfield, 1986; Macks, 1988).

Role Blurring

The overlapping roles and functions of doctors, nurses, chaplains, and social workers require dialogue and the development of agreement about social work's role and function, both internally within the social work profession, and with other disciplines, about social work's role and function (Davidson, 1990). For many years, social workers introduced a point of view about the psychosocial component of care that was shared by few other professionals. Now that others emphasize those care components, the primacy of the social worker's role is challenged. In response, social workers need to focus on bringing knowledge and skills in family and group dynamics, community organizing, cultural mediation, conflict resolution, resource location, staff support, and decision making to interdisciplinary team work. In making their role more visible, social workers can participate on teams, despite the context of time shortages and institutional pressures and imperatives.

Social workers on oncology units have various stresses related to the particular characteristics of the setting. They are on an interdisciplinary team and are working with dying patients. However, their domain varies with respect to direct service to patients and families. They may find themselves in turf battles with nurses. They may have conflict with the values of the treatment unit and may have their own viewpoint on the value of aggressive treatment. Often, there is little attention to dying patients who are no longer candidates for treatment. On the other hand, some patients will be treated beyond the point where their quality of life is preserved or bettered. The social worker's highlighting of the disparity between the doctor's recommendation for aggressive treatment and the patient's wish to die may sometimes alienate the worker from medical colleagues and from distressed families. Social workers have to be mindful that they too can be influenced by the powerful impact of institutional philosophy. The development of living wills, advance directives, and health-care proxies will support the efforts of health care professionals and enhance patient participation in decision making.

Kulys and Davis (1987) have noted that social work's long-standing difficulty in reaching consensus with other health care professionals about their domain has made it possible for nurses equally to claim the psychosocial realm of care as their own. Nurses' claim to the psychosocial area has been strengthened by lack of clarity on the part of patients and families about social work's role. Often, the social worker is seen only as important in the provision of concrete services, such as financial planning, home care arrangements, or Meals-on-Wheels (Kulys & Davis, 1987). Energy, imagination, and effort can overcome the barriers to communication resulting from differences in the socialization of various disciplines and their views of interdisciplinary collaboration (Mizrahi & Abramson, 2000).

Healing the Hurt of Work with the Dying

Early in the development of hospice, the term *staff pain* was used to refer to the impact of work with dying patients on health care providers. Davidson (1985) reports social workers' concerns with identification, fear, and feelings of loss. The stresses of their work carry over from professional to personal lives, and they feel vulnerable and intensely aware of the preciousness of time. Workers report on the difficulty of watching the patient's deterioration and death, and they are troubled by sharp awareness of their identification with their clients (Davidson, 1983). More has been written about identifying stress than about how to help health care workers cope with it.

Being open to pain and grief also opens the worker to healing, through the satisfaction of caring, helping, and sharing. This is more vivid in hospice work, but the principles operate everywhere. A similar complex set of reactions is observed in social work with AIDS patients. Such work offers prestige, resources, and opportunities to undertake research and to teach. This is a partial compensation for the anguish and turmoil of exposure to chronic illness and sometimes painful death in young people. In work with AIDS patients, social workers experience many stressors, but there is gratification from their contribution and use of creative skills.

Recently, a change has occurred in the work with AIDS patients. The clarity of the issue of death and dying has been lessened by the development of high technology treatment that causes AIDS to be viewed and treated as a long-term chronic disease. Once again, social workers welcome progress in physical treatment, but the problems faced by patients with a disease both chronic and fatal is complicated. The social worker and other AIDS workers offer help with living under difficult, uncertain conditions in the constant shadow of approaching death.

Helping Colleagues

As a colleague, and often a friend of those offering physical treatment, the social worker understands and respects their determination to treat. Their ethic is to do all that they know how to do, as long as life lasts. However, the social worker also understands and is responsible for helping the patient who knows that life will soon be over and wants to consider, with help, having aggressive treatment stopped. To know and understand this conflict is to live with a painful and unavoidable dilemma. How can the worker deal with this conflict? First comes honest acceptance of the dilemma. As part of the treating institution, the social worker is responsible for helping the patient with needs, other than medical, that exist because of the disease and its treatment. Second is interdisciplinary work, calling on other professionals to meet the patient's needs. Third is the recognition that, if cure and care are not a dichotomy, while the effort to cure goes on, social well-being must also be preserved. What does the patient want, and how can the social worker help? When the patient wants above all else to go home to die, a difficult conflict can arise, if other health care providers are unaware of this desire. When the patient wants to attend to legal and financial matters in preparation for death, and the social worker helps with this, interdisciplinary peers may disapprove.

To try to find ways of communicating the patient's and the social worker's viewpoint to medical colleagues is a heavy responsibility. Concern about these matters, without the perceived ability to influence administrative and medical decisions, is difficult to handle. Being seen by team members as valuable because one helps patients and families, which is part of the total team approach, is of value so far as it goes. It does not offset the sadness deriving from differences in power, perceptions, and values, when the nature of service for final days of life for the patient is the issue at hand. Teamwork has elements of both support and frustration, as team members help each other with their painful work, but also on occasion disagree about their approaches.

The worker's role as a provider of support for other staff varies. This exemplifies how the lack of a clearly defined role as helper, both to clients and staff, increases stress. When social workers take on the task of support to other team members who find it hard to cope with dying patients, it is helpful if that role can be recognized and valued. The form may be a structured support group, or it may be informal availability to staff to talk about the feelings and experiences they have had with patients. Social workers may provide training to help staff cope with anger and other strong emotions in their work (Monroe, 1998). There are rewards, whether this work is formal or informal, but, because education and a sense of helpfulness are known to lessen stress, institutionalizing this role can help social workers gain gratification from being recognized as knowledgeable as well as helpful. Otherwise, despite the gratification of offering support to others, there is isolation for the social worker who wonders, Who is there for me to talk to? One worker asks, "Where do I go? We give a depressed doctor a chance to talk, but the social worker is left without help. Consultation and supervision are not used that way" (Davidson, 1983). Our knowledge of ways to offset stress needs to be brought to bear on, and influence, our own planning structures.

Programs That Enhance Worker Satisfaction

In work with dying patients, teamwork and exchange of skills take on special meaning, as staff members are touched by loss, and by seeing pain, suffering, and disruption of lives. They must tackle their own feelings of fear, frustration, and helplessness in the face of it all. They must resolve the conflict between impulses to avoid what is distressing and a sense of responsibility to meet the needs of clients and colleagues. Social workers need to identify whether their own needs are being met and find ways to experience greater satisfaction. Supervisory and peer support programs help social workers recognize and cope with their own reactions to life-threatening illness, death, and bereavement, so that patient care remains a priority and the work is more satisfying (Mor & Laliberte, 1984). As we seek to understand the effects of human loss and to unearth resources to triumph over it, we are continually made aware of our own unresolved and still painful feelings of past losses and traumas. In discussing these with peers or mentors, we create that sharing, supporting community that can continue to be alongside our patients and families in sickness and anxiety, in despair and hope, and through bereavement (Earnshaw-Smith, 1988, p. 121).

Another example of a staff support program is the formation of a peer group that emphasizes mutual aid, exchange of information, and coping skills (Davidson, 1983). As such a group provides support and offers continued learning, it can empower staff through the common theme of sustaining the ability to be helpful to patients, families, and colleagues from other health disciplines. Ongoing learning and support can help workers feel their difficulties are common to other workers and to become better able to cope, as a result of the support received. Such groups can heighten self-awareness and help staff modify aspects that adversely affected their work, learning alternate ways to cope from other group members.

Programs to provide support and guidance require that social work managers advocate for and establish peer support groups and multidisciplinary mutual aid groups. Social workers need to be placed on teams, to reduce isolation and provide opportunities for mentoring and professional development. In hospice programs, staff meet with visiting professionals and teach informally, as well as in formal classes and seminars. The sense of achievement, competence, and practical expertise, which is fostered by teaching about their work, is a valuable source of support to staff.

The current growth of opportunities for social workers in work with the dying is exemplified in the work of Chachkes and Foster (2001), who note a "catalytic mushrooming of important projects and new initiatives." They point to the work of NHCPO's Social Work Section, under the leadership of Mary Raymer, in producing extensive material dealing with competency, practice standards, and outcome measures. Also, the developing networks of shared communication and information are inspiring major new endeavors. They note that foundation funding expands as successes are noted and that the achievements of social workers in the area of end-of-life care form a model for social work's potential contribution to the broader health care system.

Conclusion

We have experienced both pain and commensurate growth during the past 35 years, as we have worked with the dying and their loved ones, as we have taught students and workers, and as we have tried to communicate courage and joy to those who want to learn about this work. The window that opens into the inner life of the client facing death offers a way to help them, but it also opens the social worker to mourning, grief, the reawakening of past losses, and unresolved conflicts. To protect ourselves from empathy with the dying is to hide ourselves from a part of life that concerns us all, and that offers healing along with pain.

Discussion Questions

1. What would you want to see happen in your own setting to improve care of dying patients and their loved ones?
2. How could you further develop the expertise that you are demonstrating in the area of end-of-life care, to bring you to a level of leadership?

References

Altilio, T. (1999). Building a pain management program: Background and basics. *Oncology Issues,* Vol. 14, No. 5. Special pain management supplement, p. 7–8.

Beresford, L., & Connor, S. R. (1999). History of the National Hospice Organization. In I. Corless & Z. Foster (Eds.), *The hospice heritage: Celebrating our future* (pp. 15–31). Binghamton, NY: Haworth Press.

Chachkes, E., & Foster, Z. (2003). Taking charge: Social work leadership in end-of-life care. In J. Berzoff (Ed.), *End-of-life care for social workers.* New York: Columbia University Press.

Christ, G., & Sormanti, M. (1999). Advancing social work practice in end-of-life care. *Social Work in Health Care, 30*(2), 81–99.

Clarke, S. (1983). Hyman J. Weiner's use of systems and population approaches: Their relevance to social work practice in health care today. *Social Work in Health Care, 9*(21), 5–14.

Committee on Care at the End of Life, Division of Health care services, Institute of Medicine. (1997). *Approaching death: Improving care at the end of life* (M. J. Field & C. K. Cassel, Eds.). Washington, DC: National Academy Press.

Connor, S. R. (1999). New initiatives transforming hospice care. In I. Corless & Z. Foster (Eds.), *The hospice heritage: Celebrating our future* (pp. 193–203). Binghamton, NY: Haworth Press.

Davidson, K. (1983). *Development of a support program for social workers serving cancer patients*. Unpublished dissertation, City University of New York, New York.

Davidson, K. (1985). Social work with cancer patients: Stresses and coping patterns. *Social Work in Health Care, 10*(4), 73–82.

Davidson, K. (1990). Role blurring and the hospital social worker's search for a clear domain. *Health and Social Work, 15*(3), 228–234.

Davidson, K., & Clarke, S. (1990). *Social work in health care: A handbook for practice*. Binghamton, NY: Haworth Press.

Dunkel, J., & Hatfield, S. (1986). Countertransference issues in working with persons with AIDS. *Social Work, 31*(2), 114–117.

Earnshaw-Smith, E. (1988). *Annual report and yearbook*. London: St. Christopher's Hospice.

Foster, Z. (1965). How social work can influence hospital management of fatal illness. *Social Work, 10*(4), 30–35.

Foster, Z. (1979). Standards for hospice care: Assumptions and principles. *Health and Social Work, 4*(1), 118–127.

Glajchen, M. (2001). Chronic pain: Barriers and strategies for clinical practice. *Journal of the American Board of Family Practice 14*(3), 211–218.

Glajchen, M., Blum, D., & Calder, K. (1995). Cancer pain management and the role of social work: Barriers and interventions. *Health and Social Work, 20,* 200–206.

Hallenbeck, J. (2001). Best practices in the care of the dying. *Annals of Long-term Care, 8*(7), 39–44.

Johnson, H., Atkins, S., Battle, S., Hernandez-Arata, L., Hesselbrock, M., Libassi, M., & Parish, M. (1990). Strengthening the "Bio" in the biopsychosocial paradigm. *Journal of Social Work Education, 26*(2), 109–123.

Kastenbaum, R. (1999). The moment of death: Is hospice making a difference? In I. Corless & Z. Foster (Eds.), *The hospice heritage: Celebrating our future* (pp. 253–270). Binghamton, NY: Haworth Press.

Koocher, G. (1979). Adjustment and coping strategies among the caretakers of cancer patients. *Social Work in Health Care, 5*(2), 145–150.

Kulys, R., & Davis, M. (1987). Nurses and social workers: Rivals in the provision of social services. *Health and Social Work, 12*(2), 101–112.

Loscalzo, M., & Bucher, J. (1999). The COPE model: Its clinical usefulness in solving pain-related problems. *Journal of Psychosocial Oncology, 15*(3/4), 93–117.

Macks, J. (1988). Women and AIDS: Countertransference issues. *Social Casework, 69*(6), 340–347.

Melzack, R. (1990). The tragedy of needless pain. *Scientific American, 26*(2), 27–33.

Mizrahi, T., & Abramson, J. (2000). Collaboration between social workers and physicians: Perspectives on a shared case. *Social Work in Health Care, 31*(3), 1–24.

Monroe, B. (1998). Social work in palliative care. In D. Doyle, G. W. Hanks, & N. McDonald (Eds.), *Oxford text of palliative medicine* (2nd ed.) (pp. 867–880). New York: Oxford University Press.

Mor, V., & Laliberte, L. (1984). Burnout among hospice staff. *Health and Social Work,* 9(4), 274–283.

Project on Death in America Newsletter. (2000). Soros Social Work Leadership Awards, 1(4).

Pilsecker, C. (1979). Terminal cancer: A challenge for social work. *Social Work in Health Care,* 4(1), 369–379.

Pilsecker, C. (1987). A patient dies—a social worker reviews his work. *Social Work in Health Care,* 13(2), 35–45.

Reid, K. (1977). Nonrational dynamics of the client–worker interaction. *Social Casework,* 58(10), 600–606.

Rhymes, J. A. (1996). Barriers to palliative care. *Cancer Control Journal,* 3(3), ___.

Rusnack, B., Schaefer, S., & Moxley, D. (1988). "Safe passage": Social work roles and functions in hospice care. *Social Work in Health Care,* 13(3), 3–19.

Saunders, C. (1999). Origins: International perspectives, then and now. In I. Corless & Z. Foster (Eds.), *The hospice heritage: Celebrating our future* (pp. 1–7). Binghamton, NY: Haworth Press.

Saunders, C., & Baines, M. (1989). *Living with dying: The management of terminal disease* (2nd ed.). New York: Oxford University Press.

Sherman, D. W. (1999). End-of-life care: Challenges and opportunities for health care professionals. In I. Corless & Z. Foster (Eds.), *The hospice heritage. Celebrating our future* (pp. 109–121). Binghamton, NY: Haworth Press.

Taylor-Brown, S., Johnson, K., Hunter, K., & Rockwitz, R. (1981). Stress identification for social workers in health care: A preventive approach to burn-out. *Social Work in Health Care,* 7(2), 91–100.

Seventeen

Palliative Care Competencies for Physical Therapists

Theresa H. Michel

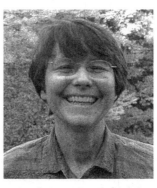

Terry Michel is an associate clinical professor of physical therapy at the MGH Institute of Health Professions at the Massachusetts General Hospital. She works part time as a cardiopulmonary clinical specialist in Physical Therapy Services of MGH. She was board-certified by the American Physical Therapy Association in 1989, and recertified in 1997 as a cardiopulmonary clinical specialist.

For the past 13 years, T. Michel has been engaged in teaching an interdisciplinary course on pain, at the MGH Institute of Health Professions. Students from the graduate programs in nursing and physical therapy have taken this course together, with occasional occupational therapists and social workers also registering from time to time.

She has been teaching a component of a Harvard Medical School course called "Pain: Exploring Issues from Sensory Receptors to Societal Concerns," over a 3-year period. The course director was Ruth L. Fischbach, from the Division of Medical Ethics, Department of Social Medicine.

T. Michel has helped lead discussion sections for the MGH Cares About Pain Initiative for 3 consecutive years (2000–2002), sponsored by May Day Pain Resource Center.

Recent research endeavors have involved a study investigating aerobic conditioning in chronic low back pain patients. She has conducted qualitative research in the area of defining the physical therapy role in palliative care. She is the physical therapist in charge of the exercise component of the life-style arm of the Diabetes Prevention Project, a project funded through the National Institutes of Health and directed by Dr. David Nathan, of the MGH.

She is currently enrolled in a doctoral program in clinical physical therapy. This study was done in partial fulfillment of that degree.

Physical therapists are often involved in end-of-life care of patients with chronic diseases and with terminal illness. Practice settings, where these patients are seen by physical therapists, include hospices, acute care settings, home care settings, and rehabilitation centers, where oncology or palliative care floors include a team of rehabilitation health care workers. Palliative care has recently become a specialty within the field of medicine, and has become a focus for the development of standards of care for the nursing profession (C. Dahlin, personal communication, June 11, 2000). Very little has been written for the physical therapist who wishes to prepare for work in this challenging area of practice.

As early as 1972, Purtilo published an article on dealing with dying patients, in which she identified Kübler-Ross's stages of grief (1969), and discussed the difficulties that physical therapists have in dealing with dying patients. She emphasized the death-denying society of the Western world, which fails to understand the psychological and spiritual/philosophical interpretations of the death experience, and which fails to help members of the society develop means to cope with one's own and other's feelings about death. She reiterated that the majority of people in Western society face death only suddenly, when it must be faced, without preparation (Purtilo, 1972).

Can physical therapists provide palliative care to terminally ill patients that addresses palliative care principles and themes? A recent publication for physical therapists described a qualitative study of three dying patients and identified areas needing to be addressed by physical therapists who wish to deal with dying patients (Mackey & Sparling, 2000). They restate the World Health Organization's 1990 principles of Palliative Care:

1. Affirm life and regard dying as a normal process.
2. Neither hasten nor postpone death.
3. Provide relief from pain and other distressing symptoms.
4. Integrate the psychological and spiritual aspects of patient care.
5. Offer a support system to help patients live as actively as possible until death.
6. Offer a support system to help family members cope during the patient's illness and their bereavement.

Aligned with these principles are the four themes that Mackey and Sparling gleaned from their three patients who were dying of cancer:

1. Social relationships—satisfaction with happy memories, comfort in their present support, and grief for future separations

2. Spirituality—lifelong religion-based and personal values used to guide everyday living
3. Response to personal mortality—acceptance, but with sadness for losses, and fear of the timing and manner of the dying process
4. Meaningful physical activity—longing for physical activities important to them

From the point of view of the patient, physical therapists can perform many tasks that satisfy the need for "a good death." In another study, in which relatively healthy elderly subjects were interviewed about what they believed were necessary ingredients of "a good death," five domains were identified for quality end-of-life care:

1. Receiving adequate pain and symptom management
2. Avoiding inappropriate prolongation of dying
3. Achieving a sense of control
4. Relieving the burden on loved ones
5. Strengthening relationships with loved ones (Singer, Martin, & Kelner, 1999).

An inspection of each of these five domains suggests that physical therapists are prepared to help provide a good death. For some of the symptoms that have been identified at the end of life, physical therapists bring a unique and expert skill mix to the patient. This is especially true for the symptoms of fatigue, dyspnea, and pain (Cohen & Michel, 1988). The symptoms of anxiety and depression may be indirectly approached by physical therapy techniques. It is true that many other symptoms may be equally distressing to dying patients. The physical therapist who works within a team must recognize the need for, and call on, skilled practitioners who can help patients to manage symptoms like dysphagia (speech therapist) or constipation (nurse).

The physical therapist does not have a direct role in avoiding inappropriate prolongation of dying. Decisions about providing life-support interventions are not in the hands of the physical therapist. Given that the patient and/or family must make these decisions, the physical therapist may facilitate discussions around these decisions, by being an active listener and a good communicator, and relating the patient's intent to the team.

The achievement of a sense of control is often facilitated by the physical and occupational therapist. For many patients, the greatest fear is the loss of the ability to care for themselves, and to make decisions. Tigges and

Sherman (1983) report that, out of 50 dying patients, 40 said their greatest need was to be independent in self care, and 46 said the second most important need was to resume their occupational role. The goal setting that physical therapists do with each patient, on a daily basis, clearly addresses these needs, which are based on functional tasks important to the patient and the family.

Helping patients to relieve the burden on loved ones is identified as a physical therapy task of educating the patient and family. Much of this education is in helping patients to maintain independence as long as possible in transfers, gait, and activities of daily living. It also involves teaching family members the skills for making these tasks efficient and effective. Many other kinds of burdens are feared by dying patients, however. The burden of grief and loss is addressed by all members of the team. The physical therapist may learn, through experience, that, in certain relationships with patients, they "connect," which allows for a sharing of meaningful experiences. By "presencing" and showing honest affection for patients and their family members, it is possible to minimize some of the burden of grief and loss, which is inevitable with the death of a loved one (Becker, 1993).

Strengthening the dying person's relationships with loved ones needs to be supported by all members of the palliative care team. By including family and significant others in the circle of caregiving, and facilitating conversations among them, team members can help to achieve this goal of the dying patient (Singer et al., 1999).

These studies prompt one to ask: What are physical therapist's palliative care tasks? Unfortunately, there is not much literature to guide the physical therapist. In 1984, Toot reported on the role of physical therapy in hospice. She suggested that physical therapists provide care aimed at physical well-being, play an important role in educating patients and families and fellow health professionals, and function as a team member (Toot, 1984). She defines a number of educational needs of physical therapists:

1. An appreciation by the physical therapist of his own death
2. An appreciation of what it is like to be dying
3. An appreciation of the needs of family members
4. An appreciation of the roles of other personnel and how those roles may be affected by a patient's death
5. An appreciation of the cultural aspects of death and dying

Physical therapists play a significant role in symptom management of dying patients. Toot (1984) emphasizes modalities used by physical therapists to alleviate pain, such as heat, cold, and TENS. She also describes the importance of educating patients to use efficient and safe movement patterns, partly to minimize pain, and perhaps to reduce fatigue or shortness of breath. The prevalence of specific symptoms in the final weeks of life has been identified in several studies. In general, fatigue or asthenia is the most frequently reported one, followed by anorexia, dry mouth, confusion, constipation, dyspnea, dysphagia, anxiety and depression, paralysis, and pain. Less frequently reported are sleep disturbances, cough, nausea, hemorrhage, vomiting, diarrhea, and dysuria (Conill et al., 1997). Coyle, Adelhardt, Foley, and Portenoy (1990) reported fatigue as the number one problem, followed by pain, generalized weakness, sleepiness, confusion, anxiety, weakness of legs, dyspnea, nausea, decreased hearing, depression, loss of appetite, inability to sleep, weakness of upper limb, cough, and others. Some of the differences in these reports reflect changing symptoms as death approaches. Pain seems to recede during the final days, and dyspnea and confusion become more frequent (Mercadante, Casuccio, & Fulfaro, 2000).

Examples of how physical therapists help to evaluate clinical symptoms of fatigue, dyspnea, and pain include the use of fatigue rating scales, such as the Borg Rating of Perceived Exertion (Borg, 1970). These scales are often used in conjunction with performance tests, such as functional evaluations or a 6 minute walk test. Physical therapists then develop safe and precise exercise prescriptions to permit patients the efficient use of their energies in performing meaningful tasks. Physical therapists are skilled at interpreting appropriate and inappropriate exercise responses in patients and base their treatment decisions upon these responses, so that fatigue or dyspnea are not made worse and the patient's quality of life is optimized (Cohen & Michel, 1988).

Similarly, dyspnea is a symptom that is addressed by physical therapists. They interpret pulmonary function tests, arterial blood gases, and pulse oximetry, and assess breathing patterns and breath sounds. They teach patients specific techniques, including pursed lips breathing and diaphragmatic breathing, to help relieve the symptom of dyspnea. They also titrate oxygen and assist patients in secretion clearance and cough effectiveness. These all may help patients to reduce the distressing symptom of dyspnea (Zadai & Irwin, 1992).

Pain is evaluated by physical therapists, then is addressed, based upon the origins of the pain. Bracing, positioning, and splinting can be very helpful techniques. Massage, modalities, and exercises can be useful. In dying patients, various techniques, such as distraction, imagery, and relaxation, often are found effective in providing coping strategies for pain. Anxiety and depression may also respond to these techniques (Michel, 1985).

All health care providers engaged in palliative care must have excellent communication skills, in order to assess needs and resources of patients and families, and to work effectively in a team. The special problems of working in a team must be a part of the physical therapist's skill mix. The hospice team approach involves blurring of professional roles, and functions much more as a sharing team (Toot, 1984). For this work, the physical therapist must be willing to step forward and step back, which requires sensitivity to the status of interactions among team members. Skills involved are identified as the art of active listening, the ability of clear expression, facilitation of team interactions, and extemporaneous innovations (Toot, 1984).

This review of the literature suggests a number of questions that could be pursued in order to elucidate the practice characteristics of physical therapists in the area of palliative care. However, for this report, the following question was addressed: How should a physical therapist treat a dying patient? Stemming from this question come further questions about what the knowledge base is that is needed for physical therapy care of terminally ill patients, who these patients are who are seen by physical therapists, what the skills are that therapists bring to this kind of care, how skilled physical therapy practitioners are, and how did they learn their skills and how should they learn them. The approach to answering these questions was to develop palliative care competencies for physical therapists using literature and professional experience, to ask a cohort of practitioners to rate themselves on these competencies, and then to follow up with a structured interview to elaborate on some of the answers.

Participants in the phase of rating competencies included 12 volunteer physical therapists who rated themselves on each competency. Three of these respondents volunteered for follow-up interviews. All three therapists interviewed were female and graduated from physical therapy programs at different universities. In the following, the three respondents are referred to as No. 1, No. 2, and No. 3.

Structured Interview Results

The meaning of palliative care in a physical therapy context was explored by a number of questions.

TABLE 17.1   Guiding Questions Used in the Interviews of 3 Subjects

1. Is there a different skill mix needed for patients who are near death, compared to those with chronic diseases that are terminal, but who are not actually dying?
2. Do physical therapists learn compassion and empathy, or are these natural qualities?
3. In helping patients with coping strategies, are there different styles, or is there an evolution of skills involved, moving from relying primarily on others to provide scripts or techniques on to short-term goal setting with assurances of positive reinforcement through successful goal achievement?
4. In entry-level education at the doctoral level, is it an expectation that higher level competencies involving analysis, synthesis, and evaluation should be the goal? If so, how will this be taught in the realm of palliative care?
5. Is there a better way to teach these competencies than on the job, which is characterized by trial and error learning?

What Types of Patients Do You See for Palliative Care?

The type of patients who are considered by the subjects included "anybody in an end-of-life situation," "cancer," "people with chronic diseases who are terminal, but not necessarily dying," and "anyone who needs care given to them that is not going to significantly change their diagnosis, but it might make them more comfortable."

What Type of Treatments Have You Given Patients in a Palliative Care Setting?

The type of treatments rendered by physical therapists were in the areas of symptom management and functional status maintenance.

No. 3 said: "The patients that I see are rehab patients in the acute care setting. Because of the nature of their treatment, there always seems to be some medical complication that keeps them from going on to rehab. Some of them bounce back every 10 days. So they're doing the same thing in rehab that they're doing here with me. I do a lot of functional things with them, especially when it comes to quality of life for some of them."

No. 2 emphasized meeting the patient's goals: "What's important are their goals. If the patient would like an exercise program that they can do every day because they're bed bound, then that's part of our role with that patient. Or their goal is to get home, and they need to transfer to a commode, and I think sometimes it's amazing what patient's can do who really want to get home. I think that patients kind of guide you in terms of what you're working on. And I think we're also working with a patient's family members and looking for answers from them in a bed level program or in transfers. A physical therapist could take a direction, like more impairment-based, or more functionally based, but I think you probably end up addressing impairments of strength or range, and function."

No. 1 said: "I try to think of what to do that will help this patient's symptoms, more than whether their pain is interfering with any function, so I ask what can we do about this patient's pain? Can I call the pain service, can I ask the pain service if there's something else they could do for the patient before they receive their physical therapy, or if there's a device that would help with pain?"

What Does It Mean to You When I Suggest That You "Connect with a Patient Who Is Dying?"

In response to a question about what it means for physical therapists to "connect with" a patient who is dying:

No. 3 said: "I guess it's taking into consideration the patient's emotional and psychological well-being, in the context of their functional status, and knowing their goals. The nature of just having those daily conversations with them, getting to know them, and getting to know their families, takes it into a little more personal level. You probably have a little bit more of a connection with some of these patients than you would with your just-average patients that you're seeing."

No. 1 said: "Connecting with a patient means helping a person be at peace with what they're doing before they die. We certainly don't want to take away hope that things could improve. Sometimes patients can be so frustrated, because they think they can't do something—it hurts too much. It's easier if they can be at peace with everything. Trying to help someone along in the process of finding peace is a weakness for me. I think I've gotten a little bit better at it, but it's been hard for me. There are always others helping them along. I think there are others who are better at it than me."

No. 2 said: "Connecting with a patient means allowing them to say what they need to say, and being able to respond to that in a professional way, but also in an understanding way. Allowing the patient to connect with whomever, allowing them that freedom to connect or not connect with you. I don't feel an urgency to connect with a dying patient, I kind of let them dictate that."

Do You Ever Ask About What Would Help the Patient Live Most Fully in the Time They Have Left?

In response to the question, "Do you ever ask about what would help the patient live most fully in the time they have left?" all three therapists replied that they always ask the patients what their goals are, but they never put a time frame on the question.

What Do Compassion and Empathy Mean in a Physical Therapy Context?

No. 1 felt that making the patient most comfortable was the important part. No. 2 stated that these terms apply to all patient populations, and that "knowing the patients and recognizing when patients and families need something, when they've had enough, when you need to alter your therapy accordingly" was what constitutes compassion and empathy. No. 3 said: "We try to alleviate whatever discomfort and pain the patient may be having, but at the same time we have the perspective of making the connection with the patient, considering their feelings, their needs in the context of what we're doing with them."

How Do Physical Therapists Help Patients Cope?

No. 3 said: "I think we teach some basic coping strategies, even if it's just breathing techniques. We may help them correlate these with relaxation techniques learned from the social workers or the psychologist. We may tend to identify the need and call on the social worker as a means to solving a problem, so we can keep our focus on the treatment and the functional things, letting them emotionally deal with the social workers. We may try to incorporate whatever strategies they are given into their functional skills that we are doing with them."

No. 2 replied: "I think we sometimes give patients coping strategies. Like, each day you need to get up and get out of bed, or take a shower. We kind of set up a vision of their day, so they can live day to day and not become overwhelmed and think about the big picture. We can give them a routine, something that is task- and goal-oriented, so that they can feel achievements along the way. We make sure the tasks are limited and smaller, so that they can experience some success."

No. 1 stated: "I have a pretty good relationship with a social worker on the floor, and I always am looking for what I should be doing with a patient. I ask, What should this patient do? or, What would the social worker do if the patient says such and such? Will the patient benefit from saying things a certain way or taking a certain approach? That's worked very well for me."

How Do Physical Therapists Document Patient Status in Palliative Care Situations So That We Can Justify Continuing to Work with These Patients?

In answer to a question about how physical therapists document patient status in palliative care situations, given that we must justify to insurance companies that patients are making progress, No. 1 said: "I think we can always make reasonable goals by changing the focus to family teaching. There's always something to work on right down to the end, when there's absolutely nothing to do." No. 2 said: "I have learned to make my goals more appropriate to the level of the patient. I put in my note that the goals for a given patient might vary more frequently, or that the patient's ability to meet the goals might vary. A constant goal is patient and family education." No. 3 replied: "Yes, there are problems at times, trying to give measurable goals to justify why you are there working with the patient. I try to do this in terms of caregiver education. If you can somehow justify physical therapy in terms of quality of life, and through small progress that shows, such as in gait training, then I would write about that. I have used the Guide [The Guide to Physical Therapy Practice, 2nd edition, Physical Therapy, January 2001, Vol. 81 (No. 1)] in trying to come up with goals sometimes. And I always pick other people's brains."

Do You Consider the Practice of Palliative Care an Advanced Level of Physical Therapy Practice?

Questions that centered around the level of practice in palliative care were addressed. These questions arose when a nurse educator commented that the palliative care competencies used in the self-assessment were below an entry-level expectation for nursing, and that physical therapists should be expected to practice at an equally high level, since they graduate with a master's degree (D. Wilkie, personal communication, June 11, 2000). In answer to the questions, Do you practice at a higher level? Would advanced competencies more accurately reflect what you do? the therapists responded as follows.

No. 1: "I certainly practice higher level skills today than I did 3 or 4 years ago, when I first came, and wasn't so secure. Now I synthesize and analyze things more than just describing the pain. Or I think I try to think of what to do that will help this patient more than just that their pain is interfering with therapy. Now I might think what can I do about this patient's pain. Can I call the pain service, ask the pain service if there's something else they could do for the patient? I look at the alternatives more than just describe the issues. I definitely do that a lot more than I used to, but I know I have a lot more to go."

No. 2 stated: "I think that, initially, I was identifying and describing patient needs, but now I do more of an analytic approach when I'm studying exactly what they need, from my standpoint, from the team, or from referrals or other resources that I can identify. It's more of a synthesis."

No. 3: "Yes, I think I probably do practice at a higher level. I think a lot of it comes from experience in doing it, and so, once you have been doing it, you pull more in and definitely it becomes more analytical."

The Impact of the Practice Setting

When the palliative care competencies were distributed to several rehabilitation hospital physical therapists, as a comparison group to those in the acute care hospital, the feedback from two respondents was that, in a rehab palliative care setting, palliative care goes far beyond symptom management and deals primarily with quality of life and functional/meaningful tasks for each patient. Therefore, this question was asked of the three interviewees: Does the nature of palliative care vary depending upon the practice setting: symptom management vs. functional status goals? There was general agreement among the three participants in this interview that both symptom management and functional/meaningful task goals are a part of palliative care, regardless of the setting.

Conclusions

A fascinating array of questions are generated by these interviews. Because these three therapists agreed on several questions and disagreed on a number of others, possibly their individual experiences reflect some of the differences among them. When the two publications describing symptoms of patients during the last 4 weeks of life (Coyle et al., 1990) and symptoms of patients during the final week of life (Conill et al., 1997) are compared, there is clearly a change in the symptoms experienced by dying patients as they near their deaths. Thus, if physical therapists are working with more patients who are at one of these final stages, rather than at an earlier stage, they may be confronted with different kinds of symptom management challenges. They may focus more on functional goals earlier in the trajectory of the final dying experience. Two of these three practitioners focused on functional status maintenance, which involved goal setting for exercise and for functional tasks. One therapist was more concerned with pain management. These differences could reflect the different types of patients being treated, or the nearness of death for these patients. Therapist No. 1 treats orthopedic oncology patients before and after bone transplantation. Pain may be an overwhelming issue for these patients. Therapists No. 2 and No. 3 treat neurologic oncology and bone marrow transplant patients, respectively. Functional goals were the most meaningful focus, in that these patients were more likely to regain functions (because bone marrow transplants offer a good deal of recovery of strength and function) or were likely to be involved in rehabilitation.

None of the respondents mentioned the symptoms of fatigue or dyspnea in their management of their patients. Perhaps these symptoms are not unique to palliative care, and therefore therapists were thinking more about specific tasks related to care at end of life.

The psychosocial skills of the three therapists were brought out in their responses to questions about "connecting" with a patient, and the definitions of compassion and empathy. All of them showed a willingness to be personal and humane, by having difficult conversations with patients and families and by being understanding of their needs and desires. This willingness is essential for therapists to meet the definition of *caring* proposed by Levetown and Carter (1998): "Caring is not merely a sentimental attitude toward someone or something, but an integral component of human relationships, without which the essence of humanity is lost" (p. 1107). Two of the three volunteers emphasized comfort and pain relief in their descriptions of being compassionate. The third therapist felt that being tuned in to patient/family needs and feelings was her way of showing empathy. All three participants showed their willingness to be caring.

The answer to the question about helping patients to cope yielded a continuum of responses. No. 1 referred to getting guidance from a social worker and relying on that guidance. No. 3 mentioned specific strategies she teaches patients, and using the guidance of other team members. No. 2 really described a holistic approach to helping patients cope, which involves restructuring the patient/family thinking about their day, each day they have together. These three answers seem to describe a progression of skill level, going from following a script to setting up an entire frame of reference for a patient. This may be an evolution of skill learned by physical therapists as they gain experience practicing in palliative care.

All three respondents agreed that they began their physical therapy careers practicing all of these skills at a lower level of competency, and have advanced to higher cognitive and affective levels. Much of this advancement represents a learning process gained through personal study and through asking questions of senior therapists and other members of the team. Some of this advancement came to them by trial and error learning, from a number of patients for whom they were responsible, and from their families. There was agreement that more preparation in their entry level education would have made this process more efficient and smoother.

There is a significant level of interest in palliative care practice among acute care practitioners who deal with cancer patients, and with patients with chronic, slowly fatal illnesses, such as kidney failure (patients on dialysis), congestive heart failure, chronic obstructive lung diseases, and neuromuscular diseases such as amyotrophic lateral sclerosis. This is inferred from the number of volunteers for the interview conducted for this study (6/12). The three interviewees expressed a preference for treating these kinds of patients. They all believe that they are becoming more effective in their treatments as their experience grows, and that they learn from all members of the team as they continue to work as a team member. This is encouraging from the standpoint of developing a better experience for dying patients in America, in the future.

The major limitation was the small sample size, both in the self-assessment phase of this study, in which 12 therapists responded to the original competency list, and also in the number of interviewees chosen. The major reason for the selection of only three respondents was the time constraints on both the investigator and the volunteers for this study. Interviews required 45–90 minutes, and were done either during lunch hour or after work. These results would have been more generalizable, if a broader sample of therapists could have been interviewed. In fact, six volunteered for the interviews, which indicated a surprising level of interest in this topic. The three who actually were interviewed were selected solely based on availability at convenient times.

The purpose of this exploratory study was to investigate the nature of palliative care as it is performed by physical therapists and to solicit ideas for learning and teaching palliative care in the future. Structured interviews of three volunteer physical therapists provided the data gathered for this report.

Possible directions for future studies are highlighted by this investigation. In the area of knowledge and skills required by physical therapists for practice in palliative care, however, there remain many avenues to explore. Is there a different skill mix needed for patients who are near death, compared with those with chronic diseases that are terminal, but who are not actually dying? Do physical therapists learn compassion and empathy, or are these inherent qualities? In helping patients with coping strategies, are there different styles, or is there an evolution of skills involved? Such an evolution might involve moving from relying primarily on others to provide scripts or techniques, to relying on the self to help patients with short-term goal setting, using positive reinforcement through successful goal achievement.

This investigation is enlightening in several ways. Physical therapists are choosing to work with dying patients, and choosing to learn from them and their families, and from the partnership that is derived from effective team interactions. The need for coherent, interdisciplinary plans for the care of dying patients is being recognized throughout the health care professions. It is important for physical therapists to be among those professionals who design the optimal plan for quality palliative care for the future.

Discussion Questions

1. What are the implications of the interviews reported in this chapter for teaching future professionals how to be competent practitioners for end of life care?
2. What interaction might there be between a clinician's years of experience, exposure to types of patients (e.g., orthopedic, oncology, postoperative vs. bone marrow graft recipients) and the closeness to death of these patients in terms of clinician's competence in: a) symptom management, b) "connecting" with the patient, and c) goal setting?
3. Would there likely be a difference between how clinician's "connect" with a patient among the various professions—e.g., medical doctors, registered nurse, physical therapist, occupational therapist, social worker?

References

Becker, G. (1993). Continuity after a stroke: Implications of life course disruption in old age. *Gerontologist, 33,* 148–158.

Borg, G. A. V. (1970). Perceived exertion as an indicator of somatic stress. *Scandinavian Journal of Rehabilitation Medicine, 2,* 92–98.

Cohen, M., & Michel, T. H. (1988). *Cardiopulmonary symptoms in physical therapy practice.* New York: Churchill Livingstone.

Conill, C., Verger, E., Henriquez, I., Saiz, N., Espier, M., Lugo, F., & Garrigo, A. (1997). Symptom prevalence in the last week of life. *Journal of Pain & Symptom Management, 14,* 328–331.

Coyle, N., Adelhardt, J., Foley, K. M., & Portenoy, R. K. (1990). Character of terminal illness in the advanced cancer patient: Pain and other symptoms during the last 4 weeks of life. *Journal of Pain & Symptom Management, 5,* 83–93.

Kübler-Ross, E. (1969). *On death and dying.* New York: MacMillan.

Levetown, M. L., & Carter, M. A. (1998). Child-centered care in terminal illness: An ethical framework. In D. Doyle, G. W. C. Hanks, & N. MacDonald (Eds.), *Oxford textbook of palliative medicine* (pp. 1107–1117). Oxford, UK: Oxford University Press.

Mackey, M. K., & Sparling, J. W. (2000). Experiences of older women with cancer receiving hospice care: Significance for physical therapy. *Physical Therapy, 80,* 459–468.

Mercadante, S., Casuccio, A., & Fulfaro, F. (2000). The course of symptom frequency and intensity in advanced cancer patients followed at home. *Journal of Pain and Symptom Management, 20,* 104–112.

Michel, T. H. (1985). Pain. *International Perspectives in Physical Therapy, 1,* 3–72.

Purtilo, R. B. (1972). Don't mention it: The physical therapist in a death-denying society. *Physical Therapy, 52,* 1031–1035.

Singer, P. A., Martin, D. K., & Kelner, M. (1999). Quality end-of-life care: Patient's perspectives. *Journal of the American Medical Association, 281,* 163–168.

Tigges, K. N., & Sherman, L. M. (1983). The treatment of the hospice patient. *American Journal of Occupational Therapy, 37,* 235–238.

Toot, J. (1984). Physical therapy and hospice. *Physical Therapy, 64,* 665–671.

Zadai, C. C., & Irwin, S. (1992). Exercise pathophysiology: Pulmonary impairment. In C. C. Zadai (Ed.), *Pulmonary management in physical therapy* (pp. 37–53). New York: Churchill Livingstone.

Eighteen

Thanatology: Its End and Future (with Special Reference to Euthanasia)

Larry R. Churchill

Larry R. Churchill is Stahlman Professor of Med-ical Ethics and adjunct professor of religious studies at Vanderbilt University. In 1991, Professor Churchill was elected to the Institute of Medicine, in recognition of his work on ethics and health policy. His most recent publication is a volume edited with Marion Danis and Carolyn Clancy, Ethical Dimensions of Health Policy *(Oxford, 2002).*

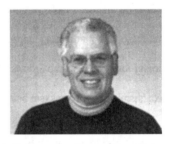

> Every art and every inquiry, and similarly every action and pursuit, is thought to aim at some good.
>
> Aristotle, *Nicomachean Ethics*

The End of Thanatology

Thanatology can be defined as the study of the phenomena of death and the attendant psychological strategies employed to cope with them (Merriam-Webster's, 1985). Such studies are very useful to health care practitioners, family, and friends of the terminally ill, and to the dying themselves—indeed, to anyone engaged with human finitude. The achievements of the past several decades in thanatology, to which this volume is additional witness, are great. But great past achievements do not guarantee a great future, or even any future at all. In fact, the factors that created the need for thanatology as a modern field of study are perhaps stronger than ever, and the diversions to which the field is susceptible are more powerful.

The factors that created the need for thanatology are well known. In the broadest sense, they are the forces of modern industrial and postindustrial urbanization and mobility. A mobile urban population is one uprooted from the land, from intimacy with the rhythms of nature, and from the witness to the life cycles evident in intergenerational households. The result is an acquisitive-possessive individualism, a notion of the good life as mostly equivalent to consumption of material commodities. In such a social ethos, both dying and aging are out of place, and the dying and aged are perceived as alien. The identification of self with material goods (or the ability to command them) leads, of course, to a truncated and stunted assessment of human abilities, so that reliance on experts of all sorts is increased. This is no less true for dealing with terminal illness than in the rest of life.

Yet my major concern is not with these cultural and psychological forces of death-denial. My chief concern is with the transformation of thanatology into a set of beliefs, techniques, and practices that will divert its true purpose, and thereby hasten its demise. My worry is not that thanatology will fail because of a frontal attack on its agenda, but because its agenda will be co-opted by, and subsumed under, other forces.

This essay is concerned with ends, in a dual sense. First, has thanatology reached its end or *finis*? Is it finished? Is thanatology dead, or will it become so because it is (or may become) subsumed under the current enthusiasm for physician-assisted suicide, or cost-containment or palliative care, or some other cause related but extrinsic to it? But this sort of talk presupposes the more important question: What is the end of thanatology, where *end* means purpose or aim (*telos*)? What should those who study and practice thanatology be striving to do? Being clear about the answer is essential. Otherwise, thanatology will forsake its end (*telos*) and become merely a means, and this, I argue, will spell its end (*finis*).

The task of identifying the purpose of thanatology is not a difficult one. The purpose of thanatology is to better understand human dying, *in order to serve the dying*. Without the moral impetus of this agenda, thanatology becomes voyeurism, necromancy, or a tool of various professional and social agendas.

One type of diversion involves using the dying to serve our needs, rather than using our work to serve theirs. A classic case is the use made of the work of Elisabeth Kübler-Ross, whose "stages" of dying (denial, anger, bargaining, depression, acceptance) have too frequently become normative expectations that health professionals place on patients. In this profession-alized, lock-step progression, the stages do not answer the needs of the dying, but rather are responses to the anxiety of caretakers, to have intellec-tual and social control, and thereby emotional control as well (Churchill, 1979). A second and more disturbing slippage occurs when thanatology changes from pursuit of knowledge about dying to pursuit of death. Here, the temptation is to see active euthanasia, or promotion of professional assistance in suicide, as a form of caring for patients *in extremis*. Because this diversion is so powerfully before us, I will spend this essay addressing it. Resisting the equation of a "good death" with mercy killing may be the most important task ahead for assuring that thanatology has a future.

The Reduction of Thanatology to Euthanasia

Marcia Angell, an editor of the *New England Journal of Medicine,* said that doctors should prepare themselves to debate the issue of active euthanasia once more (1988). There is evidence everywhere that she is right. In California, an effort to place a proposed euthanasia law on the fall, 1988, ballot failed for what most believe were organizational, not substantive, problems (Angell, 1988). The sponsoring organization, Americans Against Human Suffering—a branch of the Hemlock Society—may succeed on their next try.

Until recently, euthanasia was an illegal but widely practiced act that enjoyed broad public support, in the Netherlands. It is now legal. Although exact figures are disputed, some claim that between 6,000 and 10,000 persons are euthanized annually in the Netherlands (Harper, 1987). Four conditions must be met. The patient must be competent, must be suffering beyond tolerance, must request euthanasia repeatedly and consistently, and the act must be performed by a physician in consultation with another physician not involved in the case.

Public opinion polls show that a majority of Americans favor the legaliza-tion of euthanasia under certain circumstances (Roper Organization, 1988). Angell also cites a survey that indicates that a majority of doctors also favor legalizing euthanasia, although roughly one half of those who favor its legalization also indicated that they would not perform it (1988). Physician-assisted suicide meets with even greater public approval, with the majority of people favoring it in every survey taken over the past two decades.

If morality were merely a matter of sociology, that is, a description of what values people hold, then the debate would be over when the surveys are complete. But, of course, the ethical question is not, Do people favor euthanasia? but, Should they?

Yet, my primary interest here is not in debating the merits of active euthanasia, but in noting how the preoccupation with it may come to overshadow the study of and care for the dying. If this occurs, euthanasia may be presented as an answer to the "problem" of dying, and the "management" of the incurable patient. The chances that this will occur were in fact enhanced with the publication of a horrific tale of active euthanasia reported, without attribution, in the *Journal of the American Medical Association,* and entitled "It's Over, Debbie" (Anonymous, 1988).

"It's Over, Debbie" is a bad case for debating euthanasia, but a paradigmatic case for how the pursuit of death as its own end can engulf the proper goal of thanatology service to the dying person.

> The call came in the middle of the night. As a gynecology resident rotating through a large, private hospital, I had come to detest telephone calls, because invariably I would be up for several hours and would not feel good the next day. However, duty called, so I answered the phone. A nurse informed me that a patient was having difficulty getting rest, could I please see her. She was on 3 North. That was the gynecologic-oncology unit, not my usual duty station. As I trudged along, bumping sleepily against walls and corners and not believing I was up again, I tried to imagine what I might find at the end of my walk. Maybe an elderly woman with an anxiety reaction, or perhaps something particularly horrible.
>
> I grabbed the chart from the nurses station on my way to the patient's room, and the nurse gave me some hurried details: a 20-year-old girl named Debbie was dying of ovarian cancer. She was having unrelenting vomiting apparently as the result of an alcohol drip administered for sedation. Hmmm, I thought. Very sad. As I approached the room I could hear loud labored breathing. I entered and saw an emaciated, dark-haired woman who appeared much older than 20. She was receiving nasal oxygen, had an IV, and was sitting in bed suffering from what was obviously severe air hunger. The chart noted her weight at 80 pounds. A second woman, also dark-haired but of middle age, stood at her right, holding her hand. Both looked up as I entered. The room seemed filled with the patient's desperate effort to survive. Her eyes were hollow, and she had suprasternal and intercostal retractions with rapid inspirations. She had not eaten or slept in two days. She had not responded to chemotherapy and was being given supportive care only. It was a gallows scene, a cruel mockery of her youth and unfulfilled potential. Her only words to me were, "Let's get this over with."
>
> I retreated with my thoughts to the nurses' station. The patient was tired and needed rest. I could not give her health, but I could give her rest. I asked the nurse to draw 20 mg of morphine sulfate into a syringe. Enough, I thought, to do the job. I took the syringe into the room and told the two women I was going

to give Debbie something that would let her rest and to say good-bye. Debbie looked at the syringe, then laid her head on the pillow with her eyes open, watching what was left of the world. I injected the morphine intravenously and watched to see if my calculations on its effects would be correct. Within seconds her breathing slowed to a normal rate, her eyes closed, and her features softened as she seemed restful at last. The older woman stroked the hair of the now sleeping patient. I waited for the inevitable next effect of depressing the respiratory drive. With clocklike certainty, within four minutes the breathing rate slowed even more, then became irregular, then ceased. The dark-haired woman stood erect and seemed relieved.

It's over, Debbie.

Note first the time of day, namely, the middle of the night—not a great time to consider weighty choices. Note that the physician is a physician-in-training, a resident. He is, as are most residents, sleep-deprived, impatient, dreading his call, but dutifully obedient to it. The patient is unknown to him, and he gathers a short biological, but not a social or personal history, from the nurse. His affective response is extremely truncated. He thinks only, "Very sad." We know that he identifies with this young woman's "unfulfilled potential." Her current state he describes as a "gallows scene . . . a cruel mockery."

Note that he takes a highly ambiguous request as a wish to be mercifully killed, and he announces his own intentions in an equivocal way to the patient and her female attendant. There is no move to clarify this patient's wishes, or to otherwise relieve pain. There is only a highly egocentric consideration of options, all from the perspective of what the physician could and could not do. With a moral sovereignty usually only attributed to deities, the physician describes himself as retreating to the nursing station with his thoughts. Note here the absence of an essential ingredient in ethics—conversation, explicit, deliberative reasoning, public discourse. The resident retreated to a solipsistic self-sufficiency, which doomed him to moral clumsiness and callousness from the very beginning. No doubt he felt vindicated when, after he killed the patient, everyone "seemed relieved."

Missing Agency

Others have commented on the haste, ignorance, and ineptness that mark this case. And these are all important. Yet there is something else more central here: the lack of self-conscious, moral agency. The case is described from an administrative posture, as if the resident were looking down upon and depicting his own acts in an impersonal way—as if for the medical record. But the medical record does not constitute a moral record or a human record in which the dying person is central.

The administrative posture is one in which actions are treated as occurrences, that is, as having happened, but without disclosing the interiority of the actor. We actually know very little about what this resident thought or felt. There is, to be sure, first-person language, but it describes events like actions, not personal assessment postures. "I answered the phone . . . I grabbed the chart . . . I asked the nurse . . . I took the syringe . . . I injected the morphine . . . I waited." This is a marvelous physical topography of events, but it discloses little of the moral psyche of the actor. It reads like Caesar's regal summation: "I came, I saw, I conquered." Indeed, conquest may be precisely the right metaphor, as I will discuss later. But at least "I conquered" tells us what Caesar thought he was doing, in a way "I injected" does not and cannot.

In short, this is a case bereft of moral agency, a case, if you will, of a missing agent. So the question we must put to the resident is, "What did you think you were doing when you injected this woman with a lethal dose?"—in various senses of that question. For acknowledging explicitly what we think we are doing as we do things is what separates us as moral beings from the rest of the animal kingdom. Acknowledging what we are doing as we act is how we can know what ends we seek, and whether our actions are true to those ends.

I mean to suggest that this is a bad case in several senses. It is "bad" in the sense of "morally wrong," because it describes acts that are unthinking, hasty, callous, morally clumsy, and criminal. It is also "bad" in the sense of "inadequate," because it tells us next to nothing about who did these acts. It is, in this latter sense, a very poor case to rekindle the euthanasia debate, but an illuminating case to exhibit the reduction of care of the dying to killing the dying.

If we are to read accounts of physicians who have killed their patients from motives of mercy, I hope we will find in those accounts recitations of anguish, conflictedness, stress, deep worries about their character, detailed discussions with patients, families, colleagues, and others, profound ambivalence, lack of certainty, citation of authorities on all sides of the issue, accounts of courage, or perhaps regret, and, overall, a quality of reflection worthy of the act. Anything less is demeaning to both patients and physicians alike. Anything less illustrates that death has become the end sought, rather than service to the dying.

Sovereignty

The one time we are privy to the deliberations of this resident, he is focused on a choice centered on his own capabilities: "I could not give her health," he reflects, "*but* I could give her rest." What is revealed here is a fallacy couched in a euphemism. The euphemism perpetrated by this physician on his readers, and perhaps on himself, is that "rest" is a proxy for *death*. So it should read, "I could not give her health, but I could give her death." The fallacy is black-and-white thinking. It's *either* health *or* rest, that is, health *or* death.

What is disclosed here is a picture of a frustrated physician, a physician held captive by his powerlessness, his inability to help. What is depicted are two persons in suffering and in need of mercy, one the patient who suffers physically and the other the physician who is tortured psychologically by his lack of control and inability to relieve pain. Couched in the rhetoric of pain relief or rest, he offers the only thing he has—death. So, like Caesar, the resident came, saw, and conquered, not the patient's disease, but the patient's suffering. But to do so, he conquered the patient as well. Killing this patient was, I submit, an act comprehensible as an attempt to redeem frustrated sovereignty, an act calculated to wrest control from the enemy. When restoration to health is impossible and pain control difficult, one can still offer death. Only death is not here offered, but foisted on the patient as a way to relieve the doctor. Euthanasia is then a continuation of medicine's conquest motif. If patients cannot be cured, they can at least be killed. Killing a patient, rather than letting her die a painful death, retains control. It is a way of remaining sovereign, of being active rather than (helplessly) passive; it is a way of avoiding defeat. For, just at the point of being vanquished by disease, physicians can seize the initiative and proclaim mastery over their adversary. Thus is killing patients seen as an act of great courageousness. It is, unfortunately, the courage of a bungler and a fool, an agent who has not acted, but *reacted* with simplistic and egoistic ineptness. This physician has covered the pain of his inadequacies by dispatching the patient, the object of his suffering, and everyone, we are reassured, "seemed relieved." The physician retained his sovereignty, but at a heavy price, an essential part of which is moral self-deception.

Brutalization

A moral agent who does not acknowledge personal presence in his actions, and who entertains a need for sovereignty over his actions, is particularly susceptible to being brutalized by them. Brutalization is, in fact, the natural outcome of postures of sovereignty. Aristotle, wiser than most who have followed him, said that human beings are made for social interaction, and those who do not have it are either brutes, or gods (1941). Human beings need conviviality, fellowship, social ties, and conversation. This is especially so in ethics, and it is no accident that Aristotle thought of ethical reflection as a dimension of social life, a branch of politics, of life together in a political order, not as a free-standing discipline.

We can pretend to a godlike sovereignty, if we wish, but we are human beings, and the desire to be like gods leads us to be like brutes, to brutalization, in the most rudimentary sense—our moral sensibilities become no better than (perhaps worse than) those of animals.

The posture of sovereignty I have been attributing to the resident in the Debbie case is a form of psychological distancing. It is a way of being removed and remote from full moral awareness of one's acts; it is the assumption of an administrative posture, orchestrating and observing from above. The result can be seen in the factlike recitation we noted previously: "I retreated with my thoughts, . . . I injected, . . . I waited."

I refer to the result as "brutalization," to invoke Aristotle and his notion of ethical reflection as irreducibly social, not exercised by either brute animals (who lack a convivial order) or gods (who are sovereign). More-over, I suggest that the moral retreat and distancing frequently associated with killing is a desire for sovereignty, that is, a desire for the sort of unrestrained power over events associated with gods. Human beings, how-ever, being human, fail at sovereignty and the result is we become like brutes, or if you will, brutalized. Montaigne put it somewhat differently, but was emphasizing the same dynamic. "Two things I have always observed to be in singular accord," he says, "supercelestial thoughts and subterranean conduct." Montaigne (1965) continues:

> We seek other conditions because we do not understand the use of our own, and go outside of ourselves because we do not know what it is like inside. Yet there is no use our mounting on stilts, for on stilts we must still walk on our own legs. And on the loftiest throne in the world we are still sitting only on our own rump. (p. 865)

The Future of Thanatology

If we are to resist the temptation to reduce thanatology to euthanasia, we will have to be clear about what thanatology stands for. If we are to be convincing that mercifully killing patients perverts its purposes, we will have to say what the true purposes are.

Here it will be helpful to remember that thanatology—the study of dying—is essentially a humanities discipline. It, of course, uses a variety of tools drawn from social science disciplines and health care fields, but these are all instrumentalities in the service of what is fundamentally a humanistic enterprise.

The humanities are the study of the human situation through the sustained effort to hear, record, and faithfully interpret the human voice. Humanities disciplines (philosophy, literature, the classics, history, religion) are the formalized efforts to do so. But no less important are the neighboring fields of study that undertake their work in a less canonized, but no less important way. Thanatology is one of those neighboring, adjacent fields of study. The methods and traditions are perhaps more eclectic, but the mission—the hearing, recording, and faithful interpretation of the human voice—is the same. In thanatology, the task is more specialized, because the voices to be heard are mostly voices in crisis and voices of loss, but the driving impetus to engage is no different. In thanatology, the study is often preliminary, a first step to taking action to improve the lot of the dying and their caregivers. But what motivates the study is the same as what drives students and teachers of Shakespeare, Plato, Cicero, William Carlos Williams, Martin Luther King, Jr., or Toni Morrison. It is the passion to hear the authentically human, the remarkable, varied, and novel stories of human beings living their lives. Thanatology simply does this in a more specialized way.

The essence of humanistic inquiry is that these voices are, as much as possible, allowed to speak for themselves. The sustaining characteristic of the humanities is its effort to let be—on its own terms, and for its own sake—the human realities it studies. The first hint of techniques of manipulation, of "using" the voices for one's own purposes, to make a point, or to make a career, or to boost professional standing, or remove a troubling problem, or further a political agenda, subverts the task of attending.

The reduction of thanatology to mercy killing (or to the political effort to legalize euthanasia) is nowhere more vividly portrayed than in the Debbie case. The voice of the dying patient is completely subsumed under professional preoccupations. What I earlier characterized as the loss of agency, the effort at sovereignty, and the resulting brutalization, are all ways of expressing this reduction. The reduction not only diminishes the field of study. It also diminishes the humanity of those involved. In this gruesome scenario, in which all actions were performed in the name of mercy, both doctor and patient were belittled as human beings.

What follows from this is that the end or purpose of thanatology must include ingredients that were absent or distorted in the Debbie case: first, an explicit claim of our own moral and intellectual agency in our interaction with the dying; second, a humility in studying the dying and their experiences, which will obviate the need to control them or "fix the problem"—in thanatology, we are always studying something beyond ourselves, problems we can only partially grasp; and third, a sustained recognition of the self-deception and brutalization involved in killing the dying.

These three items do not, of course, exhaust the ingredients that make thanatology what it is or ought to be. So these items are not sufficient, but they are necessary. I offer them as part of the agenda of thanatology for the future, as ingredients that will give intellectual clarity and moral impetus to the tasks ahead.

Discussion Questions

1. Prior to his incarceration for second-degree murder in 1999, Dr. Jack Kevorkian assisted in the deaths of over 100 persons in the United States. Only 25% of these persons were terminally ill (as determined by autopsy findings), and a disproportionately large number were women; 72% were either divorced or had never been married. What hypotheses about social vulnerabilities does this profile suggest? What remedies might be used to correct these vulnerabilities?

2. Two U.S. Supreme Court rulings in 1997 (Washington v. Glucksburg & Vacco v. Quill) found that there is no constitutional right to assisted suicide, but several justices endorsed aggressive palliative treatment. Justice O'Connor said that a person facing a painful death has no legal barriers to receiving needed medication for pain, even to the point of causing unconsciousness and hastening death—a practice referred to in the medical literature as "total sedation." What are the ethical differences between total sedation and euthanasia?

References

Angell, M. (1988). Euthanasia. *New England Journal of Medicine, 319,* 1348–1350.
Anonymous. (1988). It's Over, Debbie. *Journal of the American Medical Association, 259,* 272.

Aristotle. (1941). *Politics,* Bk. I, Ch. 2, 1253a (W. D. Ross, Trans.). In Richard McKeon (Ed.), *The basic works of Aristotle.* New York: Random House.

Churchill, L. R. (1979). Interpretations of dying: Ethical implications for patient care. *Ethics in Science and Medicine, 6*(4), 211–222.

Harper, T. (1987). Where euthanasia is a way of death. *Medical Economics,* Nov. 23, 23–28.

Merriam-Webster's collegiate dictionary (9th ed.). (1985). Springfield, MA: Merriam-Webster.

Montaigne, M. de (1965). *The complete essays of Montaigne* (D. Frame, Trans.). Stanford, CA: Stanford University Press.

Roper Organization of New York City. (1988). *The 1988 Roper poll on attitudes toward active voluntary euthanasia.* Los Angeles: National Hemlock Society.

Nineteen

The Future of Palliative Care

Derek Doyle

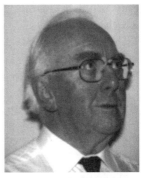

A graduate of the University of Edinburgh, Dr. Doyle spent the first 10 years of his professional life as a missionary surgeon in South Africa, before returning to Scotland for further postgraduate studies. He then worked for 10 years as a chest physician and family physician in Edinburgh, before being appointed, in 1977, as medical director of St. Columba's Hospice, Scotland's first specialist palliative care service. Between then and his retirement from clinical work in 1995, he became a member of the clinical teaching staff of Edinburgh University, the founding editor-in-chief of Palliative Medicine, *the first chairman of the Association of Palliative Medicine of Great Britain and Ireland, the first vice-chairman of the European Association of Palliative Care, and the first vice-chairman of the National Council for Hospice and Specialist Palliative Care Services of the UK. He is now the vice president of the National Council, president emeritus of the International Association for Hospice and Palliative Care, and continues as senior editor of the* Oxford Textbook of Palliative Medicine.

It has been said that we can only prepare for the future if we understand the past. That is undoubtedly true about palliative care, so we must start by looking at its brief history.

The Evolution of Palliative Care

As recently as the second half of the twentieth century, it struck many observers that patients with mortal illnesses were suffering not only appallingly, but quite unnecessarily. There were means to relieve the suffering,

357

but it often went unnoticed, and the professionals caring for such patients had never been taught how to relieve suffering. It was no coincidence that that was also the time of well-justified rejoicing about the triumphs of medicine. Great strides were being made in the fields of anesthesiology, surgery, oncology, diagnostic radiology, nuclear medicine, infection control, and immunology. There was even talk of defeating cancer, being able to replace any defective organ, and extending life in a way never thought possible before.

That people were still suffering unbearable pain and were not being offered the appropriate analgesics readily available for them, was therefore a serious indictment on both the medical and nursing professions. As more and more studies were published, it became clear that pain was not the only problem needing attention, and the sufferers were not only those with cancer, but those with cardiac, respiratory, and neurological disorders. Their dyspnea, anorexia, weakness, constipation, insomnia, fear and apprehension, depression, and profound social disruptions all seemed to cry out for attention. Many doctors and nurses appeared to have been seduced by their recent successes and were failing to see the suffering around them. Without noticing, their goal had changed from care to cure. Exciting as that was to the general public, their patients remained very conscious of their need for compassionate and highly skilled care, whatever the final outcome of treatment.

The response at that time was the establishment of *hospice care*. The name was an appropriate one, because the hospices of the Middle Ages had indeed been places of peace and healing for weary, injured, and ailing travellers on the great highways of Europe. Their modern successors were often modest buildings converted to a new purpose. Others were specially built to create an ambience and care second to none, characterized not by frenetic activity and the marvels of modern technology, but by attention to detail, skilled symptom relief, and staff in tune with every aspect of the needs of the terminally ill. Soon, teams were going out from the hospices into homes, where people said they wanted to be cared for as long as possible, then into general hospitals, where the need for better terminal care had also been identified; then student nurses and doctors were asking the hospices to train them, so woefully inadequate were they finding their training in this aspect of care.

In some countries the focus was on home care, in others hospital care. Progress was slow. Public pleasure and support were often balanced by professional skepticism and apathy, and occasionally by opposition and noncooperation. It was as if the dying were an embarrassment to some doctors (and even some nurses), an unsavory statistic, and any suggestion that their care could be improved, seen as a professional insult, an indictment. Did the problem lie in the name, rather than in the philosophy of care? Certainly, "terminal care," as it had been described, was thought by some to be too stark and frightening and certainly not a term that could be used with the patients.

The name *palliative care* was then adopted, better to reflect the nature of what was done for people with "active, progressive, far-advanced disease for whom the prognosis was short and the focus of care was the quality of life" (a definition coined by the Association for Palliative Medicine of Great Britain and Ireland), but even this was not entirely satisfactory. It was understood by doctors (although they rightly pointed out that all treatment not designed to cure is by definition palliative), but many in the general public preferred the old name of *hospice*, which by then was better understood and often generously supported.

The general public, and even some professionals, probably still regarded hospice care or palliative care, as we shall call it, as synonymous with dying and death. Although all receiving such care, whether at home, in a general hospital, or in a palliative care unit, had a mortal illness, an increasing number were able to return home from such care units, such was the quality of symptom control, psychological support, and rehabilitation. Today, more than 60% of people can be expected to return home, particularly if there is a community palliative care service available to support the family physician and the community nurses.

Not only the name of the subject and its standing were changing. When it was recognized that palliation is appropriate in all conditions, and not only for malignancy, services began to care for people with cardiac, respiratory, endocrine, and neurological conditions. Few had appreciated that cardiac and cancer patients have a similar spectrum of suffering: Almost everyone, irrespective of the underlying pathology, experiences fears about the unknown, is anxious about their loved ones, and asks similar existential questions about the meaning of life, the reasons for suffering, and what lies beyond life. Equally, their needs are similar, whatever their color, culture, creed, or country where they are cared for.

By late 1987, with palliative care services springing up in places as diverse and scattered as Australia, New Zealand, the United Kingdom, many European countries, and North America, inevitably more and more doctors and nurses would choose to make lifelong careers in this field. For that, there had to be professional recognition and accreditation, as well as a rigorous training program. In short, palliative medicine and palliative nursing had be to recognized as specialties, or at least be developed to attract career professionals.

So were born the medical specialties of palliative medicine and palliative nursing, in the UK. The benefits of such specialist status were felt immediately. Not only did patients have the right to ask to be cared for by such specialists, but universities began to incorporate the subjects into their curricula, to invite the new specialists to join their staff and soon there was a plethora of research publications, new journals, and major textbooks on the subject. In countries such as the UK, more doctors applied for specialist training than there were approved training posts for them.

One might think that, by this time, there would be no more disagreements about definitions, but they continue to this day. In those countries where palliative medicine is a specialty (UK, Australia, New Zealand, Hong Kong, and Sweden) units in which these specialist physicians work, alongside their specialist nurse colleagues, are designated specialist palliative care services. Hospices or small palliative care units where there are no specialist staff—but unquestionably devoted and skilled care—are now regarded as "generalist palliative care services," their doctors and nurses usually having undertaken advanced training to diploma rather than degree level.

Specialization brought many new challenges. The first was that of professional education and training. Few would deny that professional preparation for such caring had been woefully inadequate. Many, both doctors and nurses, had received no training whatsoever. For others, training had been a few hours usually devoted to such subjects as "breaking bad news" (something that one would assume had been done long before the patient came under palliative care) or "the use of morphine in chronic pain," again, an important but very small part of what we now know as palliative care. All that had to change. Not only did medical students need to learn about the many physical, psychosocial, and even spiritual aspects of palliative care, but junior doctors and those training in hospital specialties all needed to gain both insights and skills in this new field. More important, rigorous training programs for future specialists in palliative medicine and palliative nursing needed to be established and constantly reviewed. For doctors, this meant a further 4 years training after they had already been accredited as internists, oncologists, or radiation therapists. For nurses, it meant working for one of the many new postgraduate degrees in palliative care nursing, for which they study after years of practice in hospital or community nursing.

Across the world, a few medical schools introduced palliative care into the curriculum, but few ranked it highly enough to make it an examinable subject. Nevertheless, the profile and standing of palliative care continued to rise, with more than 20 full professorships worldwide and, at the time of writing, with more than 3,000 research projects underway.

Defining the essential knowledge base is not easy. No longer is it sufficient for palliative care workers to have an in-depth knowledge of oncology. To this must now be added experience in cardiology, neurology, respiratory medicine, and, in many countries, AIDS. Doctors are expected to have had postgraduate training in counseling, in teaching methods and research and, certainly in the UK, training in management.

Even that is not the whole story of the evolution of palliative care within the past few decades. Even in countries with a tradition—albeit it a brief one—of hospices founded and generously funded by the public, the move is now against the establishment of any more, because it has been recognized that seldom do more than 10% of terminally ill patients ever go into them. Ninety percent of the final year of life is spent at home, the professional care being given by family physicians and community nurses, and the day-to-day care being given by relatives and friends, many of whom may themselves be aged and not enjoying good health. The challenge to palliative care is to find means of enabling people to stay at home as long as they can (it has now been conclusively shown that, contrary to what has always been said, few people want to die at home) (Doyle, 1991; Hinton, 1994; Wood, 1985), and at the same time to respect the responsibility and burden this places on lay caregivers.

More people are diagnosed, treated, and cared for in general and specialist hospital units than anywhere else. If, as is always being claimed, palliative care is appropriate for them, whatever their diagnosis, wherever they are, then it must be readily available in every major hospital. To achieve this, hospital palliative care teams are being established and staffed by specialist doctors and nurses, with access to social workers, physiotherapists, occupational therapists, and pastoral care workers. No longer can there be any excuse for not knowing how to relieve pain or dyspnea, how to answer searching and upsetting questions, or how to give pastoral care and answer existential questions. There are experts in the hospital, at the end of a phone, accessible 24 hours a day. No longer need we depend exclusively on university courses to teach these skills. They can now be gained at the bedside. Although the clinical, educational, and economic benefits of such teams seem obvious, they are uncommon outside the UK. There, it is now government policy to encourage them, with a statutory requirement of all cancer units to have such teams. Evidence shows that they not only improve patient care, but also facilitate earlier discharge and better rehabilitation—music to the ears of hospital managers.

What Exactly Is Palliative Care?

Any reader previously unfamiliar with palliative care could be excused for thinking that it is a pretentious title for pain and symptom management. This is certainly a central feature of it. Others might feel it is better described as comfort care, and, again, this is a feature of it. Yet others would latch onto the description so often given—that it is holistic care—and assume that it is highly emotional, somewhat unorthodox, and spiced with alternative and unproven therapies. They would be wrong. As has come to be widely recognized in recent years, palliative care is not new, though its title may be. It is as old as care itself, possibly as old as humans themselves. Whenever humans have suffered, until recently with little likelihood of cure, others have tried to relieve that suffering. Palliative care continues that tradition, using the most modern drugs, equipment, diagnostic techniques, and understanding of psychology and psychiatry, occasionally augmented by proven complementary (but not alternative) approaches.

None of this would be possible if it were not also interdisciplinary care—skills freely shared in an atmosphere of mutual respect and support, without professional bickering and territorialism—a picture so different from the defensive hierarchy often encountered in modern care systems.

What makes palliative care unique, different from other care? The answer is simple: It is neither new nor different. It describes what should characterize all good clinical care—responsiveness to the deepest needs of patients, irrespective of whether they are predominantly physical, emotional, or social, irrespective of whether the patients will live or die, whether they have days or years of life left to them, or whether they can pay for care or not—"caring for the sake of caring."

Palliative care is concerned with three things: the quality of life, the value of life, and the meaning of life. None of them is easy to define or to describe. Quality of life (as perceived by the patient, and not by his or her professional attendants) encompasses freedom from suffering, respect for dignity and autonomy, and the freedom we all need to "be ourselves." So much of life is spent trying to give impressions that we are what we patently are not—clever, confident, capable, calm, loving and loveable, and so on. With the relentless advance of a mortal illness, people have not the energy or the inclination to continue life's charades. They want their frailty to be recognized, their fears to be ventilated, their natures and characters to be accepted: They want to be seen and accepted for what they are, rather than the Walter Mitty they have always tried to be. Quality of life, however we try to define or measure it, is vastly more than pain and symptom management, the promise of cure or the possibility of a "worthwhile remission," as doctors now choose to term it. Any doctor or nurse who sees it only as that is little more than a symptomatologist.

We live in an age when, in spite of all the claims made by political and religious leaders, life seems to have little real value. Not only do people die in their thousands in natural and human-made disasters, but many in our cities wonder if anyone needs them, if their lives contribute anything to the world, if they would be missed if they died tonight. Their sense of being of little value, even of being a drain on society, is made worse by the constant reminders from politicians that caring for the elderly and chronically sick is an expensive drain on national resources, the implication being that, because they can no longer work, their lives are of limited value in our modern society. The terminally ill are acutely conscious of this. We all need to be wanted, valued, of some use to others. That need to be wanted does not lessen as death approaches. Rather does it increase. One of the tasks of palliative care is to show our patients that they matter. "You matter because you are you." "You are valuable and we value you" is a powerful message in this age.

Humans have sought to fathom the meaning of life since time began. We must always have asked why we must suffer, why some must die so young, why some must endure pain and so much sadness, while others seem to live charmed lives. These are not religious questions, though most religions would claim to have answers to some of them. They are, however, spiritual questions of the type so frequently asked by people coming to the end of their lives. Their days are long, the nights often sleepless. There is not enough energy to be active nor concentration to read much. Thinking revolves around these fundamental questions about human existence and, although they surely know humans have never found an answer to any of them, they long to talk about them with anyone who will listen. Who better than the caring doctor or nurse who has already shared their concern and their humanity in so many ways as they minister, through palliative care? Palliative care is often said to be an exercise in communication skills, but that is only true if it is appreciated that at the heart of communication is active listening.

This brings us to the fundamental question: What attribute is most necessary for a caregiver to be effective in palliative care? Can you learn it, or must you be born with it—a "gift"? Can it be taught and demonstrated, or must it be absorbed by osmosis, as students and practitioners work alongside each other? That attribute is *sensitivity*. To practice palliative care, one must have highly developed senses—to know when something is troubling a patient before they have mentioned it; when someone is frightened, before they have articulated a fear; when they are puzzled, before they have asked a question; or when they feel alone on this, the loneliest journey of life, and may never say so. One has to be sensitive to the disappointment of colleagues who had hoped to cure that patient, to others who are embarrassed in the presence of death or because of their own inadequacy or lack of faith and philosophy.

The writer is convinced that we are all born with the potential for such sensitivity, but it must be cultivated throughout our professional training, throughout our careers. Our professional education will need to change, no longer focusing exclusively on science and technology, but introducing the humanities, studies of the unmeasurable aspects of man's being, and greater credence given to the power of love and compassion in patient care. Anecdotal as it is, and therefore unacceptable to many scientific observers, one cannot help but be amazed by the number of times patients and relatives remark on the special, safe atmosphere they feel when they come into a palliative care unit—in spite of the fact that all around them are people with major life-threatening illness and, until a few hours ago, indescribable suffering and pain.

The Future of Palliative Care

In a sense, this has already been discussed or at last hinted at. The principles of palliative care are the principles of all good care, irrespective of the underlying pathology, whether they are going to live or die, whether they are at home or in hospital. That we all learn to practice palliative care is more than a clinical necessity—it is a moral imperative we cannot avoid. To allow a person to suffer unnecessarily is frankly unethical, no matter how energetic and skilled our efforts to cure or achieve worthwhile remissions. In this sense, there is really no question about the future of palliative care. It is an undeniable, intrinsic feature of all good care and must always remain so.

If palliation skills are essential for all clinicians, what a pity that palliative medicine and palliative nursing ever needed to be given specialist status. However, in countries where this has happened, no one would now challenge the decision. From being ignored or marginalized, palliative care is now respectable and accepted; from being a Cinderella subject, it is now being given space in the curriculum and—such an important point—is being seen as a means of demonstrating communication, ethical, and humanity issues to the students. In short, palliative care is restoring some of the pearls of wisdom and compassion lost with the relentless advance of scientific materialism.

Only in countries where it has such a status are the following occurring: Major advances are taking place in its provision; palliative care research is being carried out; and undergraduate and postgraduate students are themselves demanding more training in this previously neglected subject. Is it any coincidence that, in the UK, for example, there are now more palliative medicine specialists than there are oncologists, neurologists, and nephrologists?

Of course, the challenges facing palliative care cannot, must not, be denied or minimized. We live at a time when more people are living to the age when cancer is more common; when people will have to retire earlier to care both for their very old parents and their grandchildren, making home care of the dying increasingly difficult; when public expectations of health care professionals continue to rise, sometimes to unachievable heights; and when devastating new conditions are appearing, such as new-variant Creutzfeldt-Jacob disease and AIDS, and antibiotic-resistant infections, such as tuberculosis. In the future, palliative care workers will need to be trained and experienced in a wider spectrum of disease than ever before.

The future mostly depends on the caring professions themselves. They ignore the real, but often unexpressed, needs of the patients, at their peril. Palliative care has, throughout its short history, been consumer-driven; patient- rather than profession-centered; and understood and sought by consumers, long before governments and health care managers and planners knew anything about it. The professionals must take the initiative in persuading medical and nursing colleges to give it its rightful place, in demonstrating its centrality to politicians and planners. Changes in care are made easier when doctors are persuaded of the need for change, but nurses must not underestimate how influential they can be, their authority coming from their day-in, day-out proximity to patients, and their tradition of listening and understanding their deepest needs. If they ever distance themselves from the bedside, preferring to know the patient via the screens, the monitors, and the laboratory reports, the need for palliative care will be even greater than at present. However, it will then have to be provided by colleagues who must work outside the existing health care system, rather than as an integral part of it, as is now beginning to happen. The future of palliative care mostly depends on a better understanding and appreciation of it by doctors and nurses, and not on the proliferation of little hospices and hospice home care services across the country, well-intentioned as they might be. If they espouse palliative care, the politicians and health care managers will follow.

The countries where palliative care is being developed as part of mainstream medical care are not just those where specialization has taken place, or where it has been integrated into the curricula. They are succeeding because they have won the hearts and minds of politicians, public, and press. Countries such as the UK, Australia, New Zealand, Hong Kong, Taiwan and Poland have all found innovative ways to interest and involve national politicians and the media.

Perhaps the answer to our question, "What is the future of palliative care?" is easier to find than we thought. Perhaps that answer is another question: "Is it possible for palliative care to come to nothing, when there are now more than 8,000 palliative care services worldwide, and less than 40 years ago there were less than 10?" Palliative care will prosper in the future as it has in the past, but only if it is integrated into mainstream care, if it demonstrates flexibility and adaptability, if the highest caliber professionals are attracted into it, and only if they are fearless about talking about features of care that matter, but cannot as yet be measured.

A final challenging thought. Palliative care is dedicated to the care of those who have already given of their time, their skills, their loyalty, and their love, and now face increasing dependency, suffering, loneliness, and loss. A society that does not honor such people as much as it honors those still economically useful is not worthy of being called a good society. The presence of palliative care services should be seen as a measure of how caring a society is.

Discussion Questions

1. If the principles of palliative care are relevant in all clinical practice, why do they not receive more attention in nursing and medical training?
2. Are there obstacles to palliative care being adapted and developing as much in developing countries as in the developed world?
3. Why does palliative care have to be interprofessional, interdisciplinary?
4. Is it possible to conduct research in palliative care without endangering patient dignity and privacy?

References

The Association for Palliative Medicine of Great Britain and Ireland. 11 Westwood Road, Southampton, Hants., SO17 1DL, UK.

Doyle, D. (1991). A home care service for terminally ill patients in Edinburgh. *Health Bulletin, Edinburgh, 49,* 14–23.

Hinton, J. (1994). Which patients with terminal cancer are admitted from home care? *Palliative Medicine, 8,* 197–210.

Wood, A. W. H. (1985). *Home care services for the terminally ill. Medical care research unit.* United Kingdom: University of Sheffield.

Part Five

In Conclusion

Twenty

Reprise

Mary A. Pittman

Mary A. Pittman is co-editor of this book, and her biography can be found on page ii.

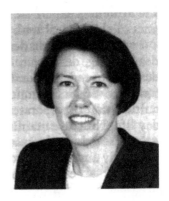

A reprise is an opportunity to recapitulate some of the ideas presented previously. I will take this opportunity to place some of these ideas in the context of public health. Death and dying is not only a topic for scholars and clinicians. Media attention is directed to the deaths of prominent public figures, particularly those of political, entertainment, and sports giants; the details of whose deaths and funerals are telecast or published around the world.

Whether as a result of natural causes or due to an accident associated with alcohol, overdose of drugs, an assassin's bullet, famine, a devastating natural disaster, or the ravages of wars, our attention is focused on death scenes in a way that is different due to the immediacy given by the electronic media. The attack on the World Trade Center in New York City and the Pentagon in Washington D.C. had a dramatic impact on all of us. The questions of how we deal with what I would call the armchair experience of death and incorporate death imagery, influences how we deal with death in our everyday lives.

"Scared to death, deathly ill, death threat, death wish, death of cold, dead wrong, dead beat, dead wood, dead end, a dead issue, death mask, death house, dead as a door nail, death rate . . . " These phrases represent but a short list of common death-related terms redolent of a language and culture that incorporates the concept of death into the speech of everyday life while maintaining an adolescent-like distance.

Although rarely examined, except by scholars, the following motifs are richly amplified as common themes coursing through the chapters in this book—the search for the truth of living and the fear and anxiety of dying, the attempts to study thanatological issues and to understand death's meaning for life, the models for caring, and the personal experiences and expressions of death, dying, and bereavement. One is always left with a question at the end of the chapter or a call for further study and inquiry or an admonition, for example, to insist on the quality of living as having equal valence with aggressive therapies (Preston, Tang, & McCorkle).

Many chapters in this book propose ways to bolster and reinforce the support network, to train and support the professional, and to explore the spiritual streams arising from death and grief. Although the papers, for the most part, are concerned with the individual, the public-health professional may also benefit from the thoughtful works presented. The health and medical community with which I have worked deal with death every day in ways described by Silverman as "stigmatized" or "spoiled." (See Silverman's chapter in *Death, Dying and Bereavement: Theoretical Perspectives . . .*). The concept of self is important in this context because the loss associated with death and the process of grieving is intrinsically linked to the transition to a new role which sheds the experience of social isolation and stigma.

Public health bridges the tough social questions that manifest themselves in medical terms. What happens to the person whose life experience is constantly associated with social stigma? What happens to the homeless drug abuser who appears in the emergency room in cardiac arrest? Who is responsible for the family whose everyday life experience incorporates traumatic death events resulting in complicated mourning that engenders feelings of vulnerability, powerlessness, guilt, and anxiety? How does one help the grieving family whose social support network is absent or experiencing the same level of distress?

Pubic health has at its foundation the incorporation of education, the prevention of the social problems affecting the disease of the individual, and the promotion of "health." Public health's roots stem from the plagues and the major "killers" in society. Following the taming of the major communicable diseases in industrialized countries and until the Human Immunodeficiency Virus (HIV)/Acquired Immunodeficiency Syndrome (AIDS) epidemic, most public-health interventions have not focused on death per se, but on the antecedents to death.

Cancer and HIV disease have heightened the awareness of the general public to hospice and other alternatives to dying in a hospital, both from the perspective of the quality of life and the preferred death scene as well as from the perspective of the economic and social costs. In part, as a result of the aging of the population, individuals in a persistent vegetative state being kept alive by technology, and more recently, gay men living with HIV disease who wanted control over their deaths, there has been a concerted effort to develop and to inform individuals of the range of options in care during a terminal illness. As Corless and Nicholas state "The ultimate contribution of hospice to how living and dying are viewed in our society may be to facilitate a greater appreciation for living as the humane possibilities for dying are actualized."

The public-health professional looks at disease patterns and the spread of disease with death as a marker, a rate, an index of where the prevention and education efforts have fallen short. One key indicator of the public's health is the rate of infant mortality.Our conflict in public health over death and dying is most often presented by the disparity in mortality rates between those who have and those who have not, the rich and the poor, the white and the black, the deserving and the undeserving.

An article on infant mortality in Washington, DC, highlighted this conflict in the city where U.S. health policy is made and directed (*Washington Post*, 27 October 1991). The article describes the way that a hospital helps the mother accept the death of her baby—a picture, a piece of the blanket the baby was wrapped in, a snippet of the hair, a sympathy card, and a rose, all placed in a basket called a *grief basket*. Such attempts by caregivers to help individuals deal with loss is an area of concern to scholars in the field of death and dying.

The public-health professional, on the other hand, working on an aggregate level focuses on the systemic exclusion of some people from basic health care. This is underscored by noting that the death rates for infants and children in developing nations are not dissimilar to those of Washington, DC. As startling as these statistics should be, as a society, we've become inured to the reality of each personal loss. The 1993 infant (0–1 year) mortality statistics for Washington, DC, indicated that there were 16.7 deaths per 1000 births, more than double the national rate of 8.2 per thousand, and well above the rate of most industrialized nations.

Health policy in the United States is heavily influenced by economics and the demographics of the population. Economic factors have been influential in identifying, segregating, and separating the so-called deserving from the undeserving for health care and social support. The demography of the population in the United States and other industrialized nations is indicative of the aging population. As a result, questions related to the quality of living in later years will focus more attention on options for dying, including attention to the legislation for active voluntary euthanasia.

It would be ironic were we to give everyone equal access to voluntary assistance with death before we gave them the same access to life.

Index